Textbook of General Pathology
for Dental Students

S. R. Prabhu

Textbook of General Pathology for Dental Students

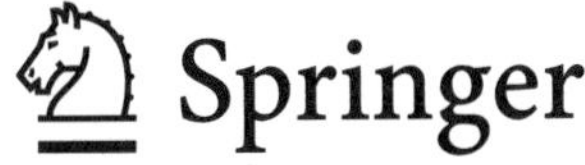 Springer

S. R. Prabhu
School of Dentistry
University of Queensland
Brisbane, QLD, Australia

ISBN 978-3-031-31246-5   ISBN 978-3-031-31244-1   (eBook)
https://doi.org/10.1007/978-3-031-31244-1

This Springer imprint is published by the registered company Springer Nature Switzerland AG
The registered company address is: Gewerbestrasse 11, 6330 Cham, Switzerland

Dedication

To

Newell W Johnson, who has inspired and motivated hundreds of students and collegues in their academic pusuits.

Foreword

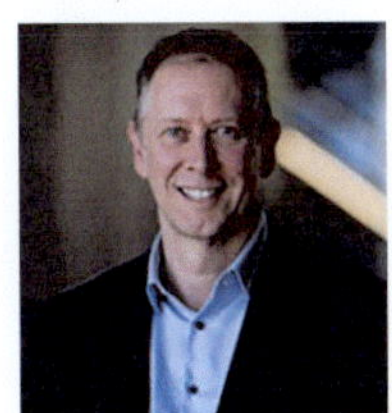

Whilst the study of general pathology is incredibly interesting, for many students, it can often be overwhelming and not always immediately relevant to clinical dental practice. Dental practitioners encounter pathology every day, and whilst, fortunately, it is not always serious, it is important that practitioners can appreciate the basic principles that underlie these presentations so that appropriate management can be implemented—as health practitioners, dentists need to understand pathology.

The importance of pathology is sometimes overlooked and at risk of being overshadowed by the various clinical disciplines and other areas that "compete" for time in dental programmes. Understanding the basic principles of pathology is essential for all dental students. It underpins a comprehensive understanding of oral and maxillofacial pathology, for which dental practitioners should be considered the experts. Furthermore, this is reinforced by the increasing understanding of the links between oral and systemic disease.

Historically, general pathology has been taught by external faculty rather than dental academics and oral pathologists. As mentioned previously, students, particularly undergraduate students, often find this approach daunting and miss the relevance of these basic pathological sciences to clinical dentistry. This textbook helps address this issue.

With clear explanations and coverage of a wide range of topics, including an overview of oral pathology, this book is an essential resource. Professor Prabhu's extensive teaching experience and deep understanding of the subject matter make this an invaluable tool for anyone looking to gain a deeper understanding of the fundamental principles of pathology at exactly the right level for dental students. I have known Professor Prabhu since my own undergraduate days and remember fondly his passion for oral pathology; it is exciting that there is now a general pathology textbook written especially for dental students, which can also be a useful reference for postgraduate students and practicing dental practitioners.

Dean and Professor of Oral and Maxillofacial Pathology   Richard Logan
The University of Adelaide Dental School
Adelaide, Australia

Preface

Understanding the basic principles of pathology is essential for students pursuing dentistry. Although excellent books on pathology are available, they are primarily targeted at medical students. Dental students often find these books too voluminous with too much basic detail, particularly from the undergraduate students' points of view. Worse, pathology books primarily targeted at dental students are hard to find. It is heartening to note that globally there is a trend developing to shoulder the responsibility of teaching general pathology topics by oral and maxillofacial pathologists. With this scenario, a need for a book on general pathology topics authored by oral and maxillofacial pathologists is real. *Textbook of General Pathology for Dental Students* is aimed at fulfilling this need.

This book deals with fundamental concepts and mechanisms underlying various human diseases in 18 chapters. Chapters on introduction to pathology, cellular pathology, homeostasis, and tissue healing set the scene for diseases and disorders of inflammatory, genetic, infectious, and neoplastic background. Because of their relevance to clinical dental practice, chapters on ageing, imbalances in fluids and electrolytes, acids and bases, haemodynamic disorders, thrombosis, infarction and shock, and environmental and nutritional pathology are included in the book. A chapter on pain is presented to provide essential basic knowledge of pain pathways. Brief details of dental, oral, and maxillofacial and salivary gland diseases are presented to introduce these topics to the preclinical dental student. Because of the strong, often bidirectional link between systemic and oral diseases, organ system-based pathology is discussed briefly as an introduction to general medicine topics taught later in the clinical years of training. Illustrations and tables are expected to reinforce the information presented in the text. Pathologic terms, most of which are new to a dental student in preclinical years, are defined in the glossary at the end of the book.

It is my earnest hope that this book will be helpful to dental students globally.

Brisbane, QLD, Australia   S. R. Prabhu
November 2022

Contents

1.1 Introduction

The history of pathology is closely intertwined with the history of medicine. Today, pathology is practised as a medical discipline and is regarded as the foundation of many aspects of patient care, including diagnostic testing, prognostication, and advice on treatment modalities. *The word pathology comes from the Greek words "pathos" and "logy." 'Patho' means suffering or disease, and 'logy' means study.* It is a speciality of medical science concerned with the cause, development, structural/functional changes, and natural history associated with diseases. Disease refers to a definable deviation from normal with observable characteristics evident via patient complaints (symptoms) and careful examination (signs) measurements. The cause of the disease is referred to as its aetiology. The process of disease development is referred to as its pathogenesis. The pathogenesis can refer to the changes in the structure or function of an organism at the gross/clinical level. Pathology, therefore, deals with nature, causes, processes, development, and consequences of diseases. The term pathophysiology is also commonly used in the study of disease to include the study of disordered function and the breakdown of homeostasis. Pathophysiology mainly focuses on alterations in function rather than alterations in structure. Pathology mainly focuses on alterations in structure. However, because structural and functional changes are closely related, a clinician must have basic knowledge of physiology and anatomy before one embarks on the study of disease. The disease is an abnormal variation in the structure or function of any part of the body. Diseases can be distinguished based on differences at the molecular, cellular, tissue, fluid chemistry, and individual organism level. A pathologist is an individual who specialises in pathology.

Pathology is divided into general and systemic pathology (systematic pathology) for pedagogical reasons. General pathology (Basic Pathology) covers the basic mechanisms of diseases, whereas systemic pathology covers conditions as they occur in the individual organ system. General pathology is the foundation of knowledge that must be acquired before studying the mechanisms involved in the pathology of various organ systems. Systemic pathology describes multiple aspects of a disease by studying its aetiology (cause), pathogenesis (mechanisms), morphologic changes (gross and microscopic structural alterations), and functional derangements (signs and symptoms).

1.2 History of Pathology

In prehistoric times, the disease was associated with religion, magic ("evil eye of the spirits"), and divine influences ("curse from God"). Herophilus, one of the great Greek physicians, along with Erasistratus, provided a beginning for anatomical pathology and autopsy. Greek philosophers Socrates, Plato, and Aristotle introduced philosophical concepts to medicine. Hippocrates was an eminent Greek Physician who disassociated medicine from magic and religion. He believed in symptoms from patients' histories and described methods of diagnosis. He is also instrumental in forming rational and ethical principles in medical practice (Hippocratic Oath). Roman physician Cornelius Celsus is credited with introducing cardinal signs of inflammation (*rubor, tumour, calor, and dolour*), and Claudius Gallen postulated humoral theory. Around 200 AD, Indian physicians Charaka and Sushruta described aspects of disease and medical and surgical remedies in books *Charaka Samhita* and *Sushruta Samhita*, respectively.

Pathology developed only as science advanced. Some prominent individuals contributed to the development of pathology in the seventeenth and eighteenth centuries. Antony van Leeuwenhoek (1632–1723) invented the first microscope, and Marcello Malpighi (1624–1694) used the microscope to study skin and lymphoid tissue in the spleen and has been credited as the father of histology. Giovanni Morgagni (1682–1771) laid the foundation for clinicopathologic methods in the study of disease. Other notable clinicians responsible for the advancement of pathology and the

© The Author(s), under exclusive license to Springer Nature Switzerland AG 2023
S. R. Prabhu, *Textbook of General Pathology for Dental Students*, https://doi.org/10.1007/978-3-031-31244-1_1

study of medicine included Sir Percival Pott (1714–1788), John Hunter (1728–1793), William Hunter (1718–1788), Edward Jenner (1749–1823), Thomas Addison (1793–1860), Thomas Hodgkin (1798–1866), Louis Pasteur (1822–1912), Paul Ehrlich (1854–1915), Christian Gram (1853–1938), D L Romanowsky (1861–1921), Robert Koch (1843–1910), Sir William Leishman (1865–1926), Rudolph Virchow (1821–1905), Karl Landsteiner (1863–1943), G N Papanicolaou (1883–1962) and Willian Boyd (1885–1979).

1.3 Making a Diagnosis

The steps involved in arriving at a diagnosis are as follows:

- Taking an appropriate clinical history of symptoms and collecting and recording relevant data
- Physical examination
- Generating a provisional and differential diagnosis. (Developing a list of the possible conditions that might produce a patient's symptoms and signs).
- Investigations (ordering, reviewing, and interpreting test results)
- Reaching a final diagnosis
- Consultation (referral to seek clarification if indicated)

Chapters 2 and 3 provide further information necessary to understand the disease process better.

1.4 Diagnostic Investigations in Pathology

Pathologists use gross, microscopic, immunologic, genetic, and molecular modalities to determine the presence of disease and frequently work closely with surgeons, radiologists, and oncologists. Pathologists can sub-specialise in different areas, such as gastroenterology, gynaecologic pathology, blood diseases, clotting disorders, microbiology, and lung and breast cancers. For every subspecialty in medicine or surgery, there is a pathologist counterpart, helping to make the correct diagnosis and guide the patient's care. In the diagnosis of disease, the following techniques are used.

1.4.1 Gross Pathology

Gross pathology refers to macroscopic disease manifestations in organs, tissues, and body cavities. Anatomical pathologists commonly use this term to refer to diagnostically useful findings made during the gross examination of specimen processing or an autopsy.

1.4.2 Biopsy

A biopsy is a procedure that removes a tissue sample from a living body to provide the pathologist with a representative, viable specimen for microscopic (histopathologic) interpretation, and diagnosis. There are many different types of biopsy procedures. The most common types include (1) incisional biopsy, in which only a sample of tissue is removed; (2) excisional biopsy, in which an entire lump or suspicious area is removed; and (3) needle biopsy, in which a sample of tissue or fluid is removed with a needle. The procedure is called a core biopsy when a wide needle is used. When a thin needle is used, the process is called a fine-needle aspiration biopsy.

1.4.3 Histopathology

Histopathology refers to examining a biopsy or surgical specimen by a pathologist after the specimen has been processed and histological sections have been placed onto glass slides. The tissue specimen obtained from a biopsy or autopsy procedure undergoes five stages of preparation before the slides are viewed by a histopathologist. Steps include formalin fixation, processing, embedding, sectioning, and staining, primarily with hematoxylin and eosin. Different stains and tests may be applied to the specimen or slides when the initial diagnosis is unclear. A frozen section can be examined for immediate diagnosis of soft tissue malignancy during a surgical procedure but is less accurate than the evaluation of paraffin-embedded tissue.

1.4.4 Cytopathology

Cytopathology is the study of abnormal cells from various body sites to determine the cause or nature of the disease. The main applications of cytopathology include screening for the early detection of asymptomatic precancer or cancer, diagnosis of symptomatic cancer, cysts, inflammatory conditions, and various types of infections. It is also used for the detection of recurrence of cancer in those who have been treated for cancer. Different cytopathologic methods include fine-needle aspiration, exfoliative, and abrasive cytology.

1.4.5 Haematopathology

This branch of pathology deals with abnormalities of the blood cells, and their precursors in the bone marrow are investigated to diagnose the different kinds of diseases.

Haematological tests can help diagnose anaemia, infection, haemophilia, blood-clotting disorders, and leukaemia. Common haematological tests include complete blood count, white blood cell count (WBC count), red blood cell count (RBC count), platelet count, haematocrit red cell volume (HCT), haemoglobin concentration (Hb), differential white blood cell count, red blood cell indices, prothrombin time (PT), partial thromboplastin time (PTT), and International Normalized Ratio (INR).

1.4.6 Histochemistry

Histochemistry combines biochemistry and histology techniques to study the chemical constitution of cells and tissues. Histochemistry specifically stains constituents of cells and tissues such as mucins, lipids, nucleic acids, amyloid, microorganisms, and other proteins.

1.4.7 Immunohistochemistry (IHC)

This method is used to detect the localisation of antigens, usually proteins, in tissue sections and cells, by the use of antibodies with specificity for an antigen.

1.4.8 Immunofluorescence (IF)

This is a detection technique where the antibodies used in the assay are labelled using fluorescent dyes or fluorescent proteins for detection purposes.

1.4.9 Molecular Pathology

Molecular pathology reveals defects in the chemical structure of molecules in the gnome. Molecular pathology can manifest in disorders such as sickle cell disease, osteogenesis imperfecta, and the development of neoplasms. This technique is commonly used in the diagnosis of cancer and infectious diseases. Common methods include polymerase chain reaction (PCR) and in situ hybridisation (ISH). In the PCR test, minute amounts of nucleic acids can be amplified using oligonucleotide primers specific to the genes being studied. ISH is a technique that allows for the precise localisation of a particular nucleic acid segment within a histologic section. ISH identifies specific genes or their messenger RNA in tissue sections or cell preparations.

1.4.10 Cytogenetics (Clinical Genetics)

This method investigates inherited chromosomal abnormalities in the germ cells or acquired chromosomal abnormalities in somatic cells using molecular biology techniques.

1.4.11 Biochemical Methods

Biochemical techniques refer to assays and procedures that enable investigators to analyse the substances found in living organisms and their chemical reactions. This is a method by which the metabolic disturbances of disease are investigated by assay of various normal and abnormal compounds in the blood, urine, saliva, etc.

1.4.12 Medical Microbiology

Medical microbiology, also known as clinical microbiology, is a subdiscipline dealing with studying microorganisms (parasites, fungi, bacteria, viruses, and prions) capable of infecting and causing human diseases.

1.4.13 Microbial Culture

Microbial culture is one of the primary diagnostic methods in microbiology. Microbial culture is a method of growing a microbial organism to determine what it is, its abundance in the tested sample, or both. The tool is often used to determine the cause of infectious disease by letting the agent multiply in predetermined media in the laboratory. In the case of bacterial infections, the most appropriate antibiotic can be selected by determining the bacteria's sensitivity to various antibacterial agents.

1.4.14 Flow Cytometry

This technique is commonly used to diagnose cancers of the blood cells, such as leukaemias.

1.4.15 Electron Microscopy

The standard microscopes used by pathologists are not powerful enough to see the smallest parts that make up a cell. Some diseases can only be diagnosed at this subcellular level using an electron microscope. Examples include types of kidney disease or aggressive cancers. Electron microscope utilises beams of electrons rather than visible light to magnify the cells in a tissue sample. It can magnify up to 2 million times, whereas the maximum power of a conventional light microscope is only 1 to 2 thousand times.

1.4.16 Forensic Pathology/Autopsy

Forensic pathology is the discipline of pathology concerned with the investigation of deaths where there are medico-legal implications. It is a field of forensic science that involves the application of pathological methods in investigating a crime and of sudden, suspicious, or unexplained deaths. An autopsy examines the dead body to identify the cause of death. This can be for forensic or clinical purposes.

1.4.17 Oral and Maxillofacial Pathology

Oral and maxillofacial pathology (OMFP) refers to the diseases of the oral cavity, jaws, and related structures, including salivary glands, temporomandibular joints, facial muscles, and perioral skin. It is considered to be a speciality of dentistry and pathology.

1.5 Summary

Pathology is concerned with the cause, development, structural, and functional changes, and natural history associated with diseases. It is the foundation for clinical practice, including dentistry. Clinical pathology and diagnostic pathology are two major divisions of pathology. Biopsy and histopathology are the most commonly used diagnostic procedures in dental practice. These procedures are extensively used to diagnose mucosal, jawbone, and salivary gland diseases. Histochemical, immunological, biochemical, and molecular pathology techniques are used for the confirmation of diagnosis of diseases of immunological and neoplastic origin.

Bibliography

Funkhouser WK Jr. Pathology: the clinical description of human disease. Molecul Pathol. 2018:217–29. https://doi.org/10.1016/B978-0-12-802761-5.00011-0.

Melrose RJ, Handlers JP, Kerpel S, Summerlin DJ, Tomich CJ. American academy of oral and maxillofacial pathology. The use of biopsy in dental practice. The position of the American Academy of Oral and maxillofacial pathology. Gen Dent. 2007;55(5):457–61.

Mohan H, Mohan S. Introduction to pathology. Essential pathology for dental students. 5th ed. New Delhi: Jaypee Brothers Medical Publishers; 2017. p. 1–8.

Pena GP, Andrade-Filho JS. How does a pathologist make a diagnosis? Arch Pathol Lab Med. 2009;133(1):124–32. https://doi.org/10.5858/133.1.124. PMID: 19123724

Simon HC. Applications of pathology. In: Simon Herrington C, editor. Muir's textbook of pathology. 15th ed. London: CRC Press; 2014. p. 3–10.

Wiltse LL. Herophilus of Alexandria (325–255 BC): the father of anatomy. Spine. 1998;23:1904–14.

Homeostasis

2

2.1 Introduction

Homeostasis is a state of dynamic equilibrium characterised by steady internal, physical, and chemical conditions maintained by living systems despite changes in the external environment. The term homeostasis is derived from *homeo* (meaning similar) and *stasis* (meaning steady). Disruption of homeostasis causes disease.

2.2 Homeostasis at the Cellular, Tissue, and Organ Levels

At the cellular level, homeostasis is observable in biochemical reactions. Cellular homeostasis relates to the fluid and oxygen levels of the intracellular environment. When the intracellular fluid levels drop, the cell obtains fluid from the surrounding extracellular fluid and the blood. Thus, fluid and oxygen levels are restored within the cell to normal levels.

Homeostasis is involved in every organ system of the body. Some body systems that constantly adjust to normal levels of health include blood sugar, blood pressure, energy, acid levels, oxygen, proteins, temperature, hormones, and electrolytes.

2.3 Regulation and Mechanisms of Homeostasis

Homeostasis is regulated by negative feedback loops and positive feedback loops. Both have the same stimulus components: sensor (also referred to as receptor), control centre, and effector (Fig. 2.1). Negative feedback loops prevent an excessive response to the stimulus, whereas positive feedback loops intensify the response until an endpoint is reached. The sensor collects information from the surroundings and reports further to the control centre. The control centre monitors and processes the received information and conveys a signal to the effector. The effector produces a reaction based on the signal provided by the control centre. Control centres in the brain and other body parts monitor and react to deviations from homeostasis. The effector is an organ, gland, muscle, or another structure that acts on the signal from the control centre to move the variable back toward the set point. A set point is a physiological value around which the normal range fluctuates. As the body works to maintain homeostasis, fluctuations are normal if they do not become too extreme. The normal body temperature range is the spread of values within which such fluctuations are considered insignificant. (E.g. the normal range for an adult is about 36.5–37.5 °C (97.7–99.5 °F).

© The Author(s), under exclusive license to Springer Nature Switzerland AG 2023
S. R. Prabhu, *Textbook of General Pathology for Dental Students*, https://doi.org/10.1007/978-3-031-31244-1_2

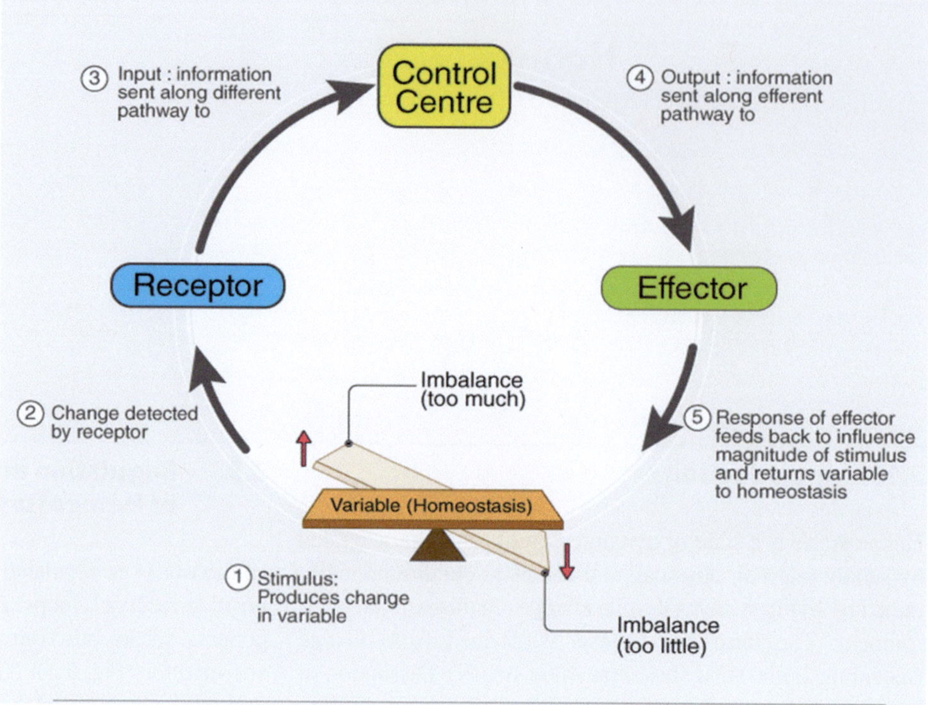

Fig. 2.1 Homeostasis is a human biological system where the self-regulating process tends to maintain the balance for survival. The regulation takes place in a defined internal environment

2.4 Homeostatic Mechanisms (Feedback Mechanisms)

The homeostatic mechanism is also known as the feedback mechanism. A feedback mechanism is a physiological regulation system in a living body that returns the body to its normal internal state (homeostasis). It is a loop system in which the system responds to perturbation either in the same direction (positive feedback) or in the opposite direction (negative feedback). Perturbation means disturbance or a change in a structure or function, usually as a result of an external influence.

2.4.1 Positive Feedback

Positive feedback amplifies changes and intensifies a response until an endpoint is reached. Childbirth and blood clotting are two examples of positive feedback mechanisms (see below).

Examples of positive feedback mechanisms:

– *Childbirth.* Positive feedback in childbirth normally begins when the head of the infant pushes against the cervix. This stimulates nerve impulses, which travel from the cervix to the hypothalamus in the brain. In response, the hypothalamus sends the hormone *oxytocin* to the pituitary gland, which secretes it into the bloodstream so that it can be carried to the uterus. *Oxytocin* stimulates uterus contractions, which push the baby harder against the cervix. In response, the cervix dilates in preparation for the baby's passage. This positive feedback cycle continues with increasing levels of *oxytocin*, more muscular uterine contractions, and wider cervix dilation until the baby is pushed through the birth canal and out of the uterus (Fig. 2.2).

– *Blood clotting (Haemostasis).* The mechanism of haemostasis can be divided into four stages: (1) Constriction of the blood vessel. (2) Formation of a temporary "platelet plug." (3) Activation of the coagulation cascade. (4) Formation of "fibrin plug" or the final clot. Haemostasis facilitates a series of enzymatic activations that lead to clot formation with platelets and fibrin polymer. This clot seals the injured area and controls and prevents further bleeding while tissue regeneration occurs. Once the injury starts to heal, the plug slowly remodels, and it dissolves with the restoration of normal tissue at the site of the damage.

– *Menstrual cycle.* The ovaries release the hormone *oestrogen* at the start of the menstrual cycle. The oestrogen operates as a positive feedback loop stimulation. The information is delivered to the brain, which prompts the hypothalamus to release the gonadotropin-releasing hormone and the pituitary to release the luteinising hormone. The control unit releases these hormones in response to the stimulation. These hormones then cause the ovaries to release oestrogen,

Fig. 2.2 Homeostasis. Childbirth mechanism during positive feedback mechanism. Image credit: Source: OpenStax College, Anatomy & Physiology, CC BY 4.0

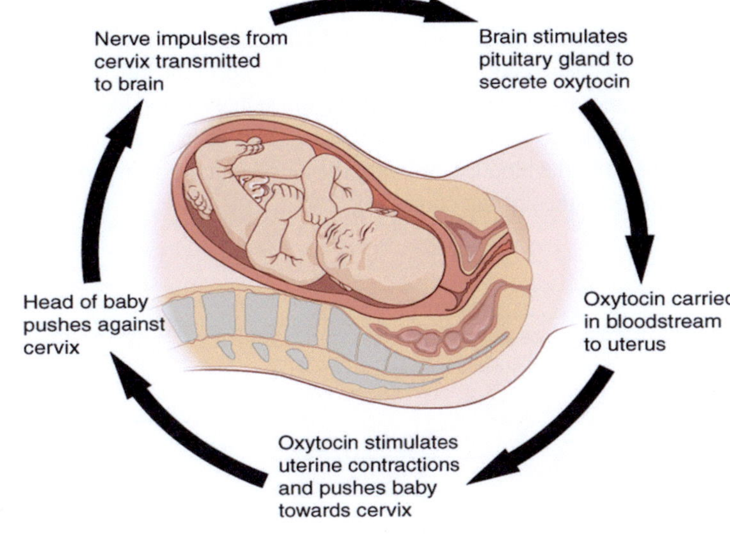

Fig. 2.3 Negative Feedback mechanism. The maintaining of body temperature is an example of a negative feedback loop. Image credit: OpenStax College, Biology, CC BY 4.0

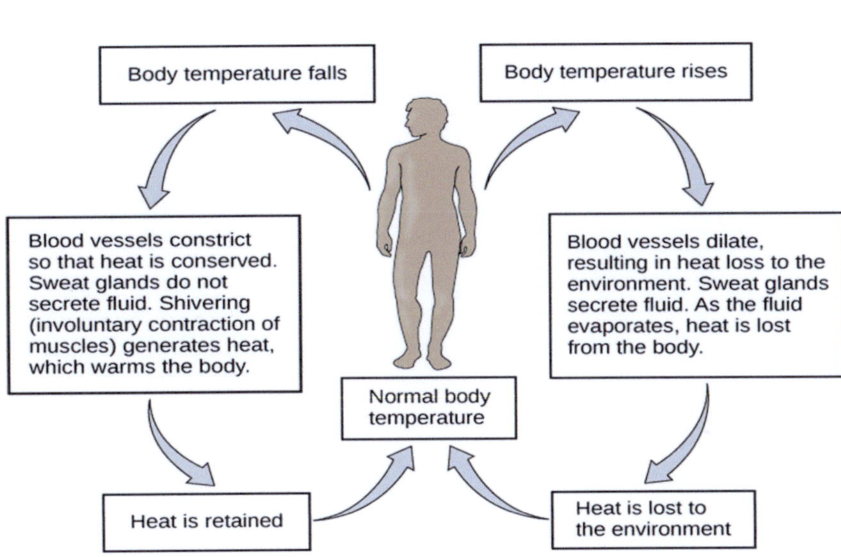

and the cycle repeats itself until the levels of these hormones are high enough to trigger the release of *follicle-stimulating hormone*. After the release of follicle-stimulating hormone, ovulation occurs, and the menstrual cycle begins. The rise in one element causes the output to move in the same direction until the task is done, which is an example of a positive feedback process.

2.4.2 Negative feedback

Negative feedback is a mechanism that reverses a deviation from the set point. Thus, negative feedback maintains body parameters within their normal range. The maintenance of homeostasis by negative feedback goes on throughout the body at all times. Some examples are given below.

Examples of negative feedback mechanisms:

– *Regulating body temperature (thermoregulation)*. A typical negative feedback mechanism in the human body is regulating body temperature. When the body's temperature rises above normal, the brain sends signals to various organs, including the skin, to release heat in the form of sweat. These physiological actions cause the temperature to drop to the point where the negative feedback mechanism's pathways are shut down. When the body's temperature drops below normal, the blood flow to the skin decreases, and the person might start shivering so that the muscles generate heat and warm the body. (Fig. 2.3).

– *Blood sugar regulation:* Blood glucose concentration rises after a meal (the stimulus). The pancreas releases the hormone *insulin* and speeds up glucose transport from the blood into selected tissues (the response). Blood glucose concentration then decreases, which in turn reduces the original stimulus and causes a reduction in the secretion of insulin into the blood, thus maintaining blood glucose regulation. If the blood glucose level falls below the normal range, pancreatic alpha cells release the hormone glucagon into the bloodstream. Glucagon signals cells to break down stored glycogen to glucose and release the glucose into the bloodstream until the blood glucose level increases to the normal range (Fig. 2.4).

– *Pain reflex:* When the hand unintentionally touches a sharp or hot object, it is immediately withdrawn due to the withdrawal reflex. This is called the pain withdrawal reflex arc (Fig. 2.5). A pain stimulus is detected by a receptor (nociceptor), and a nerve impulse is initiated in a sensory neuron. The sensory neuron enters the spinal cord via the dorsal root and synapses with a relay neuron in the

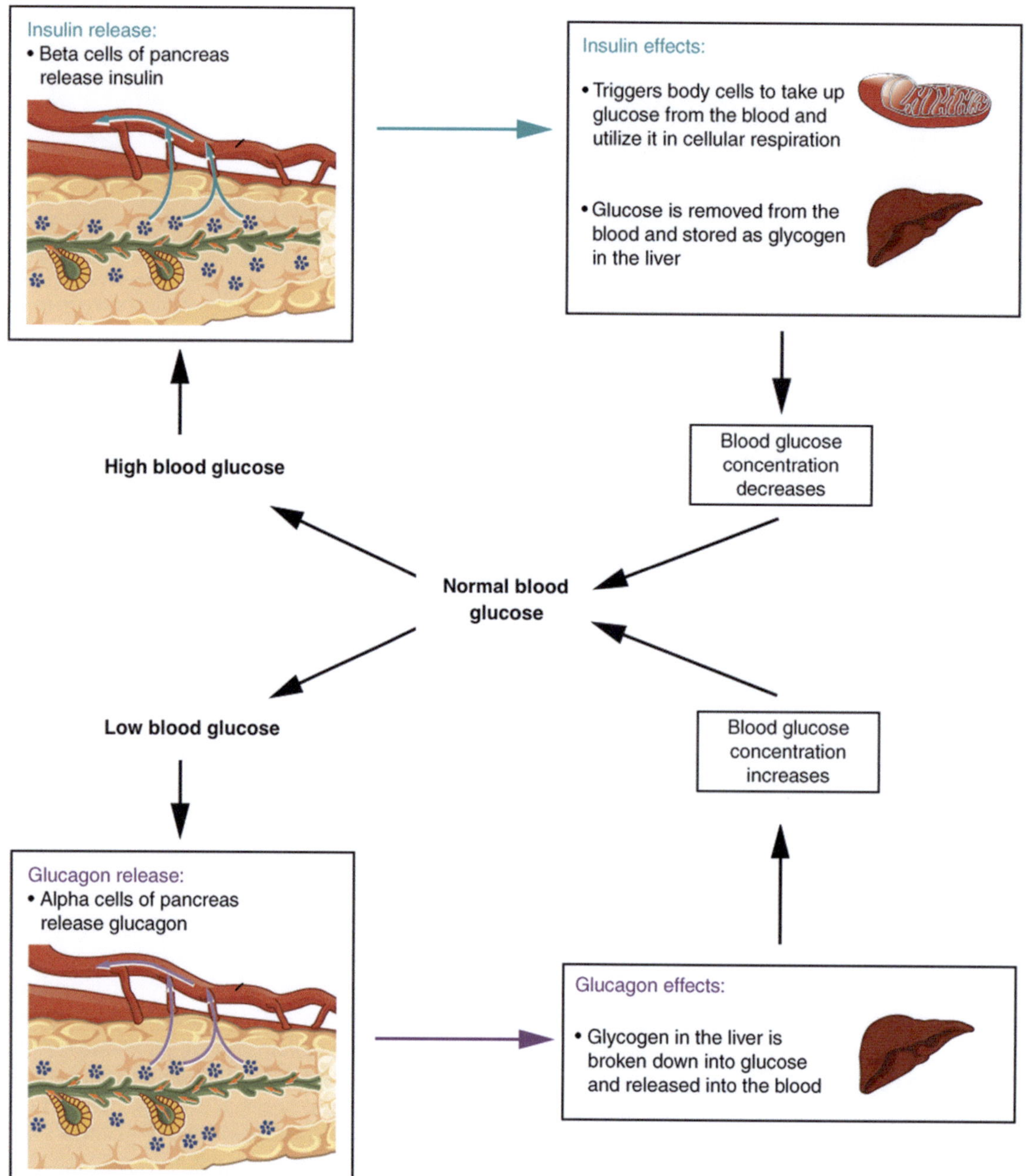

Fig. 2.4 Homeostasis. Blood sugar regulation. An example of a negative feedback mechanism. Image credit: The Endocrine Pancreas. Anatomy & Physiology, OpenStax College, CC BY 4.0

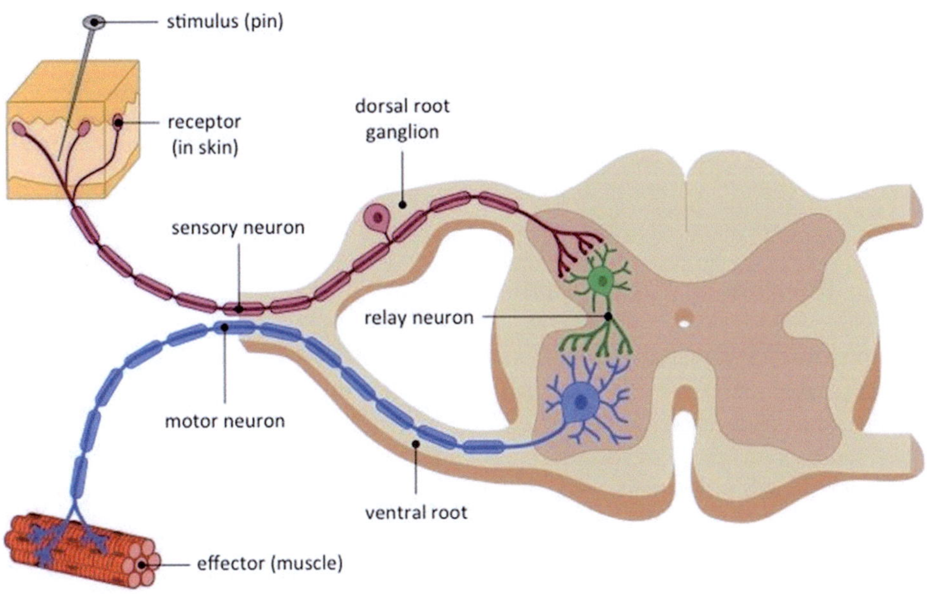

Fig. 2.5 Homeostasis. Pain withdrawal reflex arc. An example of a negative feedback mechanism

grey matter. The relay neuron synapses with a motor neuron, which leaves the spinal cord via the ventral root. The motor neuron synapses with a muscle (effector), causing it to contract and remove the limb from the pain stimulus. This reflex is extremely fast, because the nerves that go to the spinal cord detect the painful stimulus; the brain is not involved in the reflex process.

– *Thirst reflex:* Fluids are lost through urine, sweat, and other routes. The brain senses the fluid loss, triggers the thirst reflex, and makes the individual thirsty. Thirst has long been thought of as a negative homeostatic feedback response to increases in blood solute concentration or decreases in blood volume. If the lost fluid is not replaced (through fluids), hormonal signals to the kidneys are sent to reduce urine production to keep the fluid within the body. Emerging evidence suggests a clear role for thirst as a feedforward adaptive anticipatory response that precedes physiological challenges.

– *Regulation of blood calcium levels.* Another example of negative feedback is the regulation of the blood calcium level. The parathyroid glands secrete parathyroid hormone, which regulates the level of calcium in the blood. If blood calcium decreases, the parathyroid glands sense the decrease and secrete more *parathyroid hormone*. The parathyroid hormone stimulates calcium release from the bones and increases the calcium uptake into the bloodstream from the collecting tubules in the kidneys. Conversely, if blood calcium rises too much, the parathyroid glands reduce parathyroid hormone production. Both responses are examples of negative feedback, because, in both cases, the effects are negative (opposite) to the stimulus.

2.5 Oral Homeostasis

Oral homeostasis maintains a stable intra-oral environment which is achieved by (1) the epithelial barrier providing mechanical protection and as a "first line of defence" with primarily innate immune mechanisms; (2) immune exclusion with the production of secretory immunoglobulin (Ig) A or IgM by plasma cells; and (3) immune suppression through T-cell anergy. Oral resident bacteria also have pro- and anti-inflammatory activities crucial for maintaining homeostasis at heavily colonised sites in the oral cavity. The complex equilibrium between resident species in the oral cavity is responsible for maintaining a healthy state (in symbiosis) or a state associated with disease (in dysbiosis).

2.6 Homeostasis and Ageing

With ageing, the sensitivity of the hypothalamus to feedback regulators begins to decline. This results in a progressive loss of homeostasis, disruption of appropriate hormone production, and an inability of the hypothalamus to regulate its target tissues appropriately.

2.7 Nutrition and Homeostasis

Varying levels of undernutrition or overnutrition can alter homeostatic interactions between nutrition and metabolism. Undernutrition can result from inadequate ingestion of nutrients, malabsorption, impaired metabolism, loss of nutrients due to diarrhoea, or increased nutritional requirements, as occurs in cancer or infection. Chronic nutrient overload disturbs metabolic homeostasis. Cells initiate multiple protective mechanisms to adapt to elevated intracellular metabolites and restore metabolic homeostasis. Still, an irreversible injury to the cells can occur after prolonged nutrient overload. Chronic nutrient overload leads to obesity.

2.8 Environment and Homeostasis

Environmental pollutants, including herbicides and by-products from industrial chemical processes, have been implicated as responsible for the increase in chronic disorders such as cancer, cardiovascular, neurodegenerative, respiratory, renal, autoimmune, and other diseases.

2.9 Summary

In summary, homeostasis is the ability to maintain stable conditions in the body and slight changes in conditions are corrected automatically to maintain homeostasis. The homeostatic process involves positive and negative feedback mechanisms. The body's inability to maintain homeostasis leads to dysbiosis.

Bibliography

Aga Khan Academy (USA). Homeostasis. https://www.khanacademy.org/science/high-school-biology/hs-human-body-systems/hs-body-structure-and-homeostasis/a/hs-body-structure-and-homeostasis-review

Allam JP, Novak N. Mucosal homeostasis of the Oral mucosa. In: Bergmeier L, editor. Oral mucosa in health and disease. New York: Springer; 2018. https://doi.org/10.1007/978-3-319-56065-6_5.

Chen TT, Maevsky EI, Uchitel ML. Maintenance of homeostasis in the ageing hypothalamus: the central and peripheral roles of succinate. Front Endocrinol (Lausanne). 2015;6:7. https://doi.org/10.3389/fendo.2015.00007. PMID: 25699017; PMCID: PMC4313775

Craft J, Gordon C, Tiziani A. Homeostasis. In: Craft J, Gordon C, Tiziani A, et al., editors. Understanding pathophysiology. New York: Elsevier; 2011. p. 23–31.

Devine DA, Marsh PD, Meade J. Modulation of host responses by oral commensal bacteria. J Oral Microbiol. 2015;7:26941. https://doi.org/10.3402/jom.v7.26941. PMID: 25661061; PMCID: PMC4320998

Godlewski M, Kobylińska A. Programmed cell death-strategy for maintenance cellular organisms homeostasis. Postepy Hig Med Dosw (Online). 2016;70:1229.

Kilian M, Chapple I, Hannig M, et al. The oral microbiome–an update for oral healthcare professionals. Br Dent J. 2016;221:657–66.

Qiu H, Schlegel V. Impact of nutrient overload on metabolic homeostasis. Nutr Rev. 2018;76(9):693–707.

Smith SA, Travers RJ, Morrissey JH. How it all starts: initiation of the clotting cascade. Crit Rev Biochem Mol Biol. 2015;50(4):326–36.

3.1 Introduction

Often, terms such as disease, disorder, and medical condition are interchangeably used. A clear understanding of the meaning of these terms is necessary. A disease is an abnormal condition affecting the body of an organism. A disorder is a functional abnormality or disturbance, and a medical condition is a broad term that includes all diseases and disorders.

3.2 Disease: Definition and Characteristics

The WHO definition of health, formulated in 1948, describes health as "a state of complete physical, mental and social well-being and not merely the absence of disease or infirmity." *The disease can be defined as any harmful deviation from an organism's normal structural or functional state, generally associated with certain signs and symptoms.* When homeostasis fails, disease occurs.

Characteristics of any disease include aetiology (or cause), pathogenesis (or mechanism), morphological, functional, and clinical changes (or manifestations), complications and sequelae (or secondary effects), prognosis (or outcome), and epidemiology (or incidence/prevalence):

3.2.1 Aetiology

The word "aetiology" is mainly used in medicine, where it is the science that deals with the causes or origin of disease and the factors which produce or predispose toward a particular disease or disorder. This term comes from the root word prefix "aetio-" and the suffix "-ology." When the aetiology is not known or uncertain, the disease in question is called an idiopathic disease. The aetiology and pathogenesis of a disease may be combined as aetiopathogenesis.

3.2.2 Pathogenesis

The pathogenesis of a disease refers to the mechanism through which the aetiology operates to produce pathological and clinical manifestations. Some examples include inflammation, immune responses, and carcinogenesis.

3.2.3 Morphological, Functional, and Clinical Manifestations

The aetiologic agent produces morphological, functional, and clinical changes through a pathogenetic pathway. The following are some features of clinical interest:

- **Symptom:** A symptom is experienced by an individual, such as feeling feverish, having a headache, or having shortness of breath. When an illness or disease is evidenced by symptoms, it is known as symptomatic. Some conditions, including early cancers, hypertension, and infections, may be present but show no symptoms; these are asymptomatic.
- **Sign:** A sign is an objective, observable indication of a disease, injury, or abnormal physiological state that may be detected during a physical examination or diagnostic procedure.
- **Vital signs** include four clinical signs that can immediately measure the body's overall functioning and health status. They are body temperature, heart rate, breathing rate, and blood pressure. The ranges of these measurements vary with age, weight, gender, and general health.
- **Pathognomonic features:** Some diseases manifest with specifically distinctive features denoting signs and symptoms on which a diagnosis can be made. These are called pathognomonic features. Pill-rolling tremors are pathognomonic for Parkinson's disease.

- **Lesion:** An area of abnormal tissue (an ulcer, growth, etc.) caused by an aetiologic agent (trauma, infection, etc.) is called a lesion. A lesion may be purely biochemical such as defective haemoglobin in a patient with haemoglobinopathy.
- **Syndrome:** Often, the term syndrome is used by clinicians. The syndrome is a set of symptoms or conditions that occur together and suggest the presence of a particular disease. Down syndrome is an example.
- **Complications and sequelae (or secondary effects).** A complication is a medical problem that occurs during a disease or after a procedure or treatment. The complication may be caused by the disease, process, or treatment or may be unrelated. Sequelae are complications or conditions following a prior illness or disease.
- **Prognosis**. Prognosis is the likely outcome or course of a disease and the chance of recovery or recurrence.

3.3 Epidemiology

Epidemiology is the study of the distribution and determinants of health-related states or events in specified populations and the application of this study to control health problems.

3.4 Classification of the Disease

One way of solving a problem in a clinical setting is to devise systems or classifications of diseases. It is understood that no single classification provides an easy way of learning the diseases' relevant clinical and pathological features. However, the classification of diseases becomes extremely important in studying diseases. It is used in compiling statistics on causes of illness (morbidity) and causes of death (mortality). It is also essential to know what illnesses and diseases are prevalent in an area and how these prevalence rates vary with time. In the clinical setting, having gathered information through history taking, patient interviews, and clinical examination, the clinician puts the facts into various categories. This categorisation method may be called a "surgical sieve" method. It is a recognition that all the different diseases affecting patients can be categorised into a few groups according to the nature of the underlying pathology. Classifications of the disease in medicine include (1) topographic, by bodily region or system, (2) anatomic, by organ or tissue, (3) physiological, by function or effect, (4) pathological, by the nature of the disease process, (5) etiologic (causal), (6) epidemiological, and (7) statistical. The

etiologic classification of disease based on known causes is widely used in pathology. Examples of known causes can be listed as follows:

- Traumatic (e.g. mechanical, chemical, thermal, radiation trauma)
- Congenital (e.g. Heritable, and non-heritable malformations)
- Inflammatory (e.g. Trauma associated)
- Immunological (e.g. hypersensitive, immunodeficiency, and autoimmune)
- Infective (e.g. Bacterial, viral, fungal, parasitic)
- Degenerative (e.g. neurodegenerative diseases such as Alzheimer's disease)
- Neoplastic: (e.g. Benign and malignant neoplasms)
- Metabolic: (e.g. Inborn errors of metabolism, Diabetes mellitus)
- Nutritional (Nutritional deficiencies and excess)
- Environmental: (e.g. Air pollution, smoking-related)
- Iatrogenic: (induced by treatment or investigation)
- Idiopathic (Unknown cause)

Detailed information on the above classification is beyond the scope of this chapter.

3.5 Numerical Disease-Coding Systems

Understanding diseases in ways that enable prevention, treatment, and the allocation of resources requires a reliable measurement that allows valid comparisons between places and over time. Classification of diseases and related things is essential for such measurement. *The International Classification of Diseases (ICD) of the World Health Organisation is one of the main basis for comparable statistics on causes of death and non-fatal disease. Each disease or a group of diseases is designated a specific number in the ICD classification.* The World Health Assembly adopted the most recent ICD-11 in May 2019. Systematised Nomenclature of Medicine (SNOMED) is the other coded classification available. SNOMED CT stands for Systematized Nomenclature of Medicine – Clinical Terms. It is a standardised, international, multilingual core clinical healthcare terminology that can be used in electronic health records (EHRs).

ICD was adopted by the 72nd World Health Assembly in 2019 and came into effect on 1 January 2022. As a classification and terminology, ICD-11 allows the systematic recording, analysis, interpretation, and comparison of mortality and morbidity data collected in different countries or regions at different times. It ensures semantic interoperability and reusability of recorded data for different use beyond mere health statistics, including decision support, resource allocation, reimbursement, and guidelines.

3.6 Disorder (Medical Disorder)

A disorder is a functional abnormality or disturbance. *A medical disorder is a relatively distinct condition resulting from an organismic dysfunction which, in its fully developed or extreme form, is directly associated with distress, disability, or certain other types of disadvantage.* Medical disorders can be categorised into mental, physical, genetic, and emotional (behavioural) disorders.

3.6.1 Mental Disorder

Mental disorder is a medical disorder whose manifestations are primarily signs or symptoms of a psychological (behavioural) nature. A mental disorder is also referred to as a mental illness or psychiatric disorder. It is a behavioural or mental pattern that causes significant distress or impairment of personal functioning. Such features may be persistent, relapsing, remitting, or as single episodes. The causes of mental disorders are often unclear. Mental disorders are usually defined by a combination of how a person behaves, feels, perceives, or thinks. Cultural and religious beliefs, as well as social norms, should be considered when making a diagnosis. A clinical psychologist or psychiatrist may diagnose mental disorders.

3.6.2 Physical Disorder

A disease or illness described as a physical disorder likely impacts the musculoskeletal system and lacks an inciting injury. Examples may include webbed toes, and ataxia (a degenerative disease of the nervous system with symptoms mimicking being drunk, such as slurred speech and stumbling). Many disorders have been described, with signs and symptoms that vary widely.

3.6.3 Genetic Disorder

Genetic disorder is a health problem caused by one or more abnormalities in the genome. It can be caused by a mutation in a single gene (monogenic), multiple genes (polygenic), or a chromosomal abnormality. Polygenic disorders are the most common. The mutation responsible can occur spontaneously before embryonic development (a de novo mutation), or it can be inherited from two parents who are carriers of a faulty gene (autosomal-recessive inheritance) or from a

parent with the disorder (autosomal-dominant inheritance). When the genetic disorder is inherited from one or both parents, it is classified as a hereditary disease.

3.6.4 Emotional and Behavioural Disorders (EBDs)

Various terms have been used to describe irregular emotional and behavioural disorders (EBDs). Many terms, such as mental illness and psychopathology, were used until recently to describe adults with such conditions. Mental illness was a label for most people with any disorder. However, those terms are avoided when describing children as they seem too stigmatizing. Some examples of EBDs include Attention-deficit hyperactivity disorder (ADHD), Oppositional defiant disorder (ODD), Conduct disorder, Intermittent explosive disorder (IED), and Disruptive mood dysregulation disorder (DMDD). Detailed description of these is beyond the scope of this chapter.

3.7 Disability

According to the Centre for Disease Control and Prevention (CDC), a disability is any condition of the body or mind (impairment) that makes it more difficult for the person with the condition to do certain activities (activity limitation) and interact with the world around them (participation restrictions). Many types of disabilities include vision, movement, thinking, remembering, learning, communicating, hearing, and social relationships. According to the World Health Organization, disability has three dimensions: (1) Impairment in a person's body structure or function or mental functioning; examples of impairments include loss of a limb, loss of vision, or memory loss. (2) Activity limitations, such as difficulty seeing, hearing, walking, or problem-solving. (3) Participation restrictions in normal daily activities, such as working, engaging in social and recreational activities, and obtaining health care and preventive services.

Disability can be related to conditions present at birth. It may affect functions later in life, including cognition (memory, learning, and understanding), mobility (moving around in the environment), vision, hearing, behaviour, and other areas. These conditions may be disorders in single genes (e.g. muscle dystrophy); disorders of chromosomes (e.g. Down syndrome); and the result of the mother's exposure during pregnancy to infections (e.g. rubella) or substances, such as alcohol or cigarettes. Disability can be associated with developmental conditions that become apparent during childhood (e.g. autism spectrum disorder and attention-deficit/hyperactivity disorder or ADHD) or related to an injury (e.g. traumatic brain or spinal cord injury). It can also be associated with a long-standing condition (e.g. diabetes), which can cause a disability such as vision loss, nerve damage, or limb loss. Progressive (e.g. muscular dystrophy), static (e.g. limb loss), or intermittent (e.g. some forms of multiple sclerosis). Impairment is an absence of or significant difference in a person's body structure, function, or mental functioning. Impairments include structural impairments and functional impairments. Structural impairments are substantial problems with an internal or external body component. An example includes nerve damage that can occur in multiple sclerosis. Functional impairments include the complete or partial loss of function of a body part. Examples include pain that doesn't go away or joints that no longer move easily.

is any condition of the body or mind that makes it more difficult for the person with the condition to do certain activities. A medical condition is a broad term that includes all diseases and disorders. These terminologies are often misunderstood and interchangeably used in the diagnostic process.

3.8 Summary

Disease, disorder, and disability are closely related terms. A disease is an abnormal condition affecting the body. A disorder is a functional abnormality or disturbance, and a disability

Bibliography

Carton J. Basic pathology. In: Oxford handbook of clinical pathology. Oxford University Press; 2012. p. 1–14.

Centre for Disease Control and Prevention. The USA. Disability and Health. Overview. 2020. https://www.cdc.gov/ncbddd/disabilityandhealth/disability.html

Harrison JE, Weber S, Jakob R, et al. ICD-11: international classification of diseases for the twenty-first century. BMC Med Inform Decis Mak. 2021;21:206. https://doi.org/10.1186/s12911-021-01534-6.

Jutel A. Classification, disease, and diagnosis. Perspect Biol Med. 2011;54:189–205. https://doi.org/10.1353/pbm.2011.0015.

Cell Structure and Function, Cell Division and Cell Cycle, Cell Types and Stem Cells

4

4.1 Introduction

Knowledge of cells is essential for understanding human health and disease. Normal cellular functions and intercellular interactions are important aspects of human physiology, and when these processes are disrupted, human disease or disorder occurs.

Cells are the basic building blocks of living tissues and organs. Cells can be grouped into two groups: eukaryotes and prokaryotes. A eukaryote has a nucleus and membrane-bound organelles, while a prokaryote lacks these structures. Plants and animals have numerous eukaryotic cells, while many microbes, such as bacteria, consist of single cells. This chapter deals with the basics of cell structure and its functions and forms a basis for studying key processes involved in cellular pathology.

4.2 Cell Structure and Function

The human cell is a eukaryote. It has a plasma membrane, cytoplasm, nucleus, ribosomes, and other membrane-bound organelles that allow for the compartmentalisation of functions (Fig. 4.1, Table 4.1).

4.2.1 The Plasma Membrane

Plasma membrane is a trilaminar membrane made up predominantly of lipids. It also contains several proteins and carbohydrates (Fig. 4.2). It separates the cell from the external environment: controls the passage of organic molecules, ions, water, oxygen, and wastes into and out of the cell. The membrane is highly permeable to oxygen and water but limited to sodium and potassium ions. Some of the large molecules enter the cell by endocytosis. They also bear specific receptors for specific enzymes or hormones. Some cells are also specialised to engulf foreign materials through phagocytosis. The process of engulfing small molecules of fluid is called pinocytosis.

4.2.2 Cytoplasm

Cytoplasm provides structure to the cell. It is the site of many metabolic reactions and is a medium in which organelles are

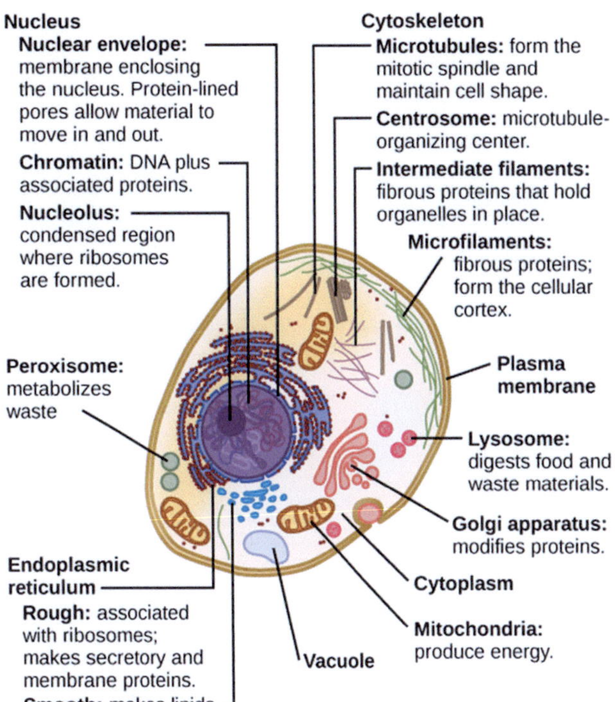

Fig. 4.1 The human cell (Source: Concepts of Biology–1st Canadian Edition by Charles Molnar and Jane Gair. Licensed under a Creative Commons Attribution 4.0 International License). Molnar, C., & Gair, J. (2015). Concepts of Biology – 1st Canadian Edition. BCcampus. Retrieved from https://opentextbc.ca/biology/ Chapter 3.3. Eukaryotic cells. Pp 95–112. All images

© The Author(s), under exclusive license to Springer Nature Switzerland AG 2023
S. R. Prabhu, *Textbook of General Pathology for Dental Students*, https://doi.org/10.1007/978-3-031-31244-1_4

Table 4.1 Summary of functions of cell components

Cell component	Function
Cytoplasm	Provides structure to cell; site of many metabolic reactions; medium in which organelles are found
Nucleus	A cell organelle that houses DNA and directs the synthesis of ribosomes and proteins
Ribosomes	Protein synthesis
Mitochondria	ATP production/cellular respiration
Peroxisomes	Oxidises and breaks down fatty acids and amino acids and detoxifies poisons
Vesicles and vacuoles	Storage and transport; digestive function in plant cells
Centrosome	Unspecified role in cell division in animal cells; organising centre of microtubules in animal cells
Lysosomes	Digestion of macromolecules; recycling of worn-out organelles
Endoplasmic reticulum	Modifies proteins and synthesises lipids
Golgi apparatus	Modifies, sorts, tags, packages, and distributes lipids and proteins
Cytoskeleton	Maintains cell's shape, secures organelles in specific positions, allows cytoplasm and vesicles to move within the cell, and enables unicellular organisms to move independently

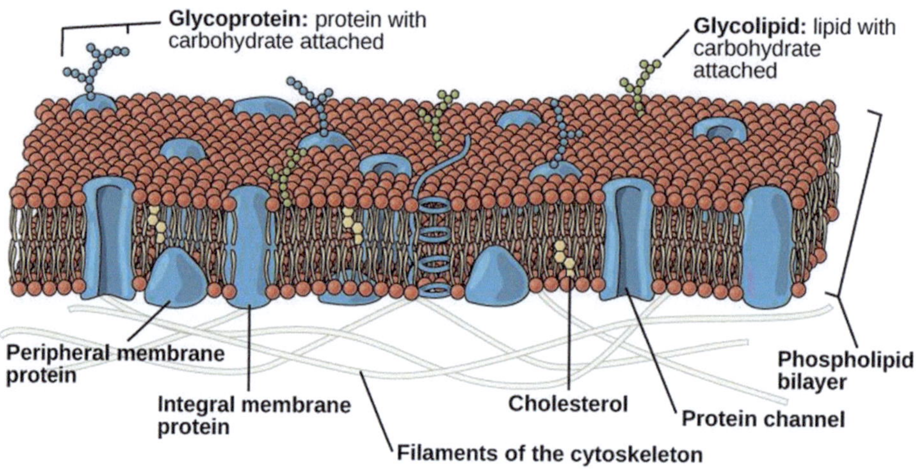

Fig. 4.2 Plasma membrane. (Source: Concepts of Biology–1st Canadian Edition by Charles Molnar and Jane Gair. It is licensed under a Creative Commons Attribution 4.0 International License). Molnar, C., & Gair, J. (2015). Concepts of Biology—1st Canadian Edition. BCcampus. Retrieved from https://opentextbc.ca/biology/ Chapter 3.3. Eukaryotic cells. Pp 95–112. All images)

found. All of the functions for cell expansion, growth, and replication are carried out in the cytoplasm of a cell. The cytosol is the gel-like material of the cytoplasm in which cell structures (organelles) are suspended. Organelles are tiny cellular structures that perform specific functions within a cell. Examples of organelles include nucleus, mitochondria, ribosomes, centrosome, lysosomes, endoplasmic reticulum, Golgi apparatus, vacuoles and vesicles, peroxisomes, and cytoskeleton.

4.2.2.1 Nucleus

All living human cells except red blood cells contain a nucleus. The nucleus has a double-layered thin membrane called a nuclear envelope (nuclear membrane) that shows perforations (Fig. 4.3). These pores are called nuclear pores, specialised to have selective permeability. At the centre of the nucleus, one or more small non-membranous bodies called nucleolus/nucleoli are present. These are made up of RNA that helps make ribosomes. They perform protein synthesis.

The nucleus is a heterogeneous structure with electron-dense (dark) and electron-lucent (light) areas. The dense region called heterochromatin consists of tightly coiled inac-

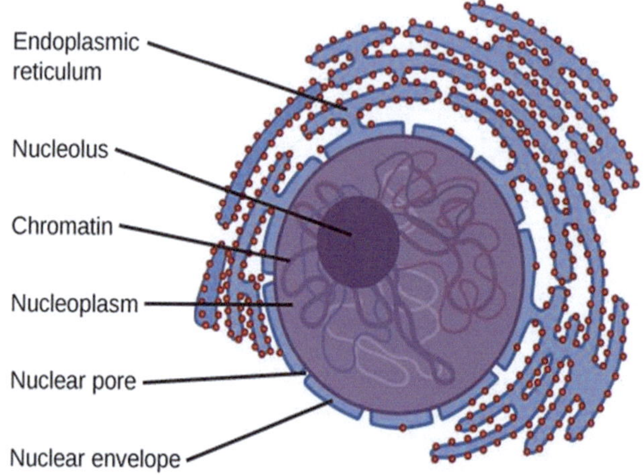

Fig. 4.3 Nucleus. The outermost boundary of the nucleus is the nuclear envelope. Notice that the nuclear envelope consists of two phospholipid bilayers (membranes)—an outer membrane and an inner membrane—in contrast to the plasma membrane, which consists of only one phospholipid bilayer. (Source: Concepts of Biology–1st Canadian Edition by Charles Molnar and Jane Gair. It is licensed under a Creative Commons Attribution 4.0 International License). Molnar, C., & Gair, J. (2015). Concepts of Biology–first Canadian Edition. BCcampus. Retrieved from https://opentextbc.ca/biology/ Chapter 3.3. Eukaryotic cells. Pp 95–112. All images)

tive chromatin found in irregular clumps, often around the periphery of the nucleus. On the other hand, the electron-lucent nuclear material is called euchromatin which represents part of DNA and is active in RNA synthesis. Heterochromatin and euchromatin are collectively called chromatin as they show affinity towards certain dyes. Chromatin contains DNA molecules, which appear as granules or threads when a cell is non-dividing, and they look like short, rod-like, tightly coiled structures when dividing and are now called chromosomes. Human cells typically contain 46 chromosomes (except mature sex cells, which have 23 chromosomes). The DNA molecules carry the master code for making all of a cell's enzymes and other proteins. Thus, they dictate both the structure and the function of the cells. The non-staining component within which the nucleoli are suspended is known as the nuclear sap.

4.2.2.2 Mitochondria

Mitochondria are oval-shaped, double-membrane organelles with ribosomes and DNA. They have two membranes: inner and outer (Fig. 4.4). The inner layer possesses many folds, and these folds are called *cristae*. Embedded within the inner membrane is granular material called the matrix, which contains the main enzymes essential for producing adenosine triphosphate (ATP). They provide all the energy a cell needs to move, divide, contract, and produce secretory products and all other functions.

4.2.2.3 Ribosomes

When viewed through an electron microscope, ribosomes appear as clusters or single tiny dots floating freely in the cytoplasm (free ribosomes) or may be attached to the cyto-

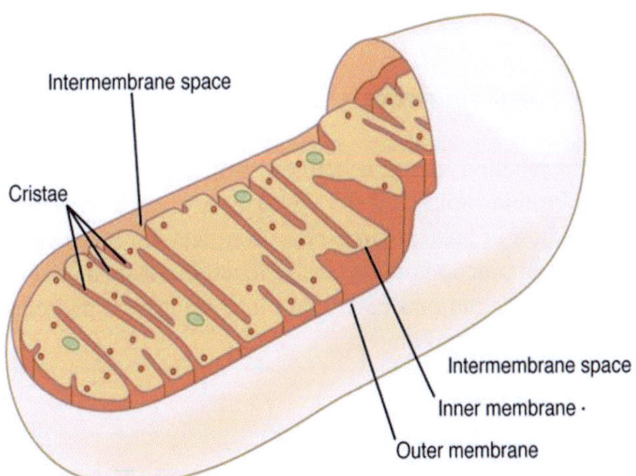

Fig. 4.4 Mitochondria. Source: Concepts of Biology–1st Canadian Edition by Charles Molnar and Jane Gair. Licensed under a Creative Commons Attribution 4.0 International License). Molnar, C., & Gair, J. (2015). Concepts of Biology–1st Canadian Edition. BCcampus. Retrieved from https://opentextbc.ca/biology/ Chapter 3.3. Eukaryotic cells. Pp 95–112. All images

plasmic side of the plasma membrane or the cytoplasmic side of the endoplasmic reticulum. Ribosomes have subunits composed of ribonucleic acid (RNA). The RNA can be rRNA (ribosomal RNA), mRNA (messenger RNA), or tRNA (transfer RNA). Ribosomes are enzyme complexes responsible for protein synthesis.

4.2.2.4 Centrosome

This is an organelle near the nucleus of a cell that contains centrioles from which the spindle fibres develop in cell division.

4.2.2.5 Lysosomes

Lysosomes are membrane-enclosed organelles that pinch off from the Golgi apparatus. They contain chemicals (*enzymes*) that help degrade and recycle cellular waste through autophagy. They have an array of enzymes that break down all biological polymers—proteins, nucleic acids, carbohydrates, and lipids. They are also said to play a role in plasma membrane repair, bone resorption, and immune response.

4.2.2.6 Endoplasmic Reticulum

The endoplasmic reticulum (ER) is a series of interconnected membranous tubules that collectively modify proteins and synthesise lipids (Fig. 4.5). ER modifies proteins and synthesises lipids. There are two types of ER: rough and smooth. The rough endoplasmic reticulum is covered by many ribosomes and helps in protein synthesis. The smooth endoplasmic reticulum synthesises specific lipids and carbohydrates.

4.2.2.7 Golgi Apparatus

Golgi apparatus is a complex of vesicles and folded membranes within the cytoplasm of most cells, involved in secretion and intracellular transport. They modify, sort, tag, package, and distribute lipids and proteins. They help in protein biosynthesis and packaging protein molecules for export from the cell. The materials from the ER will reach the Golgi bodies in the form of vesicles.

4.2.2.8 Vacuoles and Vesicles

Vacuole is a membrane-bound sac that functions in cellular storage and transport, somewhat more prominent than a vesicle. A vesicle is a small, membrane-bound sac. Its membrane can fuse with the plasma membrane and the membranes of the endoplasmic reticulum and Golgi apparatus.

4.2.2.9 Peroxisomes

Peroxisomes are tiny, round organelles enclosed by single membranes. They carry out oxidation reactions that break down fatty acids and amino acids. They also detoxify many poisons that may enter the body. Peroxisomes detoxify alcohol in liver cells. A by-product of these oxidation reactions is

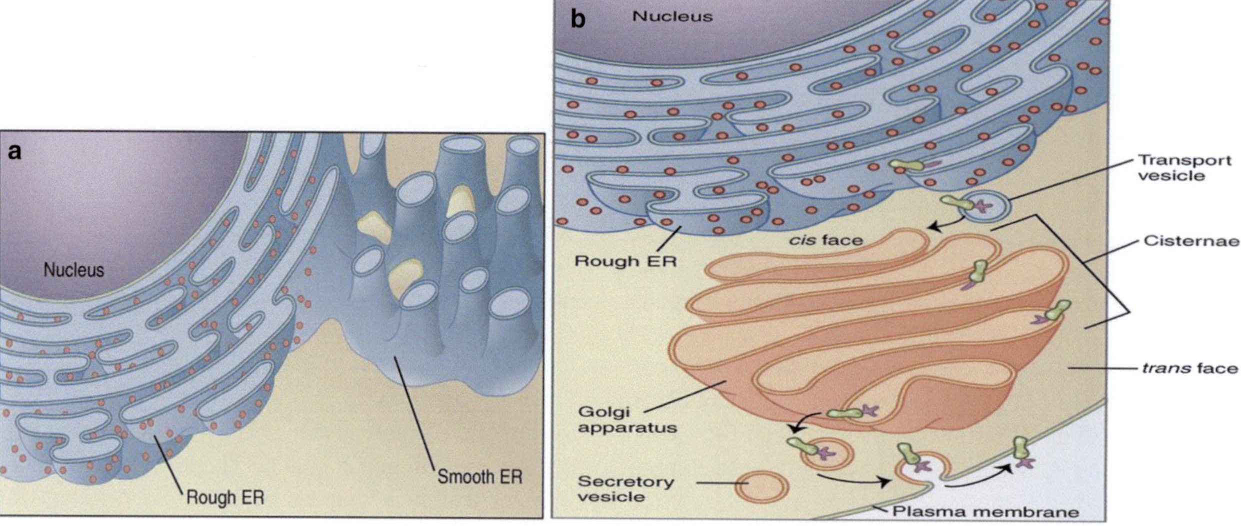

Fig. 4.5 (**a, b**) Endoplasmic reticulum. Source: Concepts of Biology– 1st Canadian Edition by Charles Molnar and Jane Gair. Licensed under a Creative Commons Attribution 4.0 International License). Molnar, C., & Gair, J. (2015). Concepts of Biology–1st Canadian Edition. BCcampus. Retrieved from https://opentextbc.ca/biology/ Chapter 3.3. Eukaryotic cells. Pp 95–112. All images

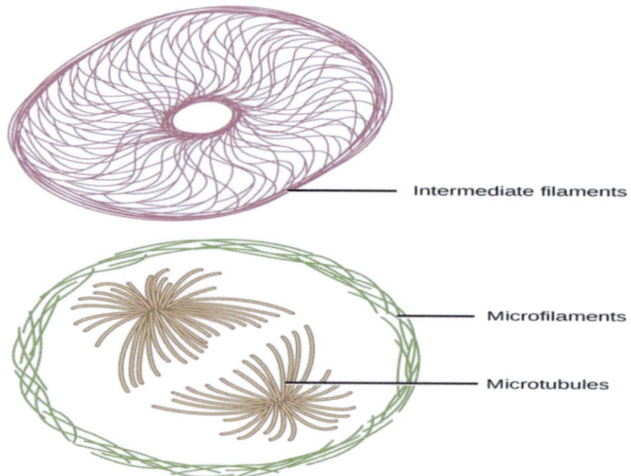

Fig. 4.6 Microfilaments, intermediate filaments, and microtubules compose a cell's cytoskeleton. Source: Concepts of Biology–1st Canadian Edition by Charles Molnar and Jane Gair. Licensed under a Creative Commons Attribution 4.0 International License). Molnar, C., & Gair, J. (2015). Concepts of Biology–1st Canadian Edition. BCcampus. Retrieved from https://opentextbc.ca/biology/ Chapter 3.3. Eukaryotic cells. Pp 95–112. All images

hydrogen peroxide, H_2O_2, which is contained within the peroxisomes to prevent the chemical from causing damage to cellular components outside of the organelle. Peroxisomal enzymes safely break down hydrogen peroxide into water and oxygen.

4.2.2.10 Cytoskeleton

The cytoskeleton is a network of fibres (Fig. 4.6). They can be divided into three types based on the composition of their protein subunits: (1) microfilaments, which are made up of actins; (2) microtubules, which are made up of tubulins; and (3) intermediate filaments, which are made of a variety of subunits. The cytoskeleton maintains the cell's shape, secures organelles in specific positions, allows cytoplasm and vesicles to move within the cell, and enables unicellular organisms to move independently.

4.3   Intercellular Junctions

Human cells communicate by direct contact, referred to as intercellular junctions. Cell contacts include tight and gap junctions and desmosomes (Fig. 4.7).

4.3.1 Tight Junctions

A tight junction is a seal between two adjacent cells (Fig. 5.2a). Proteins hold the cells tightly against each other. This tight adhesion prevents materials from leaking between the cells. Tight junctions are typically found in the epithelial tissue that lines the oral cavity and internal organs and composes most of the skin.

4.3.2 Gap Junctions

Gap junctions are channels between adjacent cells (Fig. 5.2b). They are made of connexin proteins, mediating both electrical and biochemical signals between cells and allowing for the transport of ions, nutrients, and other substances that enable cells to communicate.

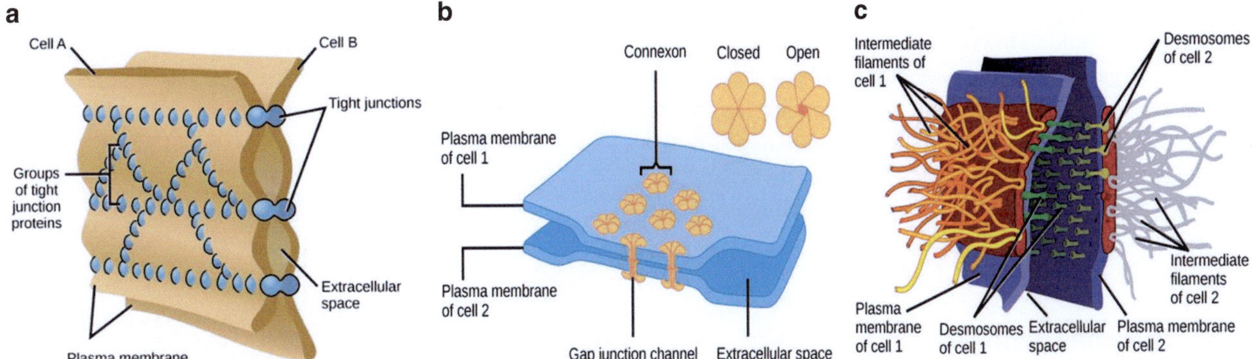

Fig. 4.7 Connections between cells. (**a**) Tight junctions join adjacent cells. (**b**) Gap junctions act as channels between cells, and (**c**) Desmosomes join two cells together. (Source: Concepts of Biology–1st Canadian Edition by Charles Molnar and Jane Gair. They are licensed under a Creative Commons Attribution 4.0 International License). Molnar, C., & Gair, J. (2015). Concepts of Biology–1st Canadian Edition. BCcampus. Retrieved from https://opentextbc.ca/biology/ Chapter 3.3. Eukaryotic cells. Pp 95–112)

4.3.3 Desmosomes/Hemidesmosomes

A linkage between adjacent epithelial cells that forms when cadherins in the plasma membrane attach to intermediate filaments (Fig. 4.7). They keep cells together in a sheet-like formation in organs and tissues that stretch, like the skin, oral epithelium, heart, and muscles. Hemidesmosomes are multi-protein complexes that facilitate the stable adhesion of basal epithelial cells to the underlying basement membrane.

4.4 Cell Communication (Cell Signalling)

Cell communication or cell signalling entails transmitting information from one cell to another cell or a group of cells. A cell can receive, process, and transmit signals to its environment and to itself. Cell communication controls a variety of functions. *Cells communicate with each other using chemicals called signalling molecules or ligands. Ligands are substances that specifically bind receptors.* A receptor is a protein expressed on the target cell that recognises and attaches to the ligand. Many ligands are proteins and fit precisely into specific receptors. Hormones and cytokines are common ligands for signalling between cells. The cell secretes these molecules out. Other cells detect the presence of the signalling molecule through receptors present on their surface, and once the signalling molecule is detected, the cells will make changes. Signalling molecules can be lipids, proteins, or gases. The disease can result when cells do not respond appropriately to their environment or do not work with other cells. Examples of disrupted cell signalling in disease include cancer cells, immunodeficiencies, and viral infections. Cancer cells have constant activation of signalling pathways instructing the cells to grow and divide. This often occurs because of mutations in receptors and changes in protein kinases or transcription factors that keep the pro-

teins in an active state. Some immunodeficiencies can occur, because immune cells lack the receptors for ligands that instruct immune cells to divide and develop or lack the specific kinases that transmit these signals. Many viruses, such as hepatitis B, produce proteins that interfere with the host cell's signalling pathways, suppress the immune system, and enhance viral reproduction.

4.5 Signalling Pathways

Signalling pathways may be classified according to the source of a signalling molecule. Depending on the ligand's origin (from the same cell, neighbour cell, or a far distance) and the receptor-ligand interaction, the cell-cell signalling pathway is classified into four different types: autocrine, endocrine, paracrine, and juxtacrine.

4.5.1 Autocrine Signalling

In autocrine signalling, the signalling molecule originates from the target cell itself. Molecules secreted by a cell affect that same cell. Cells express receptors to a ligand they secrete. For example, blood platelets secrete eicosanoids, which influence their activity. Autocrine signalling has also been observed during embryogenesis.

4.5.2 Endocrine Signalling

Endocrine signalling is an example of long-distance communication between hormone-producing cells, tissues, glands, and cells that express hormone receptor molecules. The hormones are small molecules or glycoproteins that are usually secreted into the bloodstream before being distributed throughout the body. Endocrine signals often originate from within the brain. However, glands, such as the thyroid gland, and organs, including the stomach, pancreas, liver, kidneys, and reproductive organs, also produce hormones. One endocrine signal that must travel a great distance is that of follicle-stimulating hormone (FSH), sent from the anterior pituitary gland to the testes or ovaries, stimulating germ cell maturation.

4.5.3 Paracrine Signalling

In this process, signalling occurs between cells near each other. Here, a soluble signalling molecule secreted by one cell diffuses to another. For instance, neurotransmitters secreted by neurons diffuse a few nanometers before binding to receptors on target neurons or muscle cells. Another example is the release of chemokines by neutrophils, which attract other cells through a process known as chemotaxis. Signalling molecules with minimal diffusion are rapidly degraded and taken up by other cells or trapped in the extra-cellular matrix.

4.5.4 Juxtacrine Signalling

When adjacent cells are in contact with each other, they communicate through components of their plasma membrane through a process called juxtacrine signalling. Juxtacrine signalling occurs between neighbouring cells that are in physical contact with each other. In this case, the signalling molecule is not free but is instead bound to the cell's membrane. It may then interact with a receptor on the membrane of an adjacent cell.

4.6 Interaction with Extracellular Matrix

An extracellular matrix (ECM) is a non-cellular three-dimensional macromolecular network composed of collagens, proteoglycans/glycosaminoglycans, elastin, fibronectin, laminins, and several other glycoproteins. (Fig. 4.8). *Matrix components and cell adhesion receptors bind each other, forming a complex network into which cells reside in all tissues and organs.* Cell surface receptors transduce signals into cells from ECM, which regulate diverse cellular functions, such as survival, growth, migration, and differentiation, and are vital for maintaining normal homeostasis.

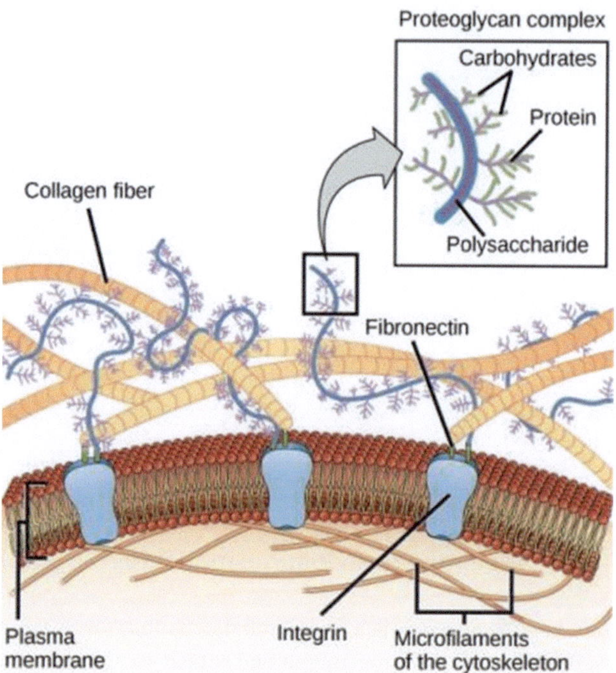

Fig. 4.8 The extracellular matrix consists of a network of substances secreted by cells. (Source: Concepts of Biology–1st Canadian Edition by Charles Molnar and Jane Gair. It is licensed under a Creative Commons Attribution 4.0 International License). Molnar, C., & Gair, J. (2015). Concepts of Biology–1st Canadian Edition. BCcampus. Retrieved from https://opentextbc.ca/biology/ Chapter 3.3. Eukaryotic cells. Pp 95–112.)

4.7 Cell Division and the Cell Cycle

From the formation of the zygote, cell division continues to occur throughout life. There are two types of cell division: one which forms the gametes, called meiosis, and the other is mitosis. The description of Meiosis is beyond the scope of this chapter.

The cell cycle has two major phases: interphase and mitotic (Figs. 4.9 and 4.10). During interphase, the cell grows, and DNA is replicated. During the mitotic phase, the replicated DNA and cytoplasmic contents are separated, and the cell divides.

4.7.1 Interphase

Many internal and external conditions must be met for a cell to move from the interphase to the mitotic phase. The three stages of interphase are called G_1, S, and G_2.

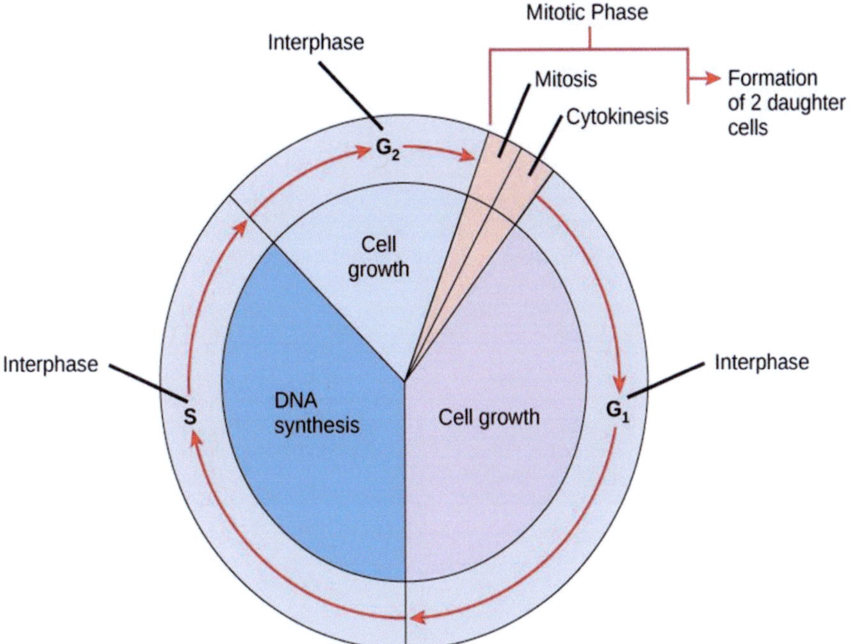

Fig. 4.9 A cell moves through a series of phases in an orderly manner. During the interphase, G1 involves cell growth and protein synthesis, the S phase involves DNA and centrosome replication, and G2 involves further development and protein synthesis. The mitotic phase follows the interphase. Mitosis is nuclear division, where duplicated chromosomes are segregated and distributed into daughter nuclei. Usually, the cell will divide after mitosis in a process called cytokinesis, in which the cytoplasm is divided, and two daughter cells are formed (Source: Concepts of Biology - 1st Canadian Edition by Charles Molnar and Jane Gair. They are licensed under a Creative Commons Attribution 4.0 International License). Molnar, C., & Gair, J. (2015). Concepts of Biology – 1st Canadian Edition. BCcampus. Retrieved from https:// opentextbc.ca/biology/ Chapter 3.3. Eukaryotic cells. Pp 95–112. All images)

G1 Phase (First gap phase). The first interphase stage is called the G_1 phase, or the first gap, because little change is visible. The cell accumulates the building blocks of chromosomal DNA and the associated proteins and accumulates enough energy reserves to complete the task of replicating each chromosome in the nucleus.

S Phase (Synthesis phase). Throughout interphase, nuclear DNA remains in a semi-condensed chromatin configuration. In the S phase (synthesis phase), DNA replication results in the formation of two identical copies of each chromosome—sister chromatids—firmly attached to the centromere region. At this stage, each chromosome is made of two sister chromatids and is a duplicated chromosome. The centrosome is repeated during the S phase. The two centrosomes will give rise to the mitotic spindle, the apparatus that orchestrates the movement of chromosomes during mitosis. The centrosome consists of a pair of rod-like centrioles at right angles. Centrioles help organise cell division. Centrioles are not present in the centrosomes of many eukaryotic species, such as plants and most fungi.

G2 Phase (Second gap phase). In the G_2 phase or second gap, the cell replenishes its energy stores and synthesises the proteins necessary for chromosome manipulation. Some cell organelles are duplicated, and the cytoskeleton is dismantled to provide resources for the mitotic spindle. There may be additional cell growth during G_2. The final preparations for the mitotic phase must be completed before the cell can enter the first stage of mitosis.

4.7.2 Mitotic Phase

The nucleus and the cytoplasm must be divided to make two daughter cells. The mitotic phase is a multistep process during which the duplicated chromosomes are aligned, separated, and moved to opposite cell poles. Then the cell is divided into two new identical daughter cells. The first portion of the mitotic phase, mitosis, is composed of five stages, which accomplish nuclear division. The second portion of the mitotic phase, cytokinesis, is the physical separation of the cytoplasmic components into two daughter cells.

Mitosis. Mitosis is divided into a series of phases—prophase, prometaphase, metaphase, anaphase, and telophase-that result in the division of the cell nucleus.

Events during prophase (the "first phase"):

- The nuclear envelope starts to break into small vesicles.
- The Golgi apparatus and endoplasmic reticulum fragment disperse to the cell's periphery.
- The nucleolus disappears.

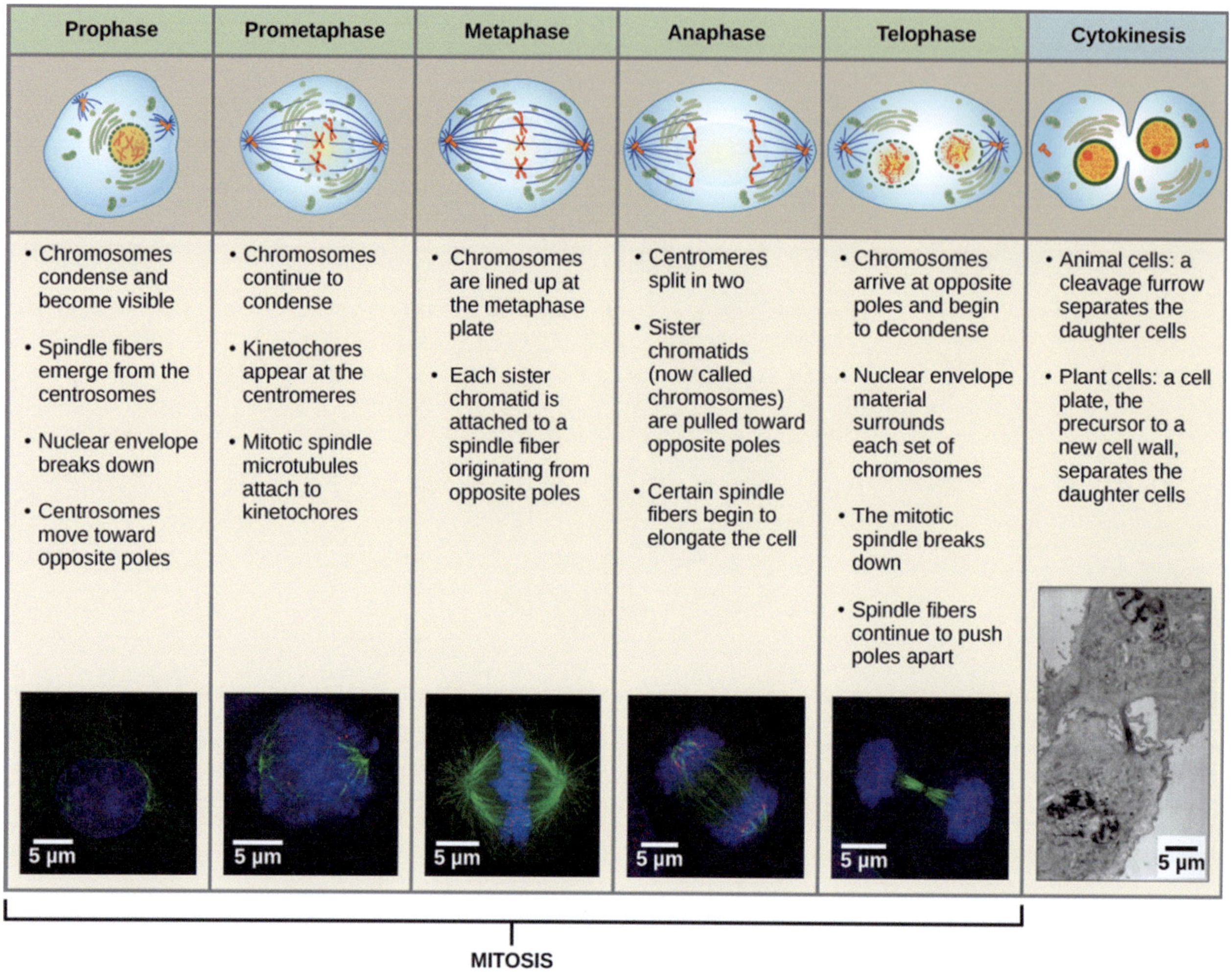

Prophase	Prometaphase	Metaphase	Anaphase	Telophase	Cytokinesis
• Chromosomes condense and become visible • Spindle fibers emerge from the centrosomes • Nuclear envelope breaks down • Centrosomes move toward opposite poles	• Chromosomes continue to condense • Kinetochores appear at the centromeres • Mitotic spindle microtubules attach to kinetochores	• Chromosomes are lined up at the metaphase plate • Each sister chromatid is attached to a spindle fiber originating from opposite poles	• Centromeres split in two • Sister chromatids (now called chromosomes) are pulled toward opposite poles • Certain spindle fibers begin to elongate the cell	• Chromosomes arrive at opposite poles and begin to decondense • Nuclear envelope material surrounds each set of chromosomes • The mitotic spindle breaks down • Spindle fibers continue to push poles apart	• Animal cells: a cleavage furrow separates the daughter cells • Plant cells: a cell plate, the precursor to a new cell wall, separates the daughter cells

MITOSIS

Fig. 4.10 Cell mitosis is divided into five stages—prophase, prometaphase, metaphase, anaphase, and telophase—visualised here by light microscopy with fluorescence. Mitosis is usually accompanied by cytokinesis, shown here by a transmission electron microscope. (Source and credit "diagrams": modification of work by Mariana Ruiz Villareal; credit "mitosis micrographs": modification of work by Roy van Heesbeen; credit "cytokinesis micrograph": modification of work by the Wadsworth Center, NY State Department of Health; donated to the Wikimedia Foundation; scale-bar data from Matt Russell) (Source: https://opentextbc.ca/biology/chapter/6-2-the-cell-cycle/)

– The centrosomes begin to move to opposite poles of the cell.
– The microtubules that form the basis of the mitotic spindle extend between the centrosomes, pushing them farther apart as the microtubule fibres lengthen.
– The sister chromatids begin to coil more tightly and become visible under a light microscope.

Events during prometaphase:

– Many processes begun in the prophase continue to advance and culminate in the formation of a connection between the chromosomes and cytoskeleton.
– The remnants of the nuclear envelope disappear.
– The mitotic spindle continues to develop as more microtubules assemble and stretch across the length of the former nuclear area.

– Chromosomes become more condensed and visually discrete.
– Each sister chromatid attaches to spindle microtubules at the centromere via a protein complex called the kinetochore.

Events during metaphase:

– All of the chromosomes are aligned in a plane called the metaphase plate, or the equatorial plane, midway between the two poles of the cell.
– The sister chromatids are still tightly attached. At this time, the chromosomes are maximally condensed.

Events during anaphase:

– The sister chromatids at the equatorial plane are split apart at the centromere.

– Each chromatid, now called a chromosome, is pulled rapidly toward the centrosome to which its microtubule is attached.
– The cell becomes visibly elongated as the non-kinetochore microtubules slide against each other at the metaphase plate where they overlap.

Events during telophase:

– All events that set up the duplicated chromosomes for mitosis during the first three phases are reversed.
– The chromosomes reach the opposite poles and begin to decondense (unravel).
– The mitotic spindles are broken down into monomers that will be used to assemble cytoskeleton components for each daughter cell.
– Nuclear envelopes form around chromosomes.

Cytokinesis. Cytokinesis is the second part of the mitotic phase, during which cell division is completed by the physical separation of the cytoplasmic components into two daughter cells.

In cells such as animal cells that lack cell walls, cytokinesis begins following the onset of anaphase—a contractile ring composed of actin filaments forms inside the plasma membrane at the former metaphase plate. The actin filaments pull the cell's equator inward, forming a fissure. This fissure, or "crack," is called the cleavage furrow. The furrow deepens as the actin ring contracts, and eventually, the membrane and cell are cleaved into two (Fig. 4.11).

Cells not actively preparing to divide are said to be in G0 Phase. The cell is in a quiescent (inactive) stage, having exited the cell cycle. Some cells enter G0 temporarily until an external signal triggers the onset of G1. Other cells that never or rarely divide, such as mature cardiac muscle and nerve cells, remain in G0 permanently (Fig. 4.12).

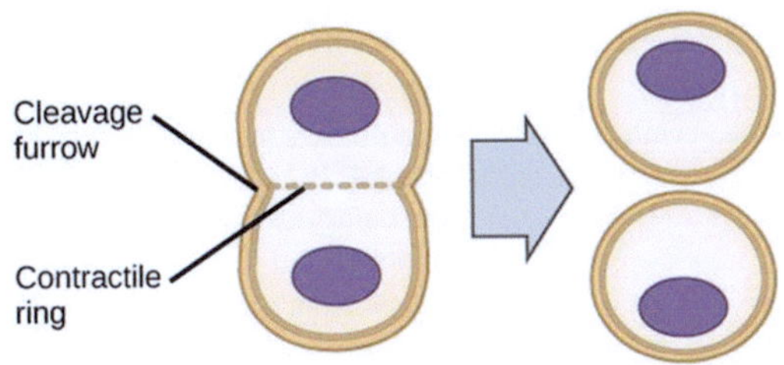

Fig. 4.11. A cleavage furrow forms at the former metaphase plate in the cell. The plasma membrane is drawn in by a ring of actin fibres contracting just inside the membrane. The cleavage furrow deepens until the cells are pinched into two. (Source: Concepts of Biology - 1st Canadian Edition by Charles Molnar and Jane Gair. It is licensed under a Creative Commons Attribution 4.0 International License). Molnar, C., & Gair, J. (2015). Concepts of Biology – 1st Canadian Edition. BCcampus. Retrieved from https://opentextbc.ca/biology/ Chapter 3.3. Eukaryotic cells. Pp 95–112. All images)

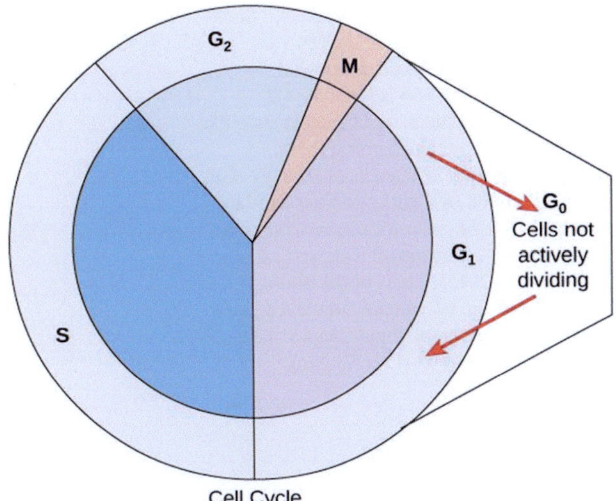

Fig. 4.12 Cells not actively preparing to divide enter an alternate phase called G0. Sometimes, this is a temporary condition until triggered to enter G1. In other cases, the cell will remain in G0 permanently. (Source: Concepts of Biology - 1st Canadian Edition by Charles Molnar and Jane Gair. It is licensed under a Creative Commons Attribution 4.0 International License). Molnar, C., & Gair, J. (2015). Concepts of Biology – 1st Canadian Edition. BCcampus. Retrieved from https://opentextbc.ca/biology/ Chapter 3.3. Eukaryotic cells. Pp 95–112. All images)

4.8   Control and Regulation of the Cell Cycle

In humans, the frequency of cell turnover ranges from a few hours in early embryonic development to an average of 2–5 days for epithelial cells or to an entire human lifetime spent in G0 by specialised cells such as cortical neurons or cardiac muscle cells. In rapidly dividing human cells with a 24-h cell cycle, the G1 phase lasts approximately 11 h. The timing of events in the cell cycle is controlled by mechanisms that are both internal and external to the cell.

Daughter cells must be exact duplicates of the parent cell. Mistakes in the duplication or distribution of the chromosomes lead to mutations that may be passed on to every new cell produced from the abnormal cell. Internal control mechanisms operate at three main cell cycle checkpoints at which the cell cycle can be stopped until favourable conditions prevent a compromised cell from continuing to divide. These checkpoints occur near the end of G1, at the G2–M transition, and during metaphase (Fig. 4.13).

The G1 Checkpoint. The G1 checkpoint determines whether all conditions are favourable for cell division to proceed. The G1 checkpoint, also called the restriction point, is the point at which the cell irreversibly commits to the cell-division process. In addition to adequate reserves and cell size, there is a check for damage to the genomic DNA at the

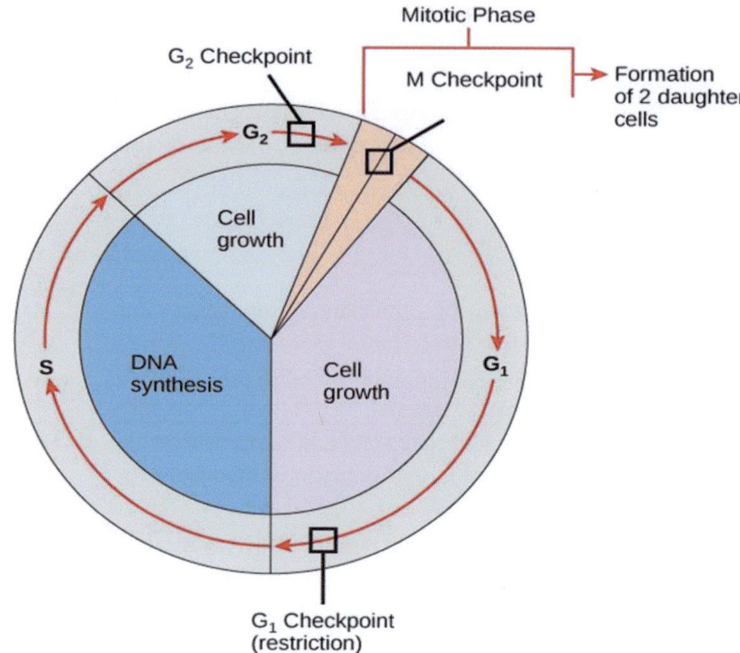

Fig. 4.13 The cell cycle is controlled at three checkpoints. The integrity of the DNA is assessed at the G1 checkpoint. Proper chromosome duplication is set at the G2 checkpoint. The attachment of each kinetochore to a spindle fibre is considered at the M checkpoint. (Source: Concepts of Biology–1st Canadian Edition by Charles Molnar and Jane Gair. It is licensed under a Creative Commons Attribution 4.0 International License). Molnar, C., & Gair, J. (2015). Concepts of Biology–1st Canadian Edition. BCcampus. Retrieved from https://opentextbc.ca/biology/ Chapter 3.3. Eukaryotic cells. Pp 95–112. All images)

G1 checkpoint. A cell that does not meet all the requirements will not be released into the S phase.

The G2 Checkpoint. The G2 checkpoint bars entry to the mitotic phase if certain conditions are not met. As in the G1 checkpoint, cell size and protein reserves are assessed. However, the most crucial role of the G2 checkpoint is to ensure that all of the chromosomes have been replicated and that the replicated DNA is not damaged.

The M Checkpoint. The M checkpoint occurs near the end of the metaphase stage of mitosis. The M checkpoint is also known as the spindle checkpoint, because it determines if all the sister chromatids are correctly attached to the spindle microtubules. Because separating the sister chromatids during anaphase is an irreversible step, the cycle will not proceed until the kinetochores of each pair of sister chromatids are firmly anchored to spindle fibres arising from opposite cell poles.

4.9   Cell Types in the Human Body

Different types of cells in the human body are listed in Table 4.2. A detailed description of cell types is available in histology books and beyond the scope of this chapter.

Table 4.2 Cell types in the human body

Tissue	Cell type
Skin /oral mucous membrane cells	Keratinocytes melanocytes Merkel cells Langerhans cells
Nerve cells	Neurons neuroglial cells
Muscle cells	Skeletal cardiac smooth
Cartilage cells	Chondrocytes
Bone cells	Osteoblasts Osteoclasts Osteocytes
Blood vessels	Endothelial
Lining body cavities	Epithelial cells
Fat cells	Adipocytes (white and brown)
Fibrous cellular tissue	Fibroblasts
Red blood cells	Erythrocytes
White blood cells	Granulocytes (neutrophils, eosinophils, basophils) Agranulocytes (monocytes, lymphocytes)
Platelets	Fragments of megakaryocytes
Sex cells	Spermatozoa Ova

4.10 Stem Cells

Stem cells are unspecialised cells of the human body. Two properties characterise stem cells: (1) the ability to self-renew and (2) differentiate into different types of cells. Stem cells exist in embryos (embryonic stem cells) and adults (adult stem cells).

Five types of stem cells exist. Totipotent, pluripotent, multipotent, unipotent, and oligopotent stem cells.

4.10.1 Totipotent Stem Cells

Totipotent stem cells can divide and differentiate into cells of the whole organism. Totipotency has the highest differentiation potential. One example of a totipotent cell is a zygote, formed after a sperm fertilises an egg. Totipotent stem cells can differentiate into the three germ layers (endoderm, ectoderm, and mesoderm), germ cells (oocyte and sperm), and placental cells.

4.10.2 Pluripotent Stem Cells (PSCs)

Pluripotent stem cells of all germ layers but not extraembryonic structures, such as the placenta. Embryonic stem cells (ESCs) are an example.

4.10.3 Multipotent Stem Cells

Multipotent stem cells have a narrower spectrum of differentiation than PSCs, but they can specialise in discrete cells of specific cell lineages. Somatic cells such as neural, bone marrow derived, or hematopoietic stem cells (HSCs) fall into this category.

4.10.4 Unipotent Stem Cells

Unipotent stem cells are characterised by the narrowest differentiation capabilities and the unique property of dividing repeatedly. They can differentiate into a single type of cell.

An example includes progenitor cells present during postnatal prostate development.

4.10.5 Oligopotent Stem Cells

Oligopotent stem cells usually consist of cells that reside in the tissue and have the ability to differentiate into cells of a specific tissue terminally. An example includes stem cells present on the mammalian ocular surface.

In embryos, foetuses, and adults, stem cells are found throughout the life cycle. Foetal and adult stem cells include umbilical cord stem cells, hematopoietic stem cells, and mesenchymal stem cells. The self-renewal and multilineage differentiation characteristics of stem cells make these cells uniquely suited for regenerative medicine, tissue repair, and gene therapy applications.

4.11 Summary

In order to understand the pathophysiology of human disease, it is important to know the basic structure and functions of the human cell. Cell division involving cell cycle is also an important aspect of pathophysiology. Stem cells exist in embryos (embryonic stem cells) and adults (adult stem cells) which can differentiate into different types of cells.

Bibliography

Basic medical Key. Cell structure and function. 2016. https://basicmedicalkey.com/cell-structure-and-function-2/.

Mitchell RN. The cell as a unit of health and disease. In: Mitchell R, Kumar V, Abbas A, Aster J, editors. Pocket companion to Robbins and Cotran pathologic basis of disease. 9th ed. Philadelphia: Elsevier; 2017. p. 3–36.

Molnar C, Gair J. Eukaryotic cells. In: Concepts of biology–1st Canadian edition. Victoria. https://opentextbc.ca/biology/: BCcampus; 2015. p. 95–112.

SEER Training. Cell Structure. (n.d.). https://training.seer.cancer.gov/anatomy/cells_tissues_membranes/cells/structure.html.

Huxley L, Walter M, Flexman R. ell Structure. In: Biology for Queensland: an Australian perspective. Oxford: Oxford University Press; 2019.

Cellular Pathology

5

5.1 Introduction

Cells are the basic unit of life. Cell survival depends on various factors: a constant supply of energy, an intact plasma membrane, safe and effective cellular activities, genomic integrity, controlled cell division, and standard internal homeostatic mechanisms.

5.2 Cell Injury

Cell injury is the functional and morphologic effects of various aetiologic agents a cell encounters resulting in changes in its internal and external environment. The term cell injury is used to indicate a state in which the capacity for physiological adaptation is exceeded. Cellular response to injury depends on the nature of the injury, duration, and severity. Consequences of injury depend on cell type.

5.3 Causes of Cell Injury

A wide range of injurious agents can cause cellular injury. Some agents include hypoxia, ischemia, mechanical trauma, temperature extremes, ionising and non-ionising radiation, electrical shock, chemicals, therapeutic and illicit drugs, Infectious agents, nutritional imbalances, genetic and metabolic defects, immunologic dysfunction, and free radicals. An injury induced unintentionally by a physician or surgeon or by medical treatment or diagnostic procedures is known as an iatrogenic injury. An injury that arises spontaneously and has no identifiable cause is known as an idiopathic injury. Some known causes of cell injury are briefly discussed below.

5.3.1 Hypoxia (Oxygen Deprivation)

Hypoxia is when oxygen is unavailable sufficiently at the tissue level to maintain adequate homeostasis. Hypoxia is the most common cause of cell injury. Hypoxic cell injury can result from reduced blood flow (e.g. myocardial ischemia), inadequate oxygenation (e.g. cardiac or respiratory failure), or reduced oxygen-carrying capacity (e.g. anaemia or carbon monoxide poisoning). As a result of hypoxia, adenosine triphosphate (ATP) levels drop, and cellular functions cannot be maintained. If the insult lasts long enough, cell death occurs.

5.3.2 Mechanical Trauma

Mechanical trauma causes cell injury, including cell death, by disrupting cells. Examples include damage due to vehicular accidents or violent physical fights.

5.3.3 Extreme Heat (Thermal Burn)

Extreme heat causes cell injury and death by denaturing enzymes and proteins.

5.3.4 Extreme Cold (Cryogenic Burn)

Extreme cold freezes cells by forming ice crystals within the cytosol and disrupts cell membranes leading to cell death.

5.3.5 Ionising Radiation

In cancer treatment, ionising radiation is used. It injures cells directly or indirectly by generating free radicals from water or molecular oxygen. It can also cause vascular dam-

© The Author(s), under exclusive license to Springer Nature Switzerland AG 2023
S. R. Prabhu, *Textbook of General Pathology for Dental Students*, https://doi.org/10.1007/978-3-031-31244-1_5

age resulting in ischemic necrosis of parenchymal cells. Ionising radiation is also mutagenic, carcinogenic, and teratogenic.

5.3.6 Non-ionising Radiation

Ultraviolet radiation from sun exposure is an example of non-ionising radiation. It releases hydroxyl and oxygen radicals and thus contributes indirectly to DNA damage. UVB (e.g. 290–320 nm wavelength) can cause mutations in the epithelial p53 tumour-suppressor gene, resulting in the dysregulation of its functions.

5.3.7 Electrical Shock

The electric current generates heat as it passes through tissues resulting in electrical burns.

5.3.8 Chemical Injury

Hazardous chemicals (gas, liquid, or solid) can be directly toxic to the cellular plasma membrane or mitochondria or metabolise into poisonous compounds. Common examples include strong acids or alkalis, alcohol, and pesticides.

5.3.9 Therapeutic and Illicit Drug Injury

Some therapeutic drugs (e.g. chemotherapeutic agents) cause cell injury. Mitochondria are critical targets for therapeutic drug toxicity, either directly or indirectly, through forming reactive metabolites. Illicit drugs (cocaine, marijuana, opioid) cause cell injury by suppressing the immune system, thereby increasing susceptibility to viral infections.

5.3.10 Injury Due to Infectious Agents

Pathogenic organisms capable of causing cell injury include bacteria, viruses, fungi, rickettsiae, and parasites. Pathogenic bacteria release endotoxins or exotoxins capable of inducing cell death. Most viruses are directly cytopathic, and some are oncogenic. Fungi can cause cell damage and disease by consuming energy and nutrients intended for the host and forming toxic metabolites (e.g. *Candida* species can produce acetaldehyde, a carcinogenic substance during metabolism).

5.3.11 Nutritional Imbalances

Nutritional deficiencies, excesses, and imbalances predispose the cell to injury. Severe malnutrition in children due to the caloric deficit (marasmus) and a diet rich in carbohydrates (Kwashiorkor) cause tissue damage. These are common in less developed countries. Malnutrition is a significant cause of immune suppression and increases host susceptibility to infectious diseases. Deficiency or excess of vitamins and minerals is also injurious to cell homeostasis. Nutritional excess can cause obesity, atherosclerosis, hypertension, and heart disease.

5.3.12 Immunologically Mediated Cell Injury

Immune responses capable of causing tissue injury and diseases are called hypersensitivity diseases. These include (1) hypersensitivity (allergic) reactions to environmental substances (antigens), (2) autoimmune disorders that occur when the immune system produces antibodies attacking the body's cells, and (3) immunodeficiency diseases that are either primary (congenital) or secondary (acquired).

5.3.13 Genetic and Metabolic Cell Injury

Genetic defects may cause cell injury because of a deficiency of functional proteins such as enzymes or an accumulation of damaged DNA or abnormal proteins. In metabolic disorders, cell injury may be direct or indirect. Metabolic cell injury occurs when cells or tissues do not receive sufficient reactants to perform normal metabolic processes critical for cellular functionality and survival.

5.3.14 Injury from Free Radicals

Free radicals and other reactive oxygen species (ROS) are derived either from normal essential metabolic processes in the human body or from external sources such as exposure to X-rays, ozone, cigarette smoking, air pollutants, and industrial chemicals. If free radicals overwhelm the body's ability to regulate them, oxidative stress ensues. Oxidative stress (oxidative damage) results when the critical balance between free radical generation and antioxidant defences is unfavourable. Free radicals thus adversely alter lipids, proteins, and DNA and trigger several human diseases. The initiation, promotion, and progression of cancer and the side effects of radiation and chemotherapy have been linked to the imbalance between ROS and the antioxidant defence system.

5.4   Mechanisms of Cell Injury

The basic mechanisms of cell injury can be categorised as plasma membrane damage, mitochondrial damage, adenosine triphosphate (ATP) depletion, cytosolic calcium derangement, and nucleic acid damage. These are briefly discussed below.

5.4.1   Plasma Membrane Damage

The cellular plasma membrane allows cells to maintain an intracellular biochemical environment. The plasma membrane can be damaged by direct chemical injury or free radical cell injury. A breakdown of membrane permeability can result in the influx of potentially toxic chemicals, the release of vital cellular nutrients and proteins, and the elimination of solute gradients across the plasma membrane. This may lead to cellular injury and cell death.

5.4.2   Mitochondrial Damage

Mitochondria are the essential organelles of cellular respiration and thus provide much of the adenosine triphosphate (ATP) for energy-dependent cellular processes. Commonly, mitochondrial damage is due to increased cytosolic calcium as well as the presence of free radicals. Damage to mitochondria results in declines in cellular ATP stores and inappropriate release of Cytochrome C, thus inducing pathways of apoptosis which can lead to cell death.

5.4.3   Adenosine Triphosphate (ATP) Depletion

Adenosine triphosphate (ATP) is an important "energy molecule" in all forms of life. Hypoxia and ischemia are the most common causes of ATP depletion. ATP depletion results in additional cell damage by causing the failure of energy-dependent enzymes.

5.4.4   Cytosolic Calcium Derangement

The cytosolic calcium concentration usually is tightly regulated and kept at low concentrations compared to the extracellular environment through ATP-dependent mechanisms. The deficiency of ATP causes slow but steady increases in cytosolic calcium due to an inability to maintain the calcium concentration gradient with the extracellular space. Additionally, damage to the plasma membrane can lead to a loss of selective calcium permeability and sharp extracellular calcium influxes. Significant increases in cytosolic calcium activate a wide variety of potent intracellular enzymes, which can cause the widespread destruction of intracellular proteins, lipids, nucleic acids, and ATP.

5.4.5   Nucleic Acid Damage

Nucleic acids, especially the genome composed of DNA, provide the basic code by which all proteins in the cell are synthesised. Nucleic acid damage can result from free radical cell injury or the activation of nucleases following increases in cytosolic calcium.

5.5   Responses to Cell Injury

The cellular stress response varies depending on host factors, such as the type of cell and tissue involved and the extent and type of cell injury. Three possible outcomes can occur when a cell is exposed to an injurious agent. These include (1) reversible injury, (2) irreversible cell injury, and (3) cellular adaptation.

5.5.1   Reversible Cell Injury

When the injury is mild to moderate (sublethal), the injured cell may recover with eventual restoration of normal or near-normal structure and function. The cellular injury is reversible if the adverse environmental responses evoke a cellular response that remains within the homeostasis range. Reversible injury is usually mild, and following the removal of the injurious agent, the cell reverts to its normal steady state. The injury has not caused severe membrane damage or nuclear dissolution at this stage. Cellular morphological changes seen in reversible injury include cellular swelling (increased influx of water into the cytoplasm and mitochondria), nuclear chromatin clumping, ribosomal detachment secondary to decreased protein synthesis, membrane blebbing, and fatty change (Fig. 5.1).

5.5.2   Irreversible Cell Injury

When the injury is persistent and severe (lethal), it causes irreversible cell damage, including cell death (necrosis). The principal targets of irreversible cell injury are the cell membranes, mitochondria, protein synthesis machinery, and DNA.

Damage to the nucleus presents in three forms: pyknosis, karyorrhexis, and karyolysis. Pyknosis is character-

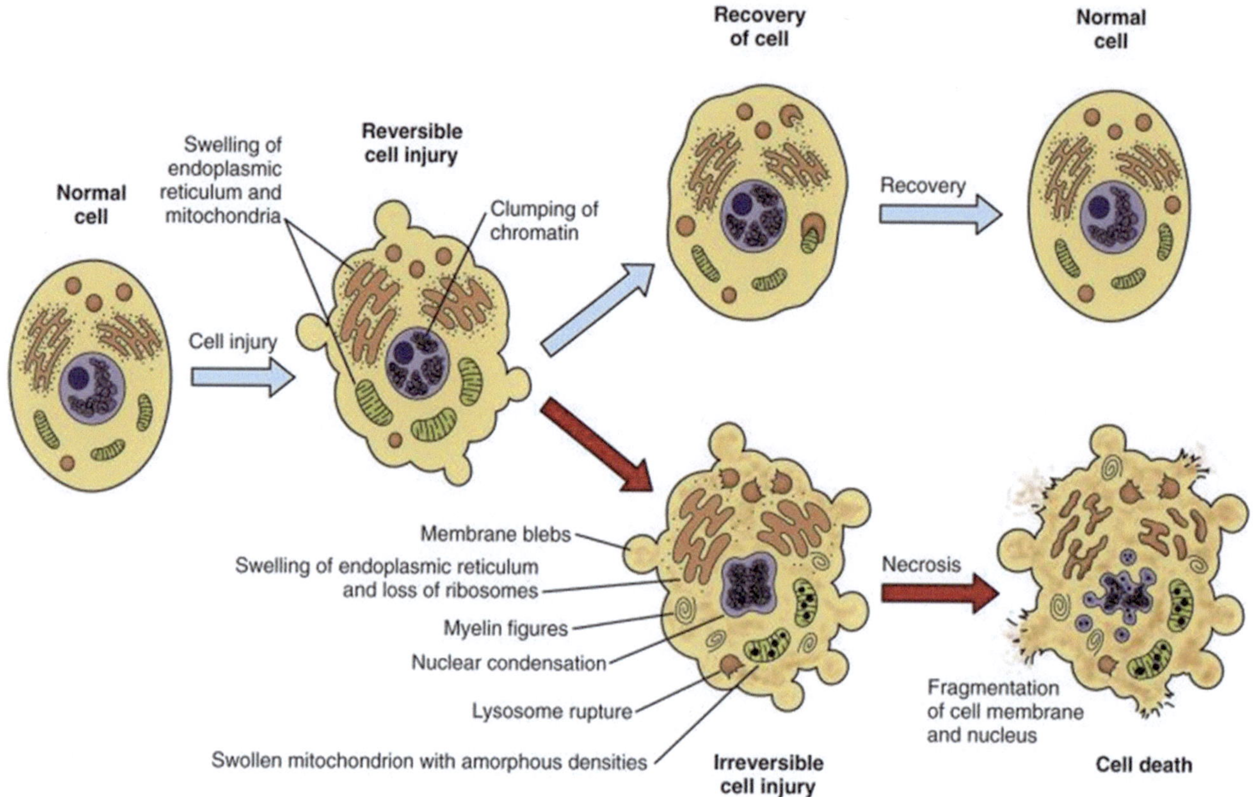

Fig. 5.1 Normal cell and the changes in reversible and irreversible cell injury. (Source: Miller, M. A., & Zachary, J. F. (2017). Mechanisms and Morphology of Cellular Injury, Adaptation, and Death. Pathologic Basis of Veterinary Disease, 2–43. e19. https://doi.org/10.1016/B978-0-323-35775-3.00001-1)

ised by the condensation of chromatin (Fig. 5.1). Karyorrhexis refers to nuclear fragmentation, and karyolysis is marked by the dissolution of the structure of the nucleus and the lysis of chromatin by enzymes such as DNase and RNase. Cytoplasmic enzymes such as aspartate aminotransferase (AST), alanine aminotransferase (ALT), and lactate dehydrogenase (LDH) are also released from the injured cells. Alcohol liver disease (ALD) is an example.

5.6 Cellular Adaptation

Cellular adaptation refers to changes made by a cell in response to adverse or varying environmental changes. The adaptation may be physiologic (normal) or pathologic (abnormal). Physiological adaptations represent tissue responses to normal stimulation by hormones or endogenous chemical mediators. Pathological adaptation means responses in which cells and tissues modulate their size, structure, and function to escape permanent injury. Four types of morphological adaptations include hypertrophy, hyperplasia, atrophy, and metaplasia. Dysplasia means "dis-

ordered cellular development." It is not considered a true adaptation, but it often accompanies or precedes metaplasia. (Fig. 5.2).

5.6.1 Hypertrophy

Hypertrophy is an increase in the size of non-dividing cells. Hypertrophy can be physiologic or pathologic and is caused either by increased functional demand or specific hormonal stimulation. This alteration in cell size results from the increased workload that leads to increased protein synthesis, size, and the number of intracellular organelles. These changes result in increased cell size (hypertrophy), leading to increased organ size. A typical example of physiological hypertrophy is muscular hypertrophy in response to a normal stressor such as exercise. Exercise stimulates skeletal and cardiac muscle fibres to increase in diameter and accumulate more structural contractile proteins. Pathologic hypertrophy occurs due to an abnormal stressor. For example, an increase in the size of the heart (hypertrophy) can occur due to aortic stenosis. Aortic stenosis occurs when the orifice of the aortic valve is significantly reduced due to the calcification of a

Fig. 5.2 Cellular adaptations

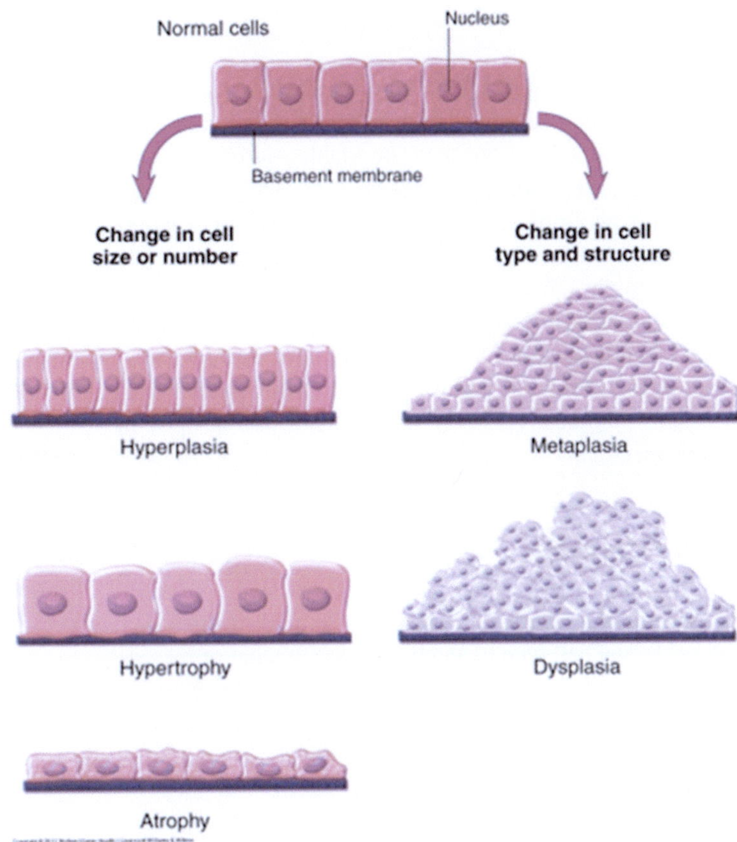

normal trileaflet aortic valve. This results in the failure of the aortic valve leaflets to open fully during systole. This condition causes the left ventricle to work harder to pump blood into the aorta, resulting in left ventricular hypertrophy and, eventually, causes symptoms of congestive heart failure.

5.6.2 Hyperplasia

Hyperplasia is an increase in the number of cells that increases the organ's size (Fig. 5.2). Hyperplasia differs from neoplastic cellular proliferation in that hyperplastic cells generally subside if the stimulus is removed, whereas, in neoplasia, cell proliferation continues even after the removal of the stimulus. The hyperplastic response can occur only in a cell population capable of cell division (mitosis). These are called labile cells, which include hematopoietic cells of the bone marrow, epithelial cells of the skin, the mouth, intestine, vagina, and cervix, urinary tract, and ductal epithelia of exocrine glands, including those of the salivary glands. Cells in these tissues quickly undergo hyperplasia in response to hormonal stimulation, inflammation, or physical trauma. Hyperplasia can be physiological or pathological. Physiological hyperplasia occurs due to a normal stressor. Examples of physiological hyperplasia include an increase in the size of the female breasts during puberty, pregnancy (hormonal hyperplasia), and liver regeneration after partial resection (compensatory hyperplasia). Examples of pathological hyperplasia include endometrial hyperplasia due to excess oestrogen hormones and benign prostatic hyperplasia due to excess androgens.

In the oral cavity, pathologic hyperplastic lesions include reactive lesions in response to a low-grade irritation or injury. These include hyperplastic pulpitis resulting from chronic pulpal inflammation due to open carious defect and mucosal lesions such as irritation fibroma, pyogenic granuloma, peripheral giant cell granuloma, epulis fissuratum, hereditary gingival fibromatosis, medication-induced gingival hyperplasia, and inflammatory papillary hyperplasia. Infection-induced hyperplastic lesions include hyperplastic candidiasis due to *Candida albicans* infection, and multifocal epithelial hyperplasia (also known as Heck's disease) occurs due to *Human papillomavirus* infection. All oral hypertrophic and hyperplastic lesions clinically present as tissue enlargements. The distinction between the two is confirmed by histopathology.

5.6.3 Atrophy

Shrinkage of the size of cells by loss of cell substances is known as cellular atrophy (Fig. 5.2). Atrophic cells may have diminished functions, but they are viable—atrophy results from decreased protein synthesis and increased protein degradation. Causes of atrophy may include decreased workload, as in immobilisation of a limb after a bone fracture (disuse atrophy), loss of innervation, diminished blood supply, inadequate nutrition, loss of endocrine stimulation, and ageing (senile atrophy). Some examples of oral atrophic diseases include atrophic glossitis, atrophic (erosive) lichen planus, oral submucous fibrosis, and oral mucosal atrophy in severe anaemia,

5.6.4 Metaplasia

Metaplasia is a reversible change of one adult epithelial or mesenchymal cell type to another adult epithelial or mesenchymal cell type in the same tissue (Fig. 5.2). Metaplasia is not known to occur during embryonic development. Generally, it results from persistent cellular trauma and is considered a protective mechanism. Metaplasia may be induced or accelerated by some abnormal stimulus, including acid or base (causing a change in pH), hormones, cigarette smoke, or alcohol. A typical example of metaplasia is the stratified squamous epithelial cells in the oesophagus becoming goblet cells when exposed to persistent acid reflux. This condition is called Barrett's oesophagus. Another example includes the occurrence of bronchial squamous metaplasia in chronic smokers. The bronchial cells convert from mucus-secreting, ciliated columnar epithelium to nonciliated, squamous epithelium incapable of secreting mucus. These transformed cells may become dysplastic or cancerous if the stimulus (e.g. cigarette smoking) is not removed. Conditions of mesenchymal metaplasia include osseous metaplasia in fibrous, cartilaginous, or myxoid tissues. Vitamin A deficiency can produce squamous metaplasia in the respiratory epithelium. Metaplasia can occur in salivary gland tumours. Osseous metaplasia is common in pleomorphic adenoma of the parotid gland.

5.6.5 Dysplasia

Cellular dysplasia refers to abnormal changes in cellular shape, size, and organisation. Dysplasia is not considered a true adaptation; it is thought to be related to hyperplasia and is sometimes called "atypical hyperplasia" (Fig. 5.2).

Tissues prone to dysplasia include cervical and respiratory epithelium, strongly associated with cancer development. It may also occur in oral mucosal potentially malignant lesions and contribute to the development of oral cancer. Although dysplasia is reversible, if causes persist, then dysplasia progresses to carcinoma in situ or invasive carcinoma.

5.7 Cellular Degeneration

Nonlethal injury to a cell may cause cell degeneration (retrogressive change), manifested as some abnormality of biochemical function, a recognisable structural change, or a combined biochemical and structural abnormality. Degeneration is reversible but may progress to necrosis if the injury persists. *Types of cellular degeneration include hydropic degeneration, fatty change, hyaline degeneration, mucoid (myxoid/myxomatous) degeneration, fibrinoid degeneration, and glycogen storage.*

5.7.1 Hydropic Degeneration (Cloudy Swelling/Vacuolar Degeneration)

Hydropic degeneration (hydropic change) means water accumulation within the cell's cytoplasm. It is characterised by the cloudy gross appearance of the affected organ (Cloudy swelling) and microscopically shows cytoplasmic (mitochondrial) vacuolisation (Vacuolar degeneration). Hydropic swelling is an entirely reversible change upon removal of the injurious agent.

The common causes of hydropic degeneration include acute and subacute cell injury from various agents such as bacterial toxins, chemicals, poisons, burns, high fever, and intravenous administration of hypertonic glucose or saline. Two major stimuli leading to hydropic change are ischemia and chemical damage. Loss of blood supply due to ischemia results in decreased oxygen tension inside the cell and ATP depletion. There is also a loss of oxidative phosphorylation, causing reduced ATP generation and failure of the Na + K+ pump. This increases intracellular sodium, water, and extracellular potassium, leading to cellular swelling (Fig. 5.3).

5.7.2 Fatty Change (Fatty Degeneration)

Fatty change (or older term fatty degeneration) is the accumulation of neutral fat (triglycerides) within parenchymal cells. Fatty change is widespread in the liver but may occur

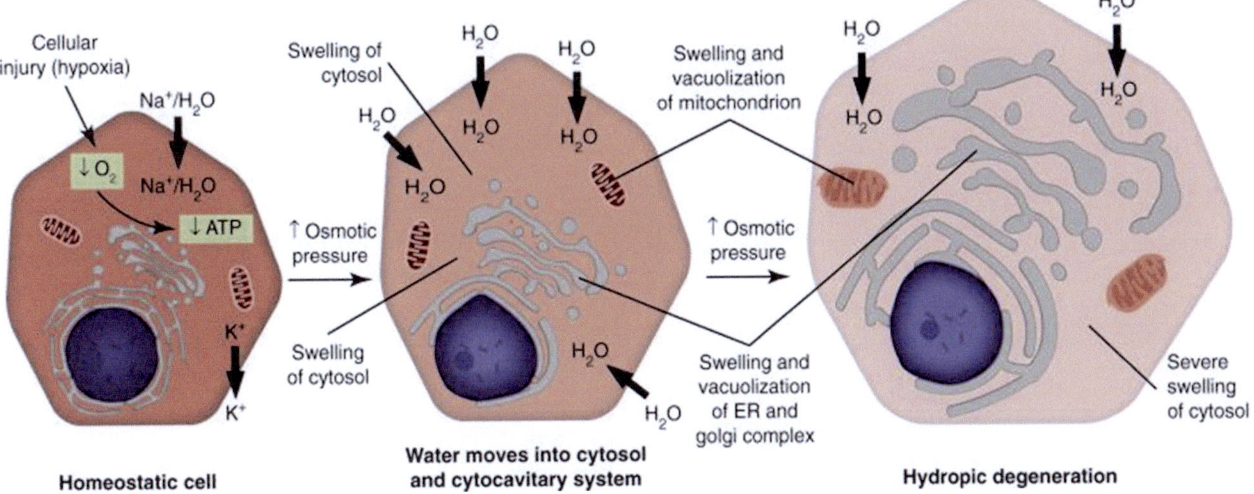

Fig. 5.3 The process of hydropic degeneration (acute cell swelling). (Miller MA, Zachary JF. Mechanisms and Morphology of Cellular Injury, Adaptation, and Death. Pathologic Basis of Veterinary Disease. 2017:2–43.e19. DOI: 10.1016/B978-0-323-35.775-3.00001-1. Epub 2017 Feb 17. PMCID: PMC7171462.)

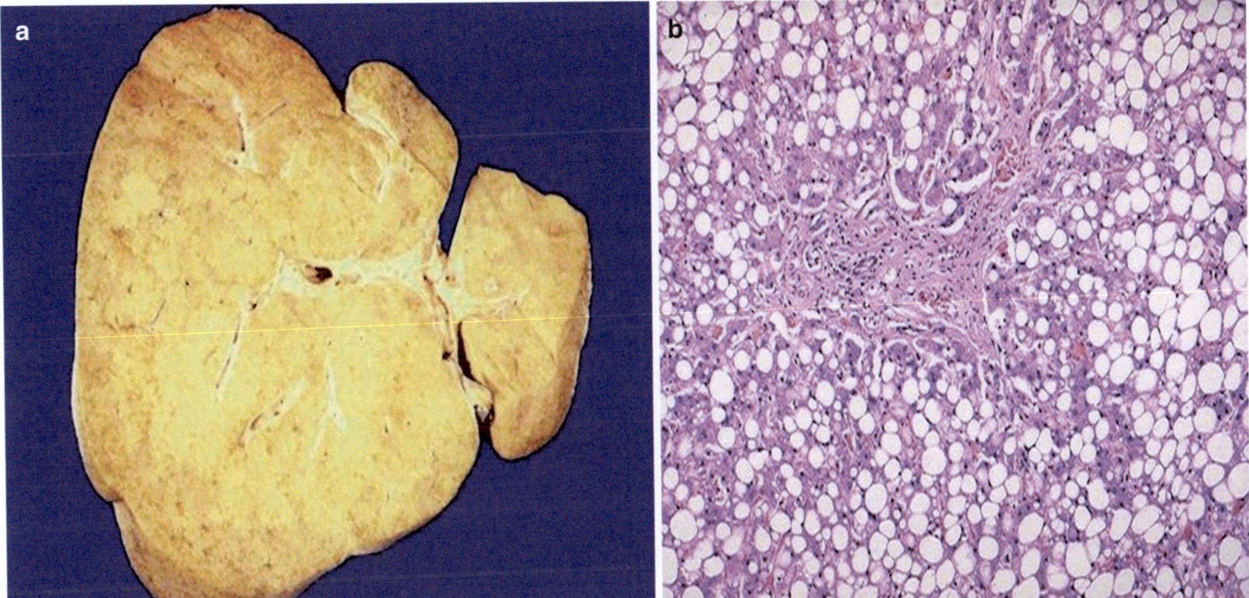

Fig. 5.4 (**a, b**) Fatty degeneration (liver). With the progressive accumulation of fat, the liver becomes increasingly yellowish in colour (**a**). Photomicrograph shows hepatic parenchymal cell cytoplasm containing clear vacuoles containing fat of varying sizes (**b**). This change displaces the nucleus towards the periphery giving a signet ring appearance (Source: (**a**) https://webpath.med.utah.edu/LIVEHTML/LIVER004.html).

in other non-fatty tissues, such as the liver, heart, skeletal muscle, and kidneys. The causes of fatty change in the liver include obesity, cirrhosis, diabetes mellitus, alcoholism, starvation, protein-calorie malnutrition, chronic illnesses (e.g. tuberculosis), hypoxia (due to anaemia, cardiac failure), and the use of hepatotoxins. The gross appearance of fatty liver is yellowish due to the deposition of lipids (Fig. 5.4a). Microscopically, many small globular intracytoplasmic clear spaces may be seen to accumulate and displace the nucleus to the periphery (Fig. 5.4b).

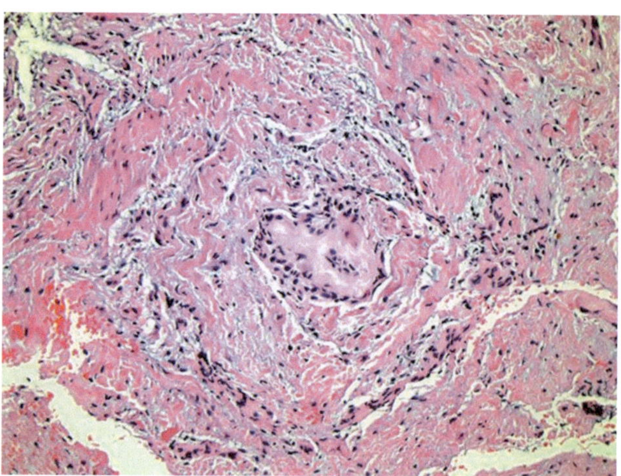

Fig. 5.5 Hyalin change. Small, circumscribed pools of eosinophilic material exhibit a corrugated periphery of condensed collagen. (Source: Pathology outlines. Public domain)

5.7.3 Hyaline Change

The word "hyaline" means glassy (halos = glass). Hyalinisation is a common descriptive histologic term for proteinaceous material's glassy, homogeneous, eosinophilic appearance in hematoxylin- and eosin-stained sections (Fig. 5.5). It does not refer to any specific substance. Hyaline change is seen in heterogeneous pathologic conditions and may be intracellular or extracellular. Intracellular hyaline is mainly seen in epithelial cells.

5.7.4 Mucoid Degeneration (Mucinous Degeneration, Myxomatous Degeneration)

Mucoid means mucus-like. The mucus is the secretory product of mucous glands and is a combination of proteins complexed with mucopolysaccharides. Mucin, a glycoprotein, is its chief constituent. Mucin is usually produced by epithelial cells of mucous membranes and glands and by some connective tissues such as ground substance in the umbilical cord. By convention, connective tissue mucin is termed myxoid.

5.7.5 Fibrinoid Degeneration (Fibrinoid Necrosis)

Fibrinoid degeneration is essentially extracellular. Two types of connective tissue degenerations occur: connective tissue fibrinoid and vascular fibrinoid. Connective tissue fibrinoid degeneration is formed by the breakdown of collagen fibres and the mucopolysaccharide ground substance between the fibres, resulting in the formation of material that has similar staining properties to fibrin.

5.8 Cellular Accumulations and Pathologic Calcification

Cells may accumulate abnormal amounts of intracellular substances in response to injury. These may be located in the cytoplasm, lysosomes, or the nucleus. These accumulations can broadly be grouped into lipids, proteins, glycogen, and pigments.

5.8.1 Abnormal Accumulations of Lipids

Abnormal accumulation of triglyceride depositions in the parenchymal cells of the liver is common. The kidney, heart, and other organs may also be affected. Fatty change is reversible; severe fatty change may cause cell death. Cholesterol depositions are due to excessive intake and defective catabolism. These accumulations may occur in macrophages (foam cells) and smooth muscle cells of blood vessels (atherosclerosis). In hyperlipidaemic syndromes, macrophages laden with cholesterol cause subepithelial connective tissue deposits on the skin or in tendons. These are called xanthomas.

5.8.2 Abnormal Accumulation of Proteins

Abnormal accumulations of protein are uncommon. These occur when proteins are presented to the cells in excess or the cells produce excessive amounts of proteins. In kidney disease (e.g. Nephrotic syndrome), when heavy protein leakage across the glomerular filter occurs, a large amount of protein is reabsorbed. This can cause pink hyaline protein cytoplasmic droplets in the renal tubular epithelium.

5.8.3 Accumulation of Glycogen

Abnormalities of metabolism of either glucose or glycogen can cause excessive intracellular accumulation of glycogen. In poorly controlled diabetes mellitus, glycogen accumulates in the renal tubular epithelium, cardiac myocytes, and β-cells of the islets of Langerhans in the pancreas. Abnormal accumulation of glycogen also occurs in glycogen storage diseases. In these diseases, glycogen synthesis or breakdown is defective.

5.8.4 Accumulation of Pigments

Intracellular accumulation of pigments can occur from exogenous or endogenous sources. Carbon is the most common exogenous pigment from polluted air. Inhaled carbon can cause *anthracosis* in the lung parenchyma. Coal dust can cause pneumoconiosis in coal mine workers. Pigments from tattooing are taken up by macrophages and persist until the cell's death. Endogenous pigments include melanin, hemosiderin, and lipofuscin.

5.8.5 Pathologic Calcification

Pathologic calcification refers to the deposition of calcium phosphates (CaP) or other calcific salts at sites that would not usually have become mineralised. Two distinct types of pathologic calcification are recognised: dystrophic calcification and metastatic calcification. Dystrophic calcification is characterised by the deposition of calcium salts in dead or degenerated tissues with normal calcium metabolism and serum calcium levels. Metastatic calcification occurs in apparently normal tissues and is associated with deranged calcium metabolism and hypercalcemia. Metastatic calcification deposition can be influenced by releasing excess calcium salts from bone, phosphate concentration, alkaline phosphatase activity, and viscera physicochemical conditions under alkalosis.

5.9 Cell Death

Cell death is a necessary event. Cell death is a complex phenomenon that is essential for life and also forms the basis for most disease processes. *There are two significant forms of cell death: apoptosis and necrosis (Fig. 5.6). The third type of cell death, called aponecrosis, has recently been suggested in which dying cells display signs of both apoptosis and necrosis.*

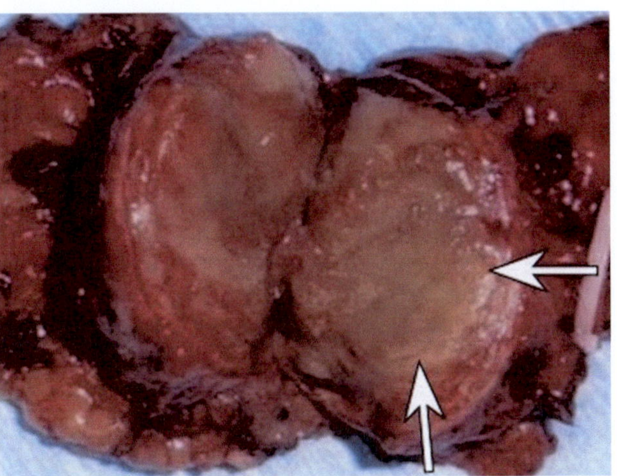

Fig. 5.6 Coagulative necrosis. Gross appearance of pheochromocytoma with coagulative necrosis (arrows). (Source: Nobumasa Ohara et al. (2016). Histopathological analysis of spontaneous large necrosis of adrenal pheochromocytoma manifested as acute attacks of alternating hypertension and hypotension: a case report; Journal of Medical Case Reports 10 (1). DOI:10.1186/s13256-016-1068-3. ISSN 1752–1947. (CC BY 4.0, https://commons.wikimedia.org/w/index.php?curid=85570578)

5.9.1 Apoptosis

Apoptosis is the normal process of coordinated and programmed cell death (PCD). It usually occurs during development and ageing and as a homeostatic mechanism to maintain tissue cell populations. During early development, apoptosis is used to eliminate unwanted cells, for example, those between the fingers of a developing hand. It also plays a vital role in the cyclic sloughing of the inner layer of the endometrium, resulting in menstruation. Apoptosis is used to get rid of the cells that have been damaged beyond repair. Apoptosis can be triggered by numerous pathologic stimuli, including ischemia, hypoxia, exposure to certain drugs and chemicals, immune reactions, infectious agents, high temperature, radiation, and various disease states.

During the early process of cellular apoptosis, cell shrinkage and pyknosis are visible by light microscopy. Pyknosis results from chromatin condensation. The apoptotic cell appears as a round or oval mass with dark eosinophilic cytoplasm and dense nuclear chromatin fragments. Extensive plasma membrane blebbing occurs, followed by karyorrhexis and the separation of cell fragments into apoptotic bodies during a process called "budding." Usually, phagocytic cells rapidly engulf apoptotic cells before apoptotic bodies occur. Apoptosis is not accompanied by inflammation.

5.9.2 Necrosis

Necrosis is a localised area of death in a living tissue accompanied by inflammation. It is characterised by enzymatic digestion and denaturation of intracellular protein in the dying cell. Necrosis occurs in response to injuries such as hypoxia, temperature extremes, toxins, physical trauma, and infection with lytic viruses. During the cell death process, chromatin clumps and the nuclear membrane is disrupted. Finally, the cell lyses, releasing its contents into the extracellular compartment, where the contents may damage neighbouring cells and induce an inflammatory response. Six distinct patterns of necrosis are identifiable: coagulative necrosis, liquefactive necrosis, caseous necrosis, gangrenous necrosis, fibrinoid necrosis, and fat necrosis.

5.9.2.1 Coagulative Necrosis
Coagulative necrosis is characterised by dead tissue's partial or complete dissolution and transformation into a liquid, viscous mass. It generally occurs due to a sudden cessation of blood flow from an obstruction, causing ischemia and infarction. It can occur in all organs except the brain. The macroscopic appearance of an area of coagulative necrosis is a pale segment of tissue contrasting against surrounding well-vascularised tissue (Fig. 5.6).

5.9.2.2 Liquefactive Necrosis
Also known as colliquative necrosis, liquefactive necrosis is usually associated with bacteria, viruses, parasites, or fungal infections. It is characteristically seen in hypoxic cell death in the brain (Fig. 5.7) and suppurative (pus or abscess-producing) bacterial infections. Liquefactive necrosis forms a viscous liquid mass as the dead cells are digested. The affected tissue is liquefied by the action of hydrolytic enzymes released from the lysosomes in the brain or released from the neutrophils in the pus/abscess. Microorganisms can

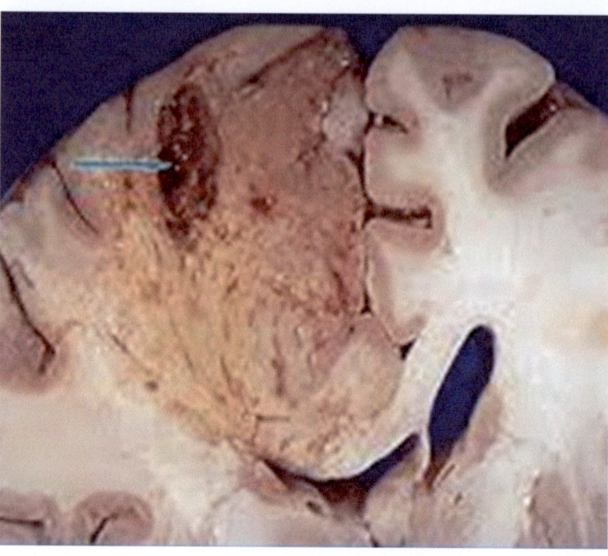

Fig. 5.7 Liquefactive necrosis. Section of the brain showing localised loss of brain tissue (arrow) due to infarction resulting in liquefactive necrosis

also release enzymes to degrade cells and initiate an immune and inflammatory response. The gross appearance of liquefaction necrosis includes a liquid-like layer (pus) and yellowing, softening, or swelling and softening (malacia) of the tissue. A cystic space is usually present for tissue resolution.

5.9.2.3 Caseous Necrosis
Caseous necrosis occurs when the immune system and body cannot successfully remove the foreign noxious stimuli, as in pulmonary tuberculosis, where there is an aberrant immune response to the mycobacteria. The immune system seals the foreign matter using fibroblasts, lymphocytes, neutrophils, natural killer (NK) cells, dendritic cells, and macrophages. A granuloma may form with fibroblast cells creating an encasing layer, leukocytes, and the formation of Langhans giant cells (fusion of epithelioid cells). Gross appearance includes a yellow-white soft cheesy sphere enclosed by a distinct border (Fig. 5.8). Microscopic appearance consists of a granuloma.

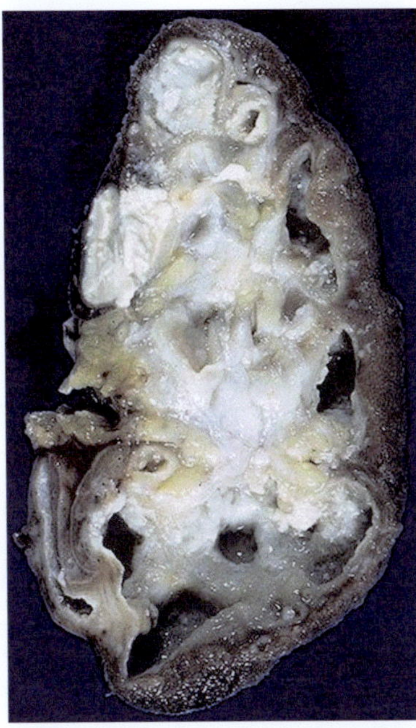

Fig. 5.8 Caseous necrosis. Renal tuberculosis showing "caseous necrosis." The "cheesy" appearance of the necrosis is due to incomplete proteolytic digestion of the necrotic tissue. (Source: Yale Rosen. USA–Wikimedia. (Creative Commons Attribution-ShareAlike License)

5.9.2.4 Gangrenous Necrosis

Gangrenous necrosis **is** a term commonly used by surgeons, this generally describes the damage to the tissues where there is severe ischemia. These extremities lack blood supply and oxygen and typically cause coagulative/liquefactive necrosis at different tissue planes. Two types of gangrene occur: Dry and wet. Dry gangrene is usually seen in the lower limb. It is non-infected ischemic coagulative necrosis of tissue. It is seen as a complication of peripheral artery diseases such as atherosclerosis and diabetes mellitus. The affected part is dry, shrunken, and dark reddish-black (Fig. 5.9a). Severe frostbite injuries can also lead to dry gangrene. When dry gangrene is infected with bacterial (putre-factive) infection, it is called wet gangrene. In wet gangrene, the coagulative necrosis of the dry gangrene is modified by the action of the bacteria into liquefactive necrosis (Fig. 5.9b). The limb becomes foul-smelling and black and starts decomposing. Wet gangrene has a poor prognosis compared to dry gangrene, because the infection can spread to the rest of the body, causing septicemia and can be life-threatening. When *Clostridium perfringens* and other clostridial species cause wound infection, it is characterised by extensive tissue necrosis and gas production by the fermentative action of the bacteria. This is gas gangrene. The gross appearance is similar to that of wet gangrene.

5.9.2.5 Fibrinoid Necrosis

Fibrinoid necrosis is associated with vascular damage caused mainly by autoimmunity, immune-complex deposition, infections, and the exudation of plasma proteins such as fibrin. Fibrinoid is not the same as fibrinous. Fibrinous denotes deposition of fibrin as occurs in inflammation and blood coagulation. The fibrinoid pattern typically occurs due to type 3 hypersensitivity, where an immune complex is formed between an antigen (Ag) with an antibody (Ab). Fibrin, a non-globular protein involved in blood clotting, is leaked out of the vessels. This creates an amorphous bright pink fibrin-like (fibrinoid) material in an H&E stain (Fig. 5.10).

5.9.2.6 Fat Necrosis

Fat necrosis occurs from acute inflammation affecting tissues with numerous adipocytes, such as the pancreas and breast tissue. Damaged cells release digestive enzymes, which break down lipids to generate free fatty acids. Fat necrosis's gross appearance includes whitish deposits due to the formation of calcium soaps. Microscopically, an infiltrate of foamy macrophages (Fig. 5.11) adjacent to adipose tissue is a predominant feature. Multinucleated giant cells, lymphocytes, and plasma cells are often present.

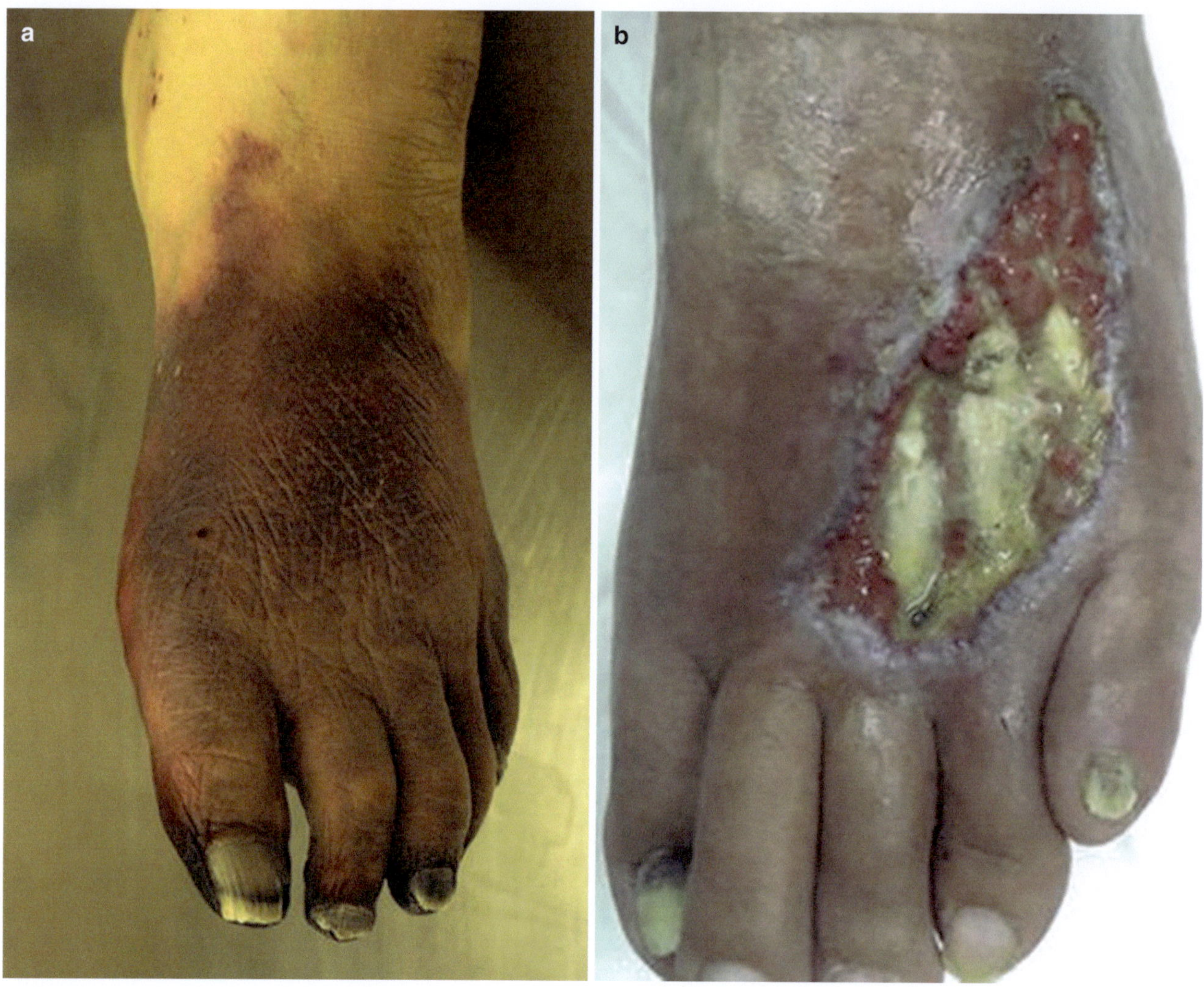

Fig. 5.9. (**a**, **b**) Dry gangrene. (**a**) Atherosclerosis-induced dry gangrene is seen in the foot. The border of the necrotic lesion is relatively sharp—wet gangrene. (**b**) The affected part becomes markedly oedematous, soft, rotten, and dark. Image shows infected deep irregular ulcers are formed in the foot (Source: Tsutsumi, Y. . Pathology of Gangrene. In: Kırmusaoğlu, S., Bhardwaj, S. B., editors. Pathogenic Bacteria [Internet]. London: IntechOpen; 2020 [cited 2022 Oct 15]. Available from: https://www.intechopen.com/chapters/73252 DOI: 10.5772/intechopen.93505. Courtesy of Drs. Mitsuhiro Tachibana and Yasuhito Kaneko at the Department of Diagnostic Pathology and Dermatology, Shimada Municipal Hospital, Shimada, Japan)

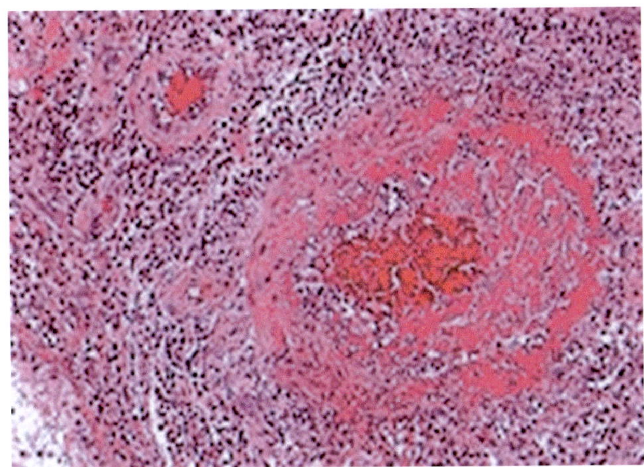

Fig. 5.10 Photomicrograph showing fibrinoid necrosis (intensely pink) in a case of vasculitis (Eosinophilic granulomatosis with polyangiitis) (Source: Wikipedia. CC BY-SA 3.0)

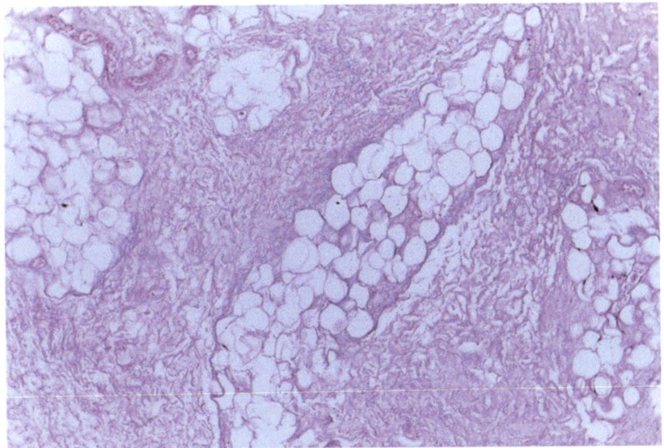

Fig. 5.11 Fat necrosis. Breast lump with an area of fat necrosis showing shadowy outlines of necrotic adipocytes surrounded by an inflammatory reaction with cholesterol clefts [H&E stain 4X] (Source: Department of Pathology, Calicut Medical College–Calicut Medical College, CC BY-SA 4.0, https://commons.wikimedia.org/w/index.php?curid=36284462)

5.10 Summary

Cells constantly interact with their environment and try to maintain homeostasis. Cell injury occurs when an adverse stimulus disrupts the normal, complex homeostatic balance of the cellular metabolism. Aetiologies of cell injury include hypoxia, temperature extremes, physical trauma, chemicals, ischemia, immunological reactions, toxins, infectious agents, genetic abnormalities, nutritional imbalances, and ageing. The main cellular mechanisms of cell injury include ATP depletion, loss of calcium homeostasis, oxidative stress, damage to mitochondria, and increased permeability of membranes. Cell injury may be reversible due to non-lethal damage, which generally can be corrected by removal of the stimulus, or irreversible due to lethal damage, causing cells to undergo cell death. Cells constantly adapt to physiological demands to maintain a homeostatic steady state. Cellular adaptations are reversible changes in the size, number, phenotype, metabolic activity, or functions of cells in response to changes in their environment. Cells are also subjected to different stresses related to metabolic alterations, which may be caused by genetic defects or be acquired. These conditions can lead to the accumulation of substances inside the cell, such as fat (steatosis), proteins, pigments, and calcium.

Bibliography

Damjanov I. Cell pathology. In: Damjanov I, editor. Pathology for the health professions. 4th ed. Missouri: Elsevier; 2012. p. 1–20.

Gordon C, Craft J. Altered cellular function. In: Craft J, Gordon C, Tiziani A, editors. Understanding pathophysiology. Sydney: Elsevier; 2011. p. 58–72.

Kumar V, Abbas AK, Fausto N, Mitchell RN. Cell injury, cell death, and adaptation. In: Kumar V, Abbas AK, Fausto N, Mitchell RN, editors. Robbins basic pathology. Philadelphia: Elsevier; 2018. p. 1–30.

Miller MA, Zachary JF. Mechanisms and morphology of cellular injury, adaptation, and death. Pathol Basis Vet Dis. 2017:2–43.e19. https://doi.org/10.1016/B978-0-323-35775-3.00001-1. Epub 2017 Feb 17. PMCID: PMC7171462

Goepel JR. Responses to cellular injury. In: Underwood JCE, Cross SS, editors. General and systematic pathology. 5th ed. London: Elsevier; 2009. p. 101–22.

Strayer DS, Rubin E. Cell adaptation, injury, and death. In: Strayer DS, Rubin E, editors. Rubin's Pathology: Clinicopathologic Foundations of Medicine. 7th ed. Philadelphia: Wolters Kluwer; 2012. p. 3–54.

Tuieng RJ, Cartmell SH, Kirwan CC, Sherratt MJ. The effects of Ionising and non-Ionising electromagnetic radiation on extracellular matrix proteins. Cell. 2021;10(11):3041. https://doi.org/10.3390/cells10113041. PMID: 34831262; PMCID: PMC8616186

6.1 Introduction

Inflammation is the protective response of the immune system to harmful stimuli. It acts by removing injurious stimuli and initiating the healing process. Inflammation is not a disease but usually a manifestation of the disease. The primary function of Inflammation is to localise and eliminate the pathogenic causative agent, limit or remove injured tissue, and allow tissue repair. It is a dynamic process involving a series of related events by mounting a neurovascular and cellular response to injury. The character of the inflammatory process largely depends on the nature of the offending agent, the duration of the insult, and the extent of tissue damage. Although the inflammatory process usually protects the body from injurious agents, it may cause tissue damage in some instances. Examples include the fatal outcome of inflammation-related high fever, loss of function due to the formation of scarring in chronically inflamed tissue, or joint destruction in septic arthritis. Important microcirculatory events during the inflammatory process include vascular permeability changes, leukocyte recruitment and accumulation, and inflammatory mediator release.

Although inflammatory response processes depend on the precise nature of the initial stimulus and its location in the body, they all share a common mechanism, which can be summarised as follows: (1) detrimental stimuli recognition by cell surface pattern receptors, (2) activation of inflammatory pathways, (3) the release of inflammatory markers, and (4) recruitment of inflammatory cells. Both cell-mediated and humoral responses of the immune system are central to inflammation. Diseases in which inflammation plays a dominant pathological role have the suffix "-itis.". For example, inflammation of the liver is called hepatitis, and inflammation of the gums is gingivitis. However, exceptions exist, such as pneumonia, typhoid fever, paronychia (nail bed inflammation due to infection), etc. This chapter deals briefly with basics of inflammatory process. For detailed information the reader is encouraged to refer to resources listed in the bibliography.

6.2 Aetiology

Inflammatory conditions are caused by infection by physical, chemical, biological, immunological, and genetic/metabolic factors. Some physical agents include mechanical injuries, temperature alterations, and radiation injuries. Chemical agents include organic, inorganic, industrial, or medicinal agents such as drugs and toxins. Biologic agents (infectious) include bacteria, viruses, fungi, and parasites. Immunologic causes include hypersensitivity reactions, autoimmunity, and immunodeficiency states. Genetic/metabolic causes include gout, diabetes mellitus, etc. Inflammation is not a synonym for infection. The sixth type of inflammation, called constitutive inflammation (listed in Table 6.1), is caused by the inborn errors of innate immunity that underlie autoinflammatory diseases.

As the body responds to harmful causes, inflammation is initially beneficial by (a) mobilising the innate and adaptive immune systems, (b) assisting the body in containing the cause of inflammation, and (c) healing damaged organs. This is the "physiologic" side of inflammation which depends on the availability of endogenous suppressors of pro-inflammatory signalling pathways. However, when physiologic suppressors fail, uncontrolled inflammation can acutely or chronically lead to apoptosis, necrosis, fibrosis, and end-stage organ destruction.

Table 6.1 The cause-based classification of inflammation

Type of inflammation	Cause of inflammation	Examples of diseases mediated by a given type of inflammation
Microbial inflammation	Bacteria, fungi, viruses, and protozoa	Abscess; pneumonia; sepsis; Ebola Haemorrhagic fever
Autoimmune inflammation	Aberrant autoimmune attack by autoantibodies and autoreactive B and T cells	Type 1 diabetes; multiple sclerosis; rheumatoid arthritis; psoriasis; systemic lupus erythematosus
Allergic inflammation	Allergens (e.g. pollen, dust mites, animal dander, fungi, insects' bites, and stings)	Atopic dermatitis/eczema; Hay fever; asthma; contact dermatitis; anaphylaxis; drug Hypersensitivity reactions
Metabolic inflammation	Excessive accumulation of metabolites (e.g. cholesteryl esters or uric acid)	Atherosclerosis; gout; phenylketonuria
Physical inflammation	Trauma, burns, or radiation	Post-traumatic injury; chemical, electric, and thermal (scalding) burns; Radiation injury
Constitutive inflammation	Inborn errors of innate immunity	Autoinflammatory diseases such as familial Mediterranean fever, Aicardi-Goutieres syndrome, NEMO mutation-linked autoinflammatory intestinal and skin disease

(Source: Jacek Hawiger and Jozef Zienkiewicz. Decoding inflammation, its causes, genomic responses, and emerging countermeasures. Scandinavian Journal of Immunology. 2019; 90:e 12,812. Available at: https://onlinelibrary.wiley.com/doi/10.1111/sji.12812 (open access. CC by 4.0))

6.3 Cardinal Signs of Inflammation

Basic local signs of inflammation are (1) Tumour. (oedema). Swelling caused by the gradual collection of fluid outside of blood vessels; (2) Dolor. (Pain) caused by the mechanical action (tissue tension, pressure on nerve endings) due to oedema and direct response to prostaglandin, serotonin, and bradykinin reactions; (3) Rubor (redness,) as a consequence of vasodilation at the damage site; and (4) Calor (Heat) caused by hyperemia, increased metabolic activity, and pro-inflammatory mediators that contribute to the rise of local and systemic temperature (fever), and (5) functio laesa (Loss of function) caused by pain and swelling. These signs are predominantly seen in acute inflammation . The infected toenail is an example of acute inflammation causing redness, swelling and pain.

Clinical responses during systemic inflammation include altered body temperature, elevated pulse rate, elevated respiratory rate, abnormal white blood cell count, and other symptoms and signs. These are more pronounced in acute inflammation. Other, mostly non-specific symptoms of inflammation include fatigue, weakness, loss of appetite, and exhaustion. These symptoms are believed to be related to the action of mediators of inflammation such as IL-1 or TNF. These are known as acute-phase reactants.

6.4 Cells of the inflammatory Response, Their Location, and Primary Role

Cells of the inflammatory response include polymorphonuclear neutrophils (PMN), eosinophils, basophils, mast cells, macrophages, lymphocytes, plasma cells, and platelets.

Polymorphonuclear Neutrophils
- PMNs are the most numerous white blood cells in blood circulation (60–70% of all circulating white blood cells).
- PMNs have a segmented nucleus, and numerous granules in the cytoplasm (hence also known as neutrophil granulocytes).
- PMNs are the predominant cell types and the first cells to appear in acute inflammation.
- PMNs are highly mobile, capable of phagocytosis, possess bactericidal activity in the cytoplasmic granules, and secrete inflammatory mediators (cytokines).

Eosinophils
- 2–3% of all circulating white blood cells.
- Contain a single nucleus divided into two lobes and cytoplasmic granules (which stain pink with eosin, hence the name).
- They are mobile, phagocytic, and bactericidal.
- Have a prominent role in allergies and parasitic infections.
- May participate in chronic infections.

Basophils
- Less than 1% of circulating white blood cells
- Most prominent cell types in allergic responses mediated by immunoglobulin E (IgE)
- Have a bean-shaped single nucleus and cytoplasmic granules
- Contain vasoactive substances (histamine)
- Precursors of mast cells (tissue basophils)

Mast cells
- Resident cells of connective tissue; contain granules rich in histamine (an inflammatory mediator) and heparin (an anticoagulant).
- Single round nucleus, cytoplasm granulated

Macrophages

- Macrophages are mononuclear tissue cells (histiocytes) derived from blood monocytes.
- Have a bean-shaped nucleus.
- Capable of phagocytosis and secreting inflammatory mediators(cytokines).
- Common cell types in chronic inflammation.

Lymphocytes

- Derived from bone marrow pre-lymphoid stem cells.
- Found in circulating blood and lymphoid tissue (spleen, tonsils, lymph nodes) and in mucosa-associated lymphoid tissues (MALT) (e.g. gastrointestinal and bronchial mucosa).
- 20–40% of the total number of white blood cells in circulating blood
- Small cells with round nuclei with minimal cytoplasm.
- Two types: T lymphocytes (matured in the thymus) and B lymphocytes (bone marrow or bursa derived).
- T cells are involved in cell-mediated immunity, whereas B cells are primarily responsible for humoral immunity (relating to antibodies).

Plasma Cells

- Derived from fully differentiated B lymphocytes
- Oval eccentrically located round nucleus with a characteristic cartwheel or clock face arrangement
- Rich in the rough endoplasmic reticulum (RER), the site of production of immunoglobulins

Platelets

- No nucleus, cytoplasm contains vacuoles and membrane-bound granules.
- Granules contain histamine, coagulation proteins, cytokines, and platelet-derived growth factor (PDGF). Histamine increases vascular permeability; degranulation of granules promotes blood clotting, and PDGF promotes the proliferation of connective tissue cells.

When pathogens enter the body, the innate immune system responds with inflammation, pathogen engulfment, and secretion of immune factors and proteins. Cells in the blood and lymph detect the specific pathogen-associated molecular patterns (PAMPs) on the pathogen's surface. PAMPs are carbohydrate, polypeptide, and nucleic acid "signatures" that are expressed by viruses, bacteria, and parasites but which differ from molecules on host cells.

6.5 Classification of Inflammation

Classification of inflammation: Inflammation can be classified as acute, subacute, and chronic. Acute inflammation is characterised by a rapid onset and short duration, whereas chronic inflammation is of prolonged duration. These two types of inflammation also differ in the cell types involved in the inflammatory process. Subacute inflammation is an intermediate between acute and chronic inflammation, exhibiting some characteristics of each. A special type of chronic inflammation called granulomatous inflammation occurs in infectious diseases such as tuberculosis, leprosy, and syphilis. Foreign body granuloma is an example of granulomatous inflammation due to a foreign body. Granulomatous inflammation is characterised by the formation of granuloma in which microscopically focal collections of macrophages, epithelioid cells, and multinucleated giant cells are seen.

These are briefly discussed below.

6.5.1 Acute Inflammation

Acute inflammation is an immediate and early response to an injurious agent. It is usually of short duration, lasting for minutes, several hours, or a few days, depending on the severity of the injury. Acute inflammation is usually non-specific. *Acute inflammation is marked by the release of fluid and blood plasma proteins and the arrival of leukocytes at the site of injury, which initially comprises neutrophils and later macrophages.*

Acute inflammation is categorised into two main responses: early vascular (microcirculatory) and late cellular responses.

6.5.1.1 Early Vascular Response

- The first change in the microcirculation is immediate and transient vasoconstriction due to neurogenic or chemical stimuli.
- This is followed by marked, active dilation of arterioles, capillaries, and venules.
- This vasodilation causes an initial marked increase in blood in the area (hyperemia).
- Hyperaemia is followed by increased vascular permeability in the post-capillary venules.
- The increased vascular permeability oozes protein-rich fluid into extravascular tissues (exudate/oedema); as a result, already dilated blood vessels are now packed with red blood cells causing sluggish blood flow and stasis.

Chemical mediators mediate the vascular events of acute inflammation.

6.5.1.2 Late Cellular Response

Usually, blood cells, particularly erythrocytes in venules, are confined to the central (axial) zone, and plasma assumes the peripheral zone. In acute inflammation, as a result of increased vascular permeability (as discussed in vascular events above), a large number of neutrophils migrate and accumulate along the peripheral zone of the endothelium.

The predominant cells of the acute inflammatory response are polymorphonuclear neutrophils (PMNs). They are attracted to the site of injury by the presence of chemical mediators. The cellular response has the following stages:

Stage.1. Margination, rolling, pavementing, and adhesion of leukocytes

Stage 2. Transmigration of leukocytes

Stage 3. Chemotaxis

Stage 4. Phagocytosis

Stage 1

Margination. In normal circulation, cells are confined to the central (axial) stream in blood vessels. In inflammation, blood flow is slow due to the loss of intravascular fluid and increased plasma viscosity; as a result, neutrophils flow in the plasmatic zone. This process causes the peripheral positioning of white cells (predominantly neutrophils) along the endothelial cells lining the blood vessels.

Rolling. Rows of leukocytes come in contact with the endothelium in a process known as rolling. The purpose of rolling and slow rolling is to bring the leukocytes into contact with the endothelial cells so that the leukocytes can be further activated by chemokines and other proinflammatory agents on the surface of the endothelial cells.

Pavementing. In normal circulation, neutrophils may randomly contact the endothelial lining but not adhere to it. In acute inflammation, neutrophils predominantly line the endothelial lining of the blood vessels. This appearance is called pavementing. This phenomenon occurs explicitly in venules.

Adhesion. The next event is leukocytes' binding (adhesion) with endothelial cells. This phenomenon is facilitated by cell adhesion molecules (CAMs) such as selectins, immunoglobulins, and integrins which result in the adhesion of leukocytes with the endothelial cells.

Stage 2

Transendothelial Migration (TEM) of Leukocytes

Transendothelial migration (TEM) is the process whereby the leukocytes squeeze in an ameboid fashion across the endothelial cells. The active ameboid movement of leukocytes occurs by extending pseudopodia through the gap created between endothelial cells and then through the basal lamina (basement membrane) into the vessel wall. This process is called diapedesis. The most important mechanism of leukocyte emigration is the widening of inter endothelial junctions after endothelial cell contractions. The basement membrane is disrupted and resealed immediately after that.

Stage 3

Chemotaxis of Neutrophils

Chemotaxis is when an extracellular gradient of chemicals determines the direction of a cell's locomotion. Newly extrav-asated leukocytes migrate to the injury site along soluble chemical mediators' gradients (Chemotactic factors). This process is known as chemotaxis. Some of these chemotactic factors are secreted by host cells at or near the injury site, while others may be microbial components. The most important chemotactic factors for neutrophils are components of the complement system (C5a), bacterial and mitochondrial products of arachidonic acid metabolism such as *leukotriene* B4, and cytokines (IL-8). All granulocytes, monocytes, and, to a lesser extent, lymphocytes respond to chemotactic stimuli. Receptors on the cell membranes of leukocytes react with the chemoattractants, resulting in the activation of phospholipase C that ultimately leads to the release of cytosolic calcium ions, which trigger cell movement towards the stimulus.

Stage 4

Phagocytosis

Phagocytosis is the process of engulfment and internalisation by specialised cells of particulate material, which include invading microorganisms, damaged cells, and tissue debris. These phagocytic cells include polymorphonuclear leukocytes (mainly neutrophils), monocytes, and tissue-resident macrophages.

Phagocytosis involves three distinct but interrelated steps. These are (1) Recognition and attachment, (2) Engulfment, and (3), Killing or degradation of the particle to be ingested by leukocytes.

Recognition and Attachment

Phagocytosis is enhanced if the material to be phagocytosed is coated with certain plasma proteins called opsonins. These opsonins promote the adhesion between the particulate material and the phagocyte's cell membrane. The three major opsonins are the Fc fragment of the immunoglobulin, components of the complement system C3b and C3bi, and the carbohydrate-binding proteins lectins. Thus, IgG binds to receptors for the Fc piece of the immunoglobulin (FcR), whereas 3cb and 3bi are ligands for complement receptors CR1 and CR2, respectively.

Engulfment

Once recognised by a neutrophil or macrophage, a foreign particle is engulfed by the phagocytic cell to form a membrane-bound vacuole called a phagosome, which fuses with lysosomes to create a phagolysosome.

Killing or Degradation

The ultimate step in phagocytosis of bacteria is killing and degradation. There are two forms of bacterial killing: Oxygen-independent and oxygen-dependent mechanisms.

- Oxygen-independent mechanism: This is mediated by the constituents of the primary and secondary granules of polymorphonuclear leukocytes. These include Bactericidal permeability-increasing (BPI) proteins, Lysozymes, Lactoferrin, and Major basic protein (MBP). The lysosomal enzymes are essential for the degradation of dead organisms within phagosomes.

- Oxygen-dependent mechanism: The oxygen-dependent killing of microorganisms is due to the formation of reactive oxygen species such as hydrogen peroxide (H_2O_2), superoxide (O_2), hydroxyl ion ($HO-$), and possibly single oxygen ($1O_2$). These species have single unpaired electrons in their outer orbits that react with molecules in the cell membrane or nucleus to cause damage. The destructive effects of H_2O_2 in the body are gauged by the action of glutathione peroxidase and catalase. There are two types of oxygen-dependent killing mechanisms: non-myeloperoxidase-dependent and myeloperoxidase–dependent mechanisms.

- Non-myeloperoxidase-dependent mechanism: The oxygen-dependent killing of microorganisms is due to the formation of reactive oxygen species such as hydrogen peroxide (H_2O_2), superoxide (O_2), and hydroxyl ion ($HO-$) and possibly single oxygen. These species have single unpaired electrons in their outer orbits that react with molecules in the cell membrane or nucleus to cause damage.

- Myeloperoxidase–dependent mechanism: The bactericidal activity of H_2O_2 involves the lysosomal enzyme myeloperoxidase, which in the presence of halide ions, converts H_2O_2 to hypochlorous acid (HOCl). This H_2O_2 – halide – myeloperoxidase system is neutrophil's most efficient bactericidal system. A similar mechanism is also effective against fungi, viruses, protozoa, and helminths.

6.5.1.3 Cell-derived Inflammatory Mediators

Chemical mediators derived from cells include histamine, lysosomal compounds, prostaglandins, leukotrienes, 5-hydroxytryptamine (serotine), and chemokines.

Histamine causes vascular dilatation and the immediate transient phase of increased vascular permeability. Mast cells are the main source of histamine.

Lysosomal compounds are derived from neutrophils. These increase vascular permeability.

Prostaglandins are derived from arachidonic acid and synthesised from many cell types. These potentiate the increase in vascular permeability.

Leukotrienes, also derived from arachidonic acid, have vasoactive properties

5-hydroxytryptamine (serotine) is present in platelets. It is a vasoconstrictor.

Chemokines. These proteins selectively attract leukocytes to the site of inflammation.

6.5.1.4 Plasma-Derived Inflammatory Mediators

Plasma contains four enzymatic cascade systems: complement system, kinin system, coagulation system, and fibrinolytic system.

The complement system, also known as the complement cascade, is a part of the immune system that enhances the ability of antibodies and phagocytic cells to clear microbes and damaged cells from an organism, promote inflammation, and attack the pathogen's cell membrane. The complement system comprises several proteins that work together to "complement" the action of antibodies in destroying bacteria. Complement proteins circulate in the blood in an inactive form. Complements are activated during inflammatory reactions. When activated, it increases pathogens' removal via opsonisation and phagocytosis. The main functions of the complement system include (1) opsonisation, (2) chemotaxis, (3) cell lysis, and (4) agglutination. Opsonisation is the process by which opsonins (such as antibody molecules) bind to the surface of the antigen so that the antigen will be readily identified and engulfed by phagocytes for destruction. Chemotaxis attracts macrophages and neutrophils via inflammation by inflammatory mediators. Cell lysis ruptures membranes due to the formation of a membrane attack complex (MAC), and agglutination causes the clustering and binding of pathogens. Activated complement proteins can also increase vascular permeability, make mast cells release histamine, and work for neutrophils as chemotactic elements.

The Kinin system consists of blood proteins that play a role in inflammation, blood pressure control, coagulation, and pain. Bradykinin and kallidin are essential mediators in inflammation and are vasodilators. Bradykinin is also the most important chemical mediator of pain in acute inflammation.

The coagulation system or clotting cascade converts soluble fibrinogen into fibrin, forming a protective protein mesh over injury sites. Coagulation factor XII (Hageman factor) activates coagulation, kinin, and fibrinolytic systems.

The Fibrinolytic system, which opposes the coagulation system, counterbalances clotting and generates several other inflammatory mediators. Lysis of fibrin by plasmin may have a local effect on vascular permeability.

6.5.2   Chronic Inflammation

A prolonged duration of inflammation characterises chronic inflammation, usually spanning weeks, months, or years. *In chronic inflammation, tissue injury, active inflammation, and the healing processes proceed simultaneously, and the predominant cell types involved include mononuclear cells including, macrophages, lymphocytes, and plasma cells.*

Products of inflammatory cells cause tissue destruction, and the reparative process involves angiogenesis and fibrosis.

Chronic inflammation can result from (1) failure to eliminate the agent causing acute inflammation, (2) exposure to a low level of a particular irritant or foreign material that cannot be eliminated by enzymatic breakdown or phagocytosis, (3) an autoimmune disorder in which the immune system recognises the normal component of the body as a foreign antigen, (4) a defect in the cells responsible for mediating inflammation leading to persistent or recurrent inflammation,(5) recurrent episodes of acute inflammation, and (6) inflammatory and biochemical inducers are causing oxidative stress and mitochondrial dysfunction.

Pathogenesis. Acute inflammation may progress to chronic inflammation when the injurious agent persists or the normal healing process is interfered with. Some chronic inflammatory conditions may occur from the onset without the preceding acute phase. Most of the features of acute inflammation continue as the inflammation becomes chronic, including vasodilation, increased blood flow and capillary permeability, and migration of neutrophils into the tissues through diapedesis. The hallmarks of chronic inflammation are the infiltration of the predominant inflammatory cells in the tissue site, including macrophages, lymphocytes, and plasma cells. These cells produce inflammatory cytokines, growth factors, and enzymes, contributing to the progression of tissue damage and secondary repair, including fibrosis and, in some infections, granuloma formation.

6.5.3 Types of Chronic Inflammation

6.5.3.1 Nonspecific Proliferative
Characterized by the presence of non-specific granulation tissue. Granulation tissue is formed by the infiltration of mononuclear cells (lymphocytes, macrophages, and plasma cells) and the proliferation of fibroblasts, connective tissue, vessels, and epithelial cells. Examples are inflammatory polyp-like nasal polyps, lung abscesses, and pyogenic granuloma (Angiogranuloma) of the gingivae.

6.5.3.2 Granulomatous Inflammation
Granulomatous inflammation is a specific type of chronic inflammation characterised by granulomas. Lesions are usually nodular formed with aggregation of activated macrophages or epithelioid cells, usually surrounded by lymphocytes. The macrophages inside the granulomas often coalesce to form giant cells (Langhans giant cells in tuberculosis) or foreign body giant cells. There are two types of granulomas: Foreign body granuloma (e.g. silicosis related) or granuloma due to T-cell-mediated immune response, for example, tuberculosis and leprosy.

6.6 Morphologic Patterns of Inflammation

6.6.1 Fibrinous Inflammation

Fibrinous Inflammation is a general morphological pattern of inflammation, whether acute or chronic. There is extensive fluid leakage from the vasculature, thus allowing for the passage of large plasma proteins, mainly fibrinogen, into tissue. This is commonly seen in bacterial infections such as streptococcal infection of the throat, bacterial pericarditis, and bacterial pneumonia. Ultimately, the organisation of the fibrinogen can occur with rigid fibrous tissue being laid down. Fibrinous inflammation should be differentiated from serous inflammation.

6.6.2 Suppurative (Purulent) Inflammation

Suppurative Inflammation is a general morphological pattern of acute or chronic inflammation. Inflammation results in a large amount of pus, which consists of neutrophils, dead cells, and fluid. Infection by pyogenic bacteria such as *Staphylococci* is characteristic of purulent inflammation. A localised collection of pus enclosed by surrounding tissues is called an abscess.

6.6.3 Serous Inflammation

Serous Inflammation is a general morphological pattern of acute or chronic inflammation. It is characterised by exudating serum generated from mildly leaky vasculature or synthesised by mesothelial cells. Examples include pneumonia, skin blisters caused by herpes virus infections or burns, serous pericarditis, pleuritis, and joint fluid in rheumatoid arthritis.

6.6.4 Ulcerative Inflammation

Inflammation occurring on an epithelial surface (skin or mucosa) can result in the necrotic loss of tissue, exposing deeper layers. Examples include gastric or duodenal ulcers. An ulcer is a general morphological pattern of inflammation, whether acute or chronic.

6.6.5 Catarrhal Inflammation

Catarrhal inflammation is a form affecting mainly mucosal surfaces, marked by a non-suppurative, copious discharge of mucus, and epithelial debris. Examples include acute rhinitis and catarrhal bronchitis.

6.6.6 Pseudomembranous Inflammation

Pseudomembranous inflammation is a form of ulcerative/exudative inflammation involving mucous and serous membranes. The exudate of fibrin, pus, cellular debris, and mucus forms a pseudomembrane on the surface of the ulcers. Examples include pseudomembranous colitis and pseudomembrane in the throat in diphtheria.

6.6.7 Granulomatous Inflammation

The formation of granulomas characterises granulomatous inflammation; they result from a limited but diverse number of diseases, such as tuberculosis, leprosy, sarcoidosis, and syphilis (see 6.5.3.2)

6.7 Summary

Inflammation is a defence mechanism that is vital to health, because it is the immune system's response to harmful stimuli and acts by removing injurious stimuli and initiating the healing process. Common aetiologic agents that cause inflammation include viruses, bacteria, fungi, chemicals, radiation, and physical trauma, such as external injuries. The inflammatory process involves immune cells, blood vessels, and molecular mediators. Inflammation can be classified as either acute or chronic. Acute inflammation is of short duration and lasts for a few days. Chronic inflammation can last for months or years. A form of chronic inflammation called granulomatous inflammation is characterised by the formation of granulomas which are the result of a limited but diverse number of chronic diseases such as tuberculosis and syphilis. In acute inflammation, neutrophils predominate, whereas in chronic inflammation, macrophages, lymphocytes, and plasma cells predominate. Cardinal clinical signs of acute inflammation include redness, heat, swelling, pain, and loss of function. Cell- and plasma-derived inflammatory mediators play an important role in the pathogenesis of inflammation.

Bibliography

Chen L, Deng H, Cui H, Fang J, Zuo Z, Deng J, Li Y, Wang X, Zhao L. Inflammatory responses and inflammation-associated diseases in organs. Oncotarget. 2017;9(6):7204–18. https://doi.org/10.18632/oncotarget.23208. PMID: 29467962; PMCID: PMC5805548

Chertov O, Yang D, Howard O, Oppenheim JJ. Leukocyte granule proteins mobilise innate host defences and adaptive immune responses. Immunol Rev. 2000;177:68–78.

Kumar V, Abbas AK, Aster JC. Chapter 3. Inflammation and repair. In: Robbins basic pathology. 10th ed. Philadelphia: Elsevier; 2018. p. 57–93.

Medzhitov R. Inflammation 2010: new adventures of an old flame. Cell. 2010;140:771–6.

Nunes AC. Introductory chapter: overview of the cellular and molecular basis of inflammatory process. In: Nunes AC, editor. Translational studies on inflammation. London: IntechOpen; 2020, [cited 2022 Aug 06]. https://www.intechopen.com/chapters/68815. https://doi.org/10.5772/intechopen.88967.

Rodríguez-Hernández H, et al. Obesity and inflammation: epidemiology, risk factors, and markers of inflammation. Int J Endocrinol. 2013;2013:678159. https://doi.org/10.1155/2013/678159.

Serhan CN, Chiang N, Dalli J, Levy BD. Lipid mediators in the resolution of inflammation. Cold Spring Harb Perspect Biol. 2015;7(2):a016311. https://doi.org/10.1101/cshperspect.a016311.

7.1 Introduction

Healing is a general term that replaces dead or injured tissue with living, healthy tissue. It involves two distinct processes: regeneration and repair. In regeneration, the lost tissue is replaced with tissue similar in type. Repair refers to replacing lost tissue with granulation tissue that matures to form a fibrous scar. To understand the healing process, it is essential to know the types of cells that can divide and proliferate to replace the lost tissue and those which lack the proliferative ability.

7.2 Types of Cells and Tissues Involved in the Healing Process

Based on the proliferative capacity of cells, there are three types of tissues in the body: Labile, stable, and permanent tissues.

- **Labile tissues** (Continuously dividing tissues): Labile tissues are made of cells that have a continuous turnover by programmed division of stem cells and by the proliferation of mature cells. They are found in the surface epithelium of the gastrointestinal treat, urinary tract, cervix, skin, and oral cavity. Non-epithelial examples of labile tissues include lymphoid and hematopoietic systems. Cells in these tissues can regenerate readily.
- **Stable tissues.** Cells of stable tissues possess a much lower level of replicative activity in their normal state, and there are few stem cells. However, the cells of such tissues can undergo rapid division in response to injury or loss of tissue mass. The parenchyma of most solid tissues, such as the liver, kidney, and pancreas, are made of cells of this type. Other examples include mesenchymal cells such as smooth muscle cells, fibroblasts, osteoblasts, and endothelial cells. Among these, the liver has an excellent capacity to regenerate after the injury compared to the regenerative capacity of other stable tissues.
- **Permanent tissues:** Cells of permanent tissues are terminally differentiated in postnatal life and non-prolifera-

tive. Examples include neurons and cardiac myocytes. These cells lack or possess insufficient proliferative capacity.

7.3 Healing by Regeneration

Regeneration is the natural process of replacing or restoring damaged or missing cells or tissues by an exactly similar cell population. Two essential conditions are required for regeneration: the damage must involve cell populations capable of dividing (labile or stable cells), and there is little or no disruption to the stromal cell framework, which provides the "scaffolding" to the new cells. *A wound where only the lining epithelium is affected heals exclusively by regeneration. Another example of regeneration includes the renewal of haematopoiesis in the bone marrow in conditions with increased loss of red blood cells due to haemorrhage.* Tissue regeneration can also occur in parenchymal organs with a stable cell population, such as the pancreas, adrenal gland, lungs, and liver. In these tissues, except the liver, regeneration is a limited process; the regenerative response in the liver is outstanding in that liver tissue can regenerate after partial hepatectomy. Surgical removal of one kidney evokes hyperplastic and hypertrophic responses in the contralateral kidney. It must be emphasised that in these situations, the residual tissue must be structurally and functionally intact for regeneration to occur. If the residual tissue is extensively damaged by infection or inflammation, regeneration may be accompanied by scar tissue.

7.4 Healing by Repair

Repair is a process in which a scar eventually replaces lost tissue. Repair by scar occurs if there is a significant disruption of the connective tissue matrix or cells involved are incapable of dividing to replace the lost tissue. Depending on the extent of the tissue damage, repair by scar formation and regeneration of cells may occur in certain situations.

S. R. Prabhu, *Textbook of General Pathology for Dental Students*, https://doi.org/10.1007/978-3-031-31244-1_7

Four sequential processes characterise repair. These include the formation of new blood vessels, migration and proliferation of fibroblasts, deposition of extracellular matrix (ECM), and maturation and reorganisation of the fibrous tissue. Within 24 h of tissue injury, repair begins: Inflammatory exudate containing polymorphs is seen in the area of tissue injury. In addition, there is platelet aggregation and fibrin deposition. This is the inflammatory phase of repair. This is followed by the demolition phase, characterised by the dead cells liberating their autolytic enzymes and other enzymes (proteolytic) from disintegrating polymorphs. There is an associated macrophage infiltration. These cells ingest particulate matter, either digesting or removing it. After 3–5 days, the phase of granulation tissue formation begins. This is characterised by the proliferation of fibroblasts and the ingrowth of new blood vessels into the area of injury with a variable number of inflammatory cells. There is also accompanying angiogenesis (neovascularisation) in the extracellular matrix (ECM). Eventually, accumulated granulation tissue forms collage and fibrous scar tissue, which undergoes maturation and reorganisation (remodelling) over time. Examples include skin wounds that extend through the basement membrane to the connective tissue, or the submucosa in the gastrointestinal tract, resulting in granulation tissue formation and eventual scarring. Lost tissues contain terminally differentiated (permanent) cells, such as neurons, and skeletal muscles heal by forming granulation tissue.

7.5 The Role of Cytokines, Growth Factors, and Extracellular Matrix

As discussed above, healing involves an orderly sequence of events which includes regeneration and migration of specialised cells, angiogenesis, the proliferation of fibroblasts and related cells, matrix protein synthesis, and, finally, cessation of these processes. Cytokines mediate these processes, and a series of low-molecular-weight polypeptides are referred to as growth factors (GFs).

Cytokines are relatively low -molecular-weight proteins secreted to influence or modulate the behaviour of immune cells and other cells. Crucial among them include interleukins, lymphokines, and other signalling molecules such as interferons and tissue necrosis factor (TNF-α). Pro-inflammatory cytokines such as interleukins 1α (IL-1α), 1β (IL-1β), and 6 (IL-6) and TNF-α play essential roles in the wound healing process by stimulating keratinocyte and fibroblast proliferation, modulating the immune response, synthesising, and breaking down extracellular matrix proteins, and promoting the chemotaxis of fibroblasts to the wound site.

Growth Factors (GFs) are naturally occurring proteins that stimulate cell division and differentiation. GFs involved in regeneration and repair include Fibroblast Growth Factor (FGF), Vascular Endothelial Growth Factor (VEGF),

Table 7.1 Role of growth factors in the healing process

Growth factor	Role of growth factors in the healing process
Fibroblast growth factor	Activates vascular endothelial cells and fibroblasts
Vascular endothelial growth factor	Induces development of blood vessels in inflammation and wound healing
Platelet-derived growth factor	Causes migration and proliferation of fibroblasts, smooth muscle cells, and monocytes. Also, has a chemotactic property.
Epidermal growth factor	Induces mitosis in epithelial cells, hepatocytes, and fibroblasts
Tumour necrosis growth factor	Causes migration and proliferation of fibroblasts and secretion of collagenase

Platelet-Derived Growth Factor (PDGF), Epidermal Growth Factor (EGF), Tumour Necrosis Factor (TNF), and Transforming Growth Factor Beta (TGF-β). They may be derived from several sources, such as platelets activated after endothelial damage, damaged epithelial/epidermal cells, circulating serum growth factors, macrophages, or lymphocytes recruited to the area of injury. The healing process ceases when lost tissue has been replaced. TGF-β also acts as a growth inhibitor for epithelial and endothelial cells and regulates their regeneration. PDGF has been established to have a chemotactic role for cells that migrate to the healing wound site, such as fibroblasts, neutrophils, and monocytes. The role of growth factors is shown in Table 7.1.

Endogenous extracellular matrix (ECM) also plays a crucial role in tissue formation and repair, serving as a scaffold for cell adhesion and proliferation, providing structure and mechanical strength to the tissue, and also binding and presenting GFs secreted by neighbouring cells to regulate cell survival, proliferation, and differentiation. The main group of enzymes responsible for the collagen and other protein degradation in extracellular matrix (ECM) is matrix metalloproteinases (MMPs). Collagen is the main structural component of connective tissue, and its degradation is a critical process in development, morphogenesis, tissue remodelling, and repair. Matrix metalloproteinases (MMPs) are involved in the inflammatory, proliferative, and remodelling phases of the wound healing process by modulating cytokine/chemokine activity by activating them enzymatically or influencing their availability by cleaving them from the cell surface. In particular, they help in the degradation of the provisional extracellular matrix, facilitate the migration of inflammatory cells to the wound site, remodel the granulation tissue, and modulate angiogenesis.

7.6 Wound Healing

A wound is any break in the continuity of the skin or mucous membrane disrupting normal anatomic structures and function. Wounds can be traumatic or surgical. *Wound healing*

Table 7.2 Normal wound-healing process

Phase	Cellular and bio-physiologic events
Haemostasis	Vascular constriction Platelet aggregation, deregulation, and fibrin formation (thrombus)
Inflammation	Neutrophil infiltration Monocyte infiltration and differentiation to macrophage Lymphocyte infiltration
Proliferation	Re-epithelialisation Angiogenesis Collagen synthesis Extra cellular matrix (ECM) formation
Remodelling	Collagen remodelling Vascular maturation and regression

Source: Mathieu D, Linke J-C, Wattel F. (2006). Non-healing wounds. In: Handbook on hyperbaric medicine, Mathieu DE, editor. Netherlands: Springer, pp. 401–427

can be divided into 4-phases: the haemostasis phase, the inflammatory phase, the proliferative or granulation phase, and the remodelling or maturation phase. Within these phases, complex and coordinated series of events take place (Table 7.2). As discussed below, healing a cutaneous or mucosal wound demonstrates epithelial regeneration and repair by scarring.

7.7 Categories of Cutaneous Wound Healing

Cutaneous wound healing involves epithelial regeneration and connective tissue scar formation. Two categories of cutaneous or mucosal wound healing occur depending on the amount of tissue damage: Healing by first intention and healing by second intention (Fig. 7.1).

7.7.1 Healing by First intention (Primary Union)

A clean incision, such as a paper cut or sutured surgical wound, heals by the primary union or the first intention. In these types of injuries, the edges of wounds are approximated.

Events in the first intention healing process are as follows (Fig. 7.1)

- The narrow incisional space is filled with clotted blood containing fibrin and blood cells.

- Dehydration of the surface clot forms the scab that covers the wound and seals it from the environment.
- Within 24 h, neutrophils appear at the margins of the incision; these move toward the fibrin clot, and the basal cells at the cut edge of the epithelium show increased mitotic activity.
- Within 24–48 h, spurs of epithelial cells from the edges of the wound migrate and grow along the cut margins of the wound and beneath the surface scab to fuse in the midline, thus producing a continuous but thin epithelial layer.
- By day 3, neutrophils largely disappear and are replaced by macrophages, and granulation tissue invades the space created by the incision. Collagen fibres appear at the margins arranged vertically. Epithelial cell proliferation continues, and a thickened epidermal covering layer results.
- By day 5, the incisional space is filled with richly vascularised granulation tissue. Collagen fibrils begin to bridge the gap created by incision. The epidermis recovers its normal thickness, followed by the differentiation of epidermal cells and surface keratinisation.
- During the second week, collagen deposition and fibroblast proliferation continue, and oedema, leukocyte infiltration, and increased vascularity diminish.
- By the end of the first month, the scar is fully formed with connective tissue cells and devoid of inflammatory cells. Covering epithelium is normal in structure.

7.7.2 Healing by Second Intention (Secondary Intention)

The second type of wound healing process is known as healing by secondary intention or by secondary intention. In this type of healing, there is an open wound with a more extensive loss of cells and tissue. Examples include inflammatory ulceration, abscess formation, and surface wounds that create large defects (Fig. 7.1). In this healing process, a large defect must be filled. Other features include:

- The clot and scab are large at the surface of the wound.
- Inflammatory cell infiltration is intense.
- Abundant granulation tissue grows in from the margin to complete the repair.
- Wound contraction caused by *myofibroblasts* is an important feature.
- Regeneration of parenchymal cells cannot completely reconstitute the original architecture.

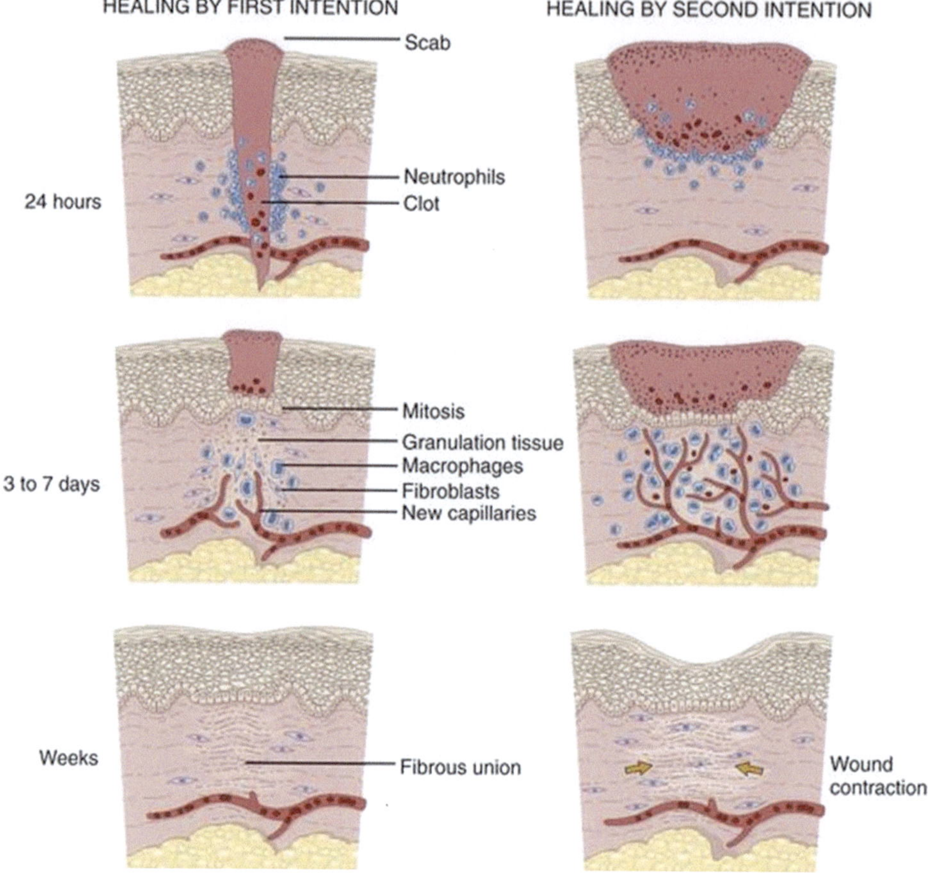

Fig. 7.1 Healing of cutaneous wound by first and second intention. Source: By kind permission of Cao Xuan cu

7.8 Healing of Oral Mucosal Wounds

Healing of oral mucosal wounds occurs with events similar to those of cutaneous wounds, except that inflammation and scar formation in the mucosal wound is minimal. Wounds in the oral cavity heal much faster than skin wounds, with rapid re-epithelialisation and re-modelling resulting in minimal scar formation. This is believed to be due to the presence of growth factors or cytokines in the saliva. Saliva contains several essential molecules, such as epidermal growth factors, lysosomes, and lactoferrin, which have antimicrobial and anti-inflammatory properties. In gingival tissues, in particular, fibroblasts play an essential role in wound healing, and extracellular matrix (ECM) significantly contributes to remodelling by synthesising ECM components, collagen, fibronectin, hyaluronan, and elastin and the secretion of matrix metalloproteinase and tissue inhibitor of metalloproteinase.

7.9 Fracture Healing

Bone is composed of calcified osteoid tissue, which consists of collagen fibres embedded in a mucoprotein matrix (Osseomucin). Depending on the arrangement of the colla-

gen fibres, there are two histological types of bone: Woven (immature or non-lamellar) bone and lamellar bone. Woven bone shows irregularity in the collagen bundles' arrangement and the osteocytes' distribution. The osseomucin is less abundant, and it also contains less calcium. The collagen bundles in lamellar or adult bone are arranged in parallel sheets.

The basic processes involved in healing bone fractures bear many resemblances to those seen in skin wound healing. *Unlike the healing of a skin wound, the defect caused by a fracture is repaired not by a fibrous "scar" tissue but by specialised bone-forming tissue so that, under favourable circumstances, the bone is restored nearly to normal.*

7.9.1 Stages in Fracture Healing (Bone Regeneration) (Fig. 7.2)

Stage 1: Haematoma formation. Immediately following the injury, there is a variable amount of bleeding from torn vessels; if the periosteum is torn, this blood may extend into the surrounding muscles. If it is subsequently organised and ossified, myositis ossificans results (Fig. 7.2).

Stage 2: Inflammation. The tissue damage excites an inflammatory response, and the exudate adds more fibrin to

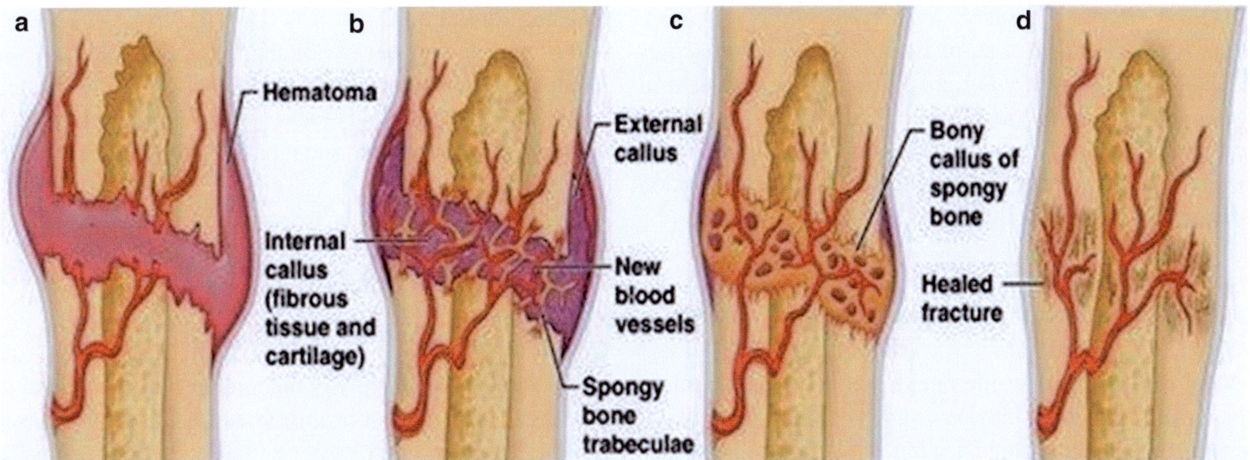

Fig. 7.2 Stages in fracture repair: the healing of a bone fracture follows a series of progressive steps: (**a**) Broken blood vessels leak blood that clots into a fracture haematoma, (**b**) Internal and external calluses form made of cartilage and bone, (**c**) Cartilage of the calluses is gradually eroded and replaced by bone, forming the hard callus. (**d**) Remodelling occurs to replace the immature bone with mature bone

the clot. The inflammatory changes differ from those seen in other inflamed tissues. There is an increased blood flow and a polymorphonuclear leucocytic infiltration. The hematoma attains a fusiform shape.

Stage 3: Demolition. Macrophages invade the clot and remove the fibrin, red cells, inflammatory exudate, and debris. Any bone fragments detached from their blood supply undergo necrosis and are attacked by macrophages and osteoclasts.

Stage 4: Formation of granulation tissue. Following this demolition phase, there is an ingrowth of capillary loops and mesenchymal cells derived from the periosteum and the endosteum of the cancellous bone. These cells have osteogenic potential and, together with the newly formed blood vessels, contribute to the granulation of tissue formation.

Stage 5: Woven bone and cartilage formation. The mesenchymal "osteoblasts" next differentiate to form woven bone or cartilage. The term "callus," derived from the Latin and meaning hard, is often used to describe the material uniting the fracture ends regardless of its consistency. When this is granulation tissue, the "callus" is soft, but as bone or cartilage formation occurs, it becomes hard (Fig. 7.2).

Stage 6: Formation of lamellar bone. Capillaries headed by osteoclasts next invade the dead calcified cartilage or woven bone. As the initial scaffolding ("provisional callus") is removed, osteoblasts lay down osteoid, which calcifies to form bone. Its collagen bundles are now arranged in an orderly lamellar fashion, for the most part concentrically around the blood vessels, and in this way, the Haversian systems are formed. Adjacent to the periosteum and endosteum, the lamellae are parallel to the surface as in the normal bone. This phase of formation of definitive lamellar bone merges with the last stage.

Stage 7: Remodelling. The final remodelling process involves the continued osteoclastic removal and osteoblastic laying down of bone, resulting in the formation of a bone that differs remarkably little from the original tissue. The external callus is slowly removed, and the intermediate callus becomes converted into compact bone containing Haversian systems. In contrast, the internal callus is hollowed out into a marrow cavity in which only a few spicules of cancellous bone remain (Fig. 7.1d).

7.10 Tooth Extraction Socket Healing

The socket healing pattern post-tooth extraction follows a bone-healing process. After the tooth extraction, the socket is filled with a blood clot. Platelets retract the clot, expressing the fluid, which results in the formation of a harder clot that shrinks below the level of the adjacent soft tissues and pulls the soft tissue inwards. Clot retraction is complete in approximately 4 h. At 4 days, new capillaries and fibroblasts appear in the blood clot from the periphery, which is now fixed to the socket wall. Macrophages migrate into the clot, which is replaced by granulation tissue. At the gingival margin, epithelium proliferates and migrates over the granulation tissue. Re-epithelisation is complete within 7–10 days. The granulation tissue with fibroblasts and collagen network formation is laid down in 18 days. At this stage, woven bone forms at the socket's periphery. By 6 weeks, woven bone fills the socket and is remodelled to the lamellar bone, and the bone remodelling process proceeds around 6 months after extraction. The socket healing process is accompanied by the loss of alveolar bone height and width due to bone remodelling, including bone formation and resorption. *The degree of bone resorption during the socket bone remodelling procedure depends on various factors, including local factors such as the quality and quantity of alveolar bone, inflammation, oral hygiene, and systemic factors such as smoking, nutrition, and medical conditions.* A periodontally compromised socket with severe bone defect by chronic pathologic lesion can result in erratic healing.

7.11 Factors that Influence Wound Healing

Several factors can alter the rate and efficiency of healing. These can be classified into local and systemic factors. These factors apply to skin wound healing, but many are likely relevant to healing at other sites.

7.11.1 Local Factors

Type, Size, and Location of the Wound
- A clean, aseptic wound produced by the surgeon's scalpel heals faster than a wound produced by blunt trauma. In blunt injury, necrosis is abundant, and wound edges are irregular.
- Small blunt wounds heal faster than more extensive wounds.
- Injuries in richly vascularised areas (e.g. the face) heal faster than those in poorly vascularised ones (e.g. the foot).
- In areas where the skin adheres to bony surfaces, as in injuries over the tibia, wound contraction and adequate apposition of the edges are difficult. Hence, such wounds heal slowly.

Vascular Supply
- Wounds with impaired blood supply heal slowly. For example, the healing of leg wounds in patients with varicose veins is prolonged.
- Ischemia, due to pressure, produces bed sores and then prevents their healing. Ischemia due to arterial obstruction, often in the lower extremities in diabetic patients, also prevents healing.

Infection
- Infection delays or prevents healing, promotes the formation of excessive granulation tissue (proud flesh), and may result in large, deforming scars.

Movement
- Early movement, mainly before tensile strength has been established, subjects a wound to persistent trauma, thus preventing or retarding healing.

Ionising Radiation
- Prior irradiation leaves vascular lesions that interfere with blood supply and result in slow wound healing. Acutely, irradiation of a wound blocks cellular proliferation, inhibits wound contraction, and retards the formation of granulation tissue.

7.11.2 Systemic Factors

Circulatory Status
- Adequate blood supply to the injured area is essential for wound healing. Poor healing is attributed to cardiovascular disorders. Old age is often due to impaired circulation.

Infection
- Systemic infections delay wound healing.

Metabolic Status
- Poorly controlled diabetes mellitus is associated with delayed wound healing. The risk of infection in clean wounds approaches fivefold the risk in non-diabetic patients; there can be impaired circulation secondary to arteriosclerosis and impaired sensation due to diabetic neuropathy. The impaired sensation renders the lower extremity to everyday hazards. Hence, in diabetic patients, wounds heal very slowly.

Nutritional Status (Deficiencies)
- Protein deficiency: Granulation tissue and collagen formation are impaired in protein depletion, resulting in delayed wound healing.
- Vitamin deficiency: Vitamin C is required for collagen synthesis and secretion. It is necessary for the hydroxylation of proline and lysine in the process of collagen synthesis. Vitamin C deficiency (scurvy) results in grossly deficient wound healing, with a lack of vascular proliferation and collagen deposition.
- Trace element deficiency: Zinc (a co-factor of several enzymes) deficiency will retard healing by preventing cell proliferation. Zinc is necessary for several DNA and RNA polymerases and transferases; hence, a deficiency state will inhibit mitosis. The proliferation (fibroplasia) is, therefore, retarded.
- Hormones: Corticosteroids impair wound healing, an effect attributed to the inhibition of collagen synthesis. However, these hormones have many other effects, including anti-inflammatory actions and a general depression of protein synthesis. It also inhibits fibroplasia and neovascularisation. Both epithelialisation and wound

contraction are impaired. Thyroid hormones, androgens, oestrogens, and growth hormones also influence healing. This effect, however, may be more due to their regulation of general metabolic status rather than to a specific modification of the healing process.

Anti-Inflammatory Drugs
– Anti-inflammatory medications do not interfere with wound healing when administered at the usual daily dosages. However, Aspirin and indomethacin inhibit prostaglandin synthesis and thus delay healing.

7.12 Complications of Wound Healing

Abnormalities in repair and regeneration can result in complications of wound healing. These include the following:

Infection. A wound may provide a portal of entry for many organisms. Infection may delay healing and, if severe, stop it completely.

Deficient Scar Formation. Inadequate formation of granulation tissue or an inability to form a suitable extracellular matrix leads to deficient scar formation and its complications. The complications of poor scar formation are wound dehiscence, incisional hernias, and ulceration

Wound Dehiscence and Incisional Hernias. Dehiscence (bursting of a wound) is of most concern after abdominal surgery. If the insufficient extracellular matrix is deposited or there is inadequate cross-linking of the matrix, weak scars result. Wound infection and increased mechanical stress on the wound from vomiting, coughing, or ileus is a factor in most cases of abdominal dehiscence. Systemic factors that predispose to dehiscence include poor metabolic statuses, such as vitamin C deficiency, hypoproteinemia, and the general inanition that often accompanies metastatic cancer.

– **An incisional hernia.** *Incisional hernia,* usually of the abdominal wall, refers to a defect caused by poor wound healing following surgery into which the intestines protrude.

Ulceration. Wounds ulcerate because of an inadequate intrinsic blood supply or insufficient vascularisation during healing. For example, leg wounds in persons with varicose veins or severe atherosclerosis typically ulcerate. Non-healing wounds also develop in areas devoid of sensation because of persistent trauma. Such trophic or neuropathic ulcers are occasionally seen in patients with leprosy, diabetic peripheral neuropathy, and tertiary syphilis from spinal involvement (in tabes dorsalis).

Excessive Scar Formation. Excessive extracellular matrix deposition at the wound site results in a keloid or hypertrophic scar.

– **Keloid** is an exuberant scar that tends to progress and recur after excision. The cause of this is unknown. Genetic predisposition, repeated trauma, and irritation caused by a foreign body, hair, keratin, etc., may play a part. It is a commonplace after burns. It is common in areas of the neck and in the ear lobes.
– **Hypertrophic scar** is structurally similar to keloid. Following excision, keloid recurs, whereas a hypertrophic scar does not.

Excessive contraction. A decrease in the size of a wound depends on the presence of myofibroblasts, the development of cell-cell contacts, and sustained cell contraction. An exaggeration of these processes is termed contracture (cicatrisation) and results in severe deformity of the wound and surrounding tissues. Contracture is also said to arise due to the late reduction in wound size. Contractures are particularly conspicuous in the healing of severe burns. Contractures of the skin and underlying connective tissue can be severe enough to compromise the movement of joints. Cicatrisation is also essential in hollow viscera such as the urethra, oesophagus, and intestine. It leads to progressive stenosis with stricture formation. In the alimentary tract, a contracture (stricture) can obstruct the passage of food in the oesophagus or block the flow of intestinal contents.

Implantation. Epithelial cells that flow into the healing wound may sometimes persist and proliferate to form an epidermoid cyst.

7.13 Summary

Regeneration is the natural process of replacing or restoring damaged or missing cells or tissues by an exactly similar cell population. Repair refers to replacing lost tissue with granulation tissue that matures to form a fibrous scar. Based on the proliferative capacity of cells, labile, stable, and permanent types of cells take part in the healing process. Several cell types, cytokines, and growth factors take part in the healing process. Cutaneous healing involves primary and secondary phases. Healing of oral mucosal wounds occurs with events similar to those of cutaneous wounds. In bone fracture healing, the defect caused is repaired not by fibrous tissue but by specialised bone-forming tissue so that, under favourable circumstances, the bone is restored nearly to normal. The process of post-extraction tooth socket healing follows similar events. The remodelling process is a key factor in both bone and tooth socket healing. Local and systemic factors play a role in the success of the complete restoration of lost tissue in the healing process.

Bibliography

Chhabra S, Chhabra N, Kaur A, Gupta N. Wound healing concepts in clinical practice of OMFS. J Maxillofac Oral Surg. 2017;16(4):403–23. https://doi.org/10.1007/s12663-016-0880-z. Epub 2016 Mar 5. PMID: 29038623; PMCID: PMC5628060

Eming SA, Martin P, Tomic-Canic M. Wound repair and regeneration: mechanisms, signalling, and translation. Sci Transl Med. 2014;6(265):265sr6. https://doi.org/10.1126/scitranslmed.3009337. PMID: 25473038; PMCID: PMC4973620

Gomes PS, Daugela P, Poskevicius L, Mariano L, Fernandes MH. Molecular and cellular aspects of socket healing in the absence and presence of graft materials and autologous platelet concentrates: a focused review. J Oral Maxillofac Res. 2019;10(3):e2. http://www.ejomr.org/JOMR/archives/2019/3/e2/v10n3e2ht.htm. https://doi.org/10.5037/jomr.2019.10302.

Gosain A, DiPietro LA. Ageing and wound healing. World J Surg. 2004;28:321–6.

Grey JE, Enoch S, Harding KG. Wound assessment. BMJ. 2006;332(7536):285–8. https://doi.org/10.1136/bmj.332.7536.285.

Krafts KP. Tissue repair: the hidden drama. Organ. 2010;6(4):225–33. https://doi.org/10.4161/org.6.4.12555. PMID: 21220961; PMCID: PMC3055648

Kumar V, Abbas AK, Fausto N, Mitchell RN. Tissue repair: regeneration, healing and fibrosis. In: Robbins basic pathology. 8th ed. Philadelphia: Saunders; 2007. p. 59–80.

Mathieu D, Linke J-C, Wattel F. Non-healing wounds. In: Mathieu DE, editor. Handbook on hyperbaric medicine. Netherlands: Springer; 2006. p. 401–27.

Reinke JM, Sorg H. Wound repair and regeneration. Eur Surg Res. 2012;49:35–43. https://doi.org/10.1159/000339613.

8.1 Introduction

A genetic disorder is a disease caused in whole or in part by a change in the DNA sequence away from the normal sequence. Genetic disorders can be caused by a mutation in one gene (monogenic disorders), by mutations in multiple genes (polygenic and multifactorial disorders), by a combination of gene mutations and environmental factors (multifactorial disorders), or by damage to chromosomes (changes in the number or structure of entire chromosomes, the structures that carry genes (chromosomal disorders). There are well over 6000 known genetic disorders described in the medical literature. Around 1 in 50 people are affected by a known single-gene disease, while about 1 in 263 are affected by a chromosomal disorder. The clinician must possess basic knowledge of chromosomes, genes, and related aspects to understand the mechanisms involved in genetic disorders. These are briefly described below.

8.2 Chromosomes and Genes

Chromosomes represent the genome of an organism that carries genetic information. They are thread-like structures composed of nucleic acid DNA. There are two types of chromosomes: autosomes and sex chromosomes. Autosomes contain genes that code for somatic characteristics. In contrast, sex chromosomes determine the gender of the individual. A normal human cell contains two sets of 23 chromosomes, of which 22 are in identical pairs numbered 1 through 22, depending on their unique features. These are called autosomes. The remaining chromosomes are called

sex chromosomes which may be either X or Y. Females have two X chromosomes, whereas males have an X and Y chromosome. One set of 23 chromosomes is inherited from the father and the other from the mother. Because all female cells, including the mother's ovum, contain only X chromosomes, the paternal chromosome (either the X or Y) determines the sex of the child. Chromosomes are found inside the nucleus of a cell and are made up of proteins and DNA organised into genes. Each chromosome contains a molecule of DNA. Most DNA is present within the nucleus as chromosomes (the nuclear DNA or nuclear genome) and a small amount in the mitochondria (the mtDNA or mitochondrial genome). Each gene has a specific location (locus), typically the same on the two homologous chromosomes. Homologous chromosomes are chromosome pairs containing a maternal and a paternal chromatid that are similar in length and gene position and are joined at the centromere.

Genes consist of deoxyribonucleic acid (DNA). DNA contains the code, or blueprint, used to synthesise a protein. Each DNA molecule is a long double helix that resembles a spiral staircase containing millions of steps. The steps of the staircase consist of pairs of four types of molecules called bases (nucleotides). In each stage, the base adenine (A) is paired with the base thymine (T), or the base guanine (G) is paired with the base cytosine (C). Each extremely long DNA molecule is coiled up inside one of the chromosomes (Fig. 8.1).

Genes vary in size, depending on the dimensions of the proteins for which they code. The genes that occupy the same locus on each chromosome of a pair (one inherited from the mother and one from the father) are called alleles. A pair of identical alleles for a particular gene is homozygosity; having a pair of nonidentical alleles is heterozygosity.

S. R. Prabhu, *Textbook of General Pathology for Dental Students*, https://doi.org/10.1007/978-3-031-31244-1_8

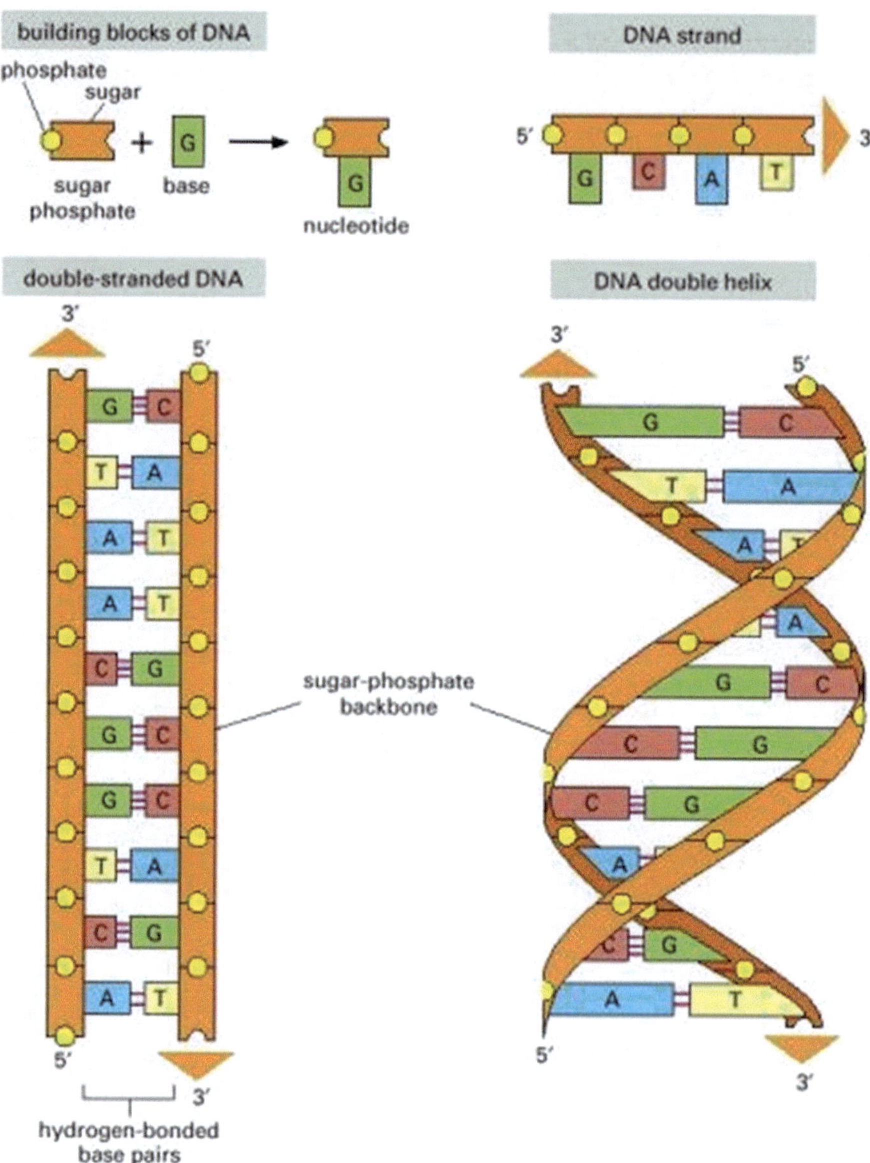

Fig. 8.1 DNA is made of four nucleotides linked covalently into a polynucleotide chain (a DNA strand) with a sugar-phosphate backbone from which the bases (A, C, G, and T) extend. A DNA molecule is composed of two DNA strands held together by hydrogen bonds between the paired bases. The *arrowheads* at the ends of the DNA strands indicate the polarities of the two strands, which run antiparallel to each other in the DNA molecule. In the diagram at the bottom left of the figure, the DNA molecule is shown straightened out; in reality, it is twisted into a double helix, as shown on the right (Source: https://www.ncbi.nlm.nih.gov/books/NBK26821/)

8.3   Genotype and Phenotype

The genotype (or genome) is a person's unique combination of genes or genetic makeup. Thus, the genotype is a complete set of instructions on how that person's body synthesises proteins and, therefore, how that body is supposed to be built and function. The phenotype is the actual structure and function of a person's body. The phenotype is how the genotype manifests in a person. The genotype, environment (including illnesses and diet), and other unknown factors determine whether and how a gene is expressed.

8.4   Inheritance Patterns

Understanding the fundamental laws of inheritance is essential to appreciate how conditions are passed on in a family. Genetic disorders can be inherited in different ways. *Four inheritance patterns include single-gene, sex-linked, mitochondrial, and multifactorial inheritance.* These are briefly discussed below.

8.4.1 Single-Gene Inheritance (Mendelian Inheritance)

Genes are responsible for transmitting traits from parents to offspring from one generation to another. The passing on of genetic traits is expressed in Mendelian inheritance patterns. Children inherit one chromosome from each parent and depending on the dominance of a gene in those chromosomes, a particular trait or disease may develop in the child. *In Mendelian genetics, genes can be autosomal dominant or recessive or linked to one of the sex chromosomes: X or Y.* In autosomal-dominant disorder, only one chromosome in the pair must have the gene defect in question for the trait to manifest. An affected parent has a 50% chance of transmitting the mutated gene to any child. When a disorder is autosomal recessive, the child must inherit one copy of the defective gene from each parent for the disorder to occur. Because each parent has one copy of the defective gene and is a carrier, there is a 25% chance that both mutant copies of the gene will be passed on to their offspring and that the child will manifest the disorder. Fifty percent of the time, the offspring will get one copy of the mutant gene from one parent and will be a carrier, and 25% of the time, the offspring will get two normal copies of the gene and will not develop the associated disorder.

8.4.2 Sex-Linked Inheritance

Sex-linked genes occur on either the X or Y chromosomes. However, only males can inherit Y-linked genes. For traits on the X chromosome, as males only have one X chromosome, a son has a 50% chance of inheriting the defective gene from his mother and manifesting the disease. If the defective gene is transmitted to a daughter, she will be carrier of the disease and may display a mild phenotype.

8.4.3 Mitochondrial Inheritance.

This is mediated by maternally transmitted mitochondrial genes inherited exclusively by maternal transmission. A mitochondrial inheritance pattern is a rare form of inheritance. This is a non-Mendelian type of inheritance.

8.4.4 Multifactorial Inheritance

Many common diseases are not inherited as a single gene defect but result from modifications in gene expression or gene-environment interactions. This includes diabetes, hypertension, bipolar disorder, non-syndromic cleft lip and palate, dental caries, and periodontal disease. These diseases involve multiple interactions between genes and environmental factors such as smoking, diet, stress, and environmental chemicals. An individual's response to environmental factors and subsequent susceptibility to disease are related to mechanisms that modify gene expression without altering the DNA sequence. Epigenetics is the mediation of gene expression without changes to the DNA sequence and may account for phenotypic variation between monozygotic twins. Epigenetic changes include DNA methylation and histone modification, non-coding RNA-associated gene silencing, and may result from age, stress, nutrition, or environmental factors that occur during developmental stages.

8.5 Genetic Disorders

One or more abnormalities cause a genetic disorder in the genome. It can be caused by a mutation in a single gene (monogenic), multiple genes (polygenic), or a chromosomal abnormality. The mutation can occur spontaneously before embryonic development (a de novo mutation), or it can be inherited from two parents who are carriers of a faulty gene (autosomal-recessive inheritance) or from a parent with the disorder (autosomal-dominant inheritance). The genetic disorder is inherited from one or both parents; it is considered a hereditary disease. Some disorders are caused by a mutation on the X chromosome and have X-linked inheritance. Genetic disorders present before birth can produce birth defects, but birth defects can also be developmental that are not hereditary. https://en.wikipedia.org/wiki/Genetic_disorder

8.5.1 Monogenic Disorders

As described above, *monogenic disorder (single-gene disorder, Mendelian disorder) results from a single mutated gene. Single-gene disorders can be passed on to subsequent generations.*

Examples of monogenic disorders include sickle cell anaemia, Cystic fibrosis, haemophilia, Huntington's disease, and most congenital metabolic disorders known as inborn errors of metabolism. Ways in which monogenic disorders can be inherited from parents include (1) autosomal-dominant inheritance, where only one copy of a faulty gene (this can be from either parent) is necessary to cause the disease, and (2) autosomal-recessive inheritance, where two copies of a faulty gene (one from each parent) are necessary to cause the disease and (3) X-linked inheritance, where the faulty gene is only present on the X-chromosome, the female chromosome.

- **Autosomal-dominant disorders**: *Autosomal-dominant traits or disorders are encoded by a gene located on one of the 22 autosomes and are dominant in relation to its allele.* This trait is fully expressed under heterozygous conditions. (i.e. even if only one copy of the gene is present) Some examples include Marfan's syndrome, Osteogenesis imperfecta, achondroplasia, familial hypercholesteremia, adult polycystic kidney disease, spherocytosis, familial polyposis coli, and neurofibromatosis.
- **Autosomal-recessive disorders**: *Autosomal-recessive traits or disorders are encoded by genes located on one of the 22 chromosomes expressed only under homozygous conditions.* (i.e. only if paired with an identical allele). In this condition, the parents of the affected homozygote are usually asymptomatic carriers of the trait or disorder. Disorders inherited as autosomal-recessive traits are more common than those inherited as autosomal-dominant traits. Some autosomal-recessive disorders include cystic fibrosis, sickle cell anaemia, thalassemia, Hurler's syndrome, Hunter's syndrome, and phenylketonuria.
- **X-linked recessive disorders**: *X-linked recessive traits are encoded by recessive genes located on the X chromosome but not found on the Y-chromosome.* The gene effect is evident only in males and very rarely in females. The gene is transmitted from the asymptomatic mother, and the sisters of an affected male are asymptomatic. Unaffected brothers do not carry the gene and do not transmit the trait. Examples include haemophilia A and B, muscular dystrophy, agammaglobulinemia, and lymphoproliferative disorders.
- **X-linked dominant disorders:** X-linked dominant disorders are uncommon relative to other types of Mendelian diseases and show an excess of affected females in a family, since women have two X chromosomes. Hypophosphatemia and incontinentia pigmenti are examples of X-linked dominant disorders.

8.5.2 Polygenic Disorders (Multifactorial Inheritance Disorders)

The vast majority of genetic diseases are polygenic disorders. Genetic variations influence these diseases in many genes. They are also often influenced by many exogenous (epigenetic) factors, such as nutrition, exercise, and environmental exposures. *Since most polygenic diseases are determined by the interactions of several genes and environmental factors called "multifactorial" diseases,* some common polygenic diseases include Coronary artery disease, Type 2 diabetes, gout, Alzheimer's disease, cancer, cleft lip/palate, anencephaly, and Schizophrenia.

8.5.3 Chromosomal Disorders (Cytogenetic Disorders)

Some disorders result from defects in chromosomes. *There are many types of chromosomal abnormalities. They can be organised into two basic groups: numerical abnormalities and structural abnormalities.*

Numerical Abnormalities: When an individual is missing one of the chromosomes from a pair, the condition is called monosomy. The condition is called trisomy when an individual has more than two chromosomes instead of a pair. An example of a condition caused by numerical abnormalities is Down syndrome, marked by mental disability, learning difficulties, a characteristic facial appearance, and poor muscle tone (hypotonia) in infancy. An individual with Down syndrome has three copies of chromosome 21 rather than two; for that reason, the condition is also known as Trisomy 21. An example of monosomy, in which an individual lacks a chromosome, is Turner syndrome. In Turner syndrome, a female is born with only one sex chromosome, an X, and is usually shorter than average and unable to have children, among other difficulties.

Structural Abnormalities: A chromosome's structure can be altered in several ways. These include the following:

- Deletions. A portion of the chromosome is missing or deleted.
- Duplications: A portion of the chromosome is duplicated, resulting in extra genetic material.
- Translocations. A portion of one chromosome is transferred to another chromosome. There are two main types of translocation. In a reciprocal translocation, segments from two different chromosomes have been exchanged. In a Robertsonian translocation, an entire chromosome has attached to another at the centromere.
- Inversions. A portion of the chromosome has broken off, turned upside down, and reattached. As a result, the genetic material is inverted.
- Rings. A portion of a chromosome has broken off and formed a circle or ring. This can happen with or without the loss of genetic material.

Most chromosome abnormalities occur as an accident in the egg or sperm. In these cases, the abnormality is present in every cell of the body. Some abnormalities happen after conception; some cells have the abnormality, and some do not. Chromosomal abnormalities can be inherited from a parent (such as a translocation) or be "de novo" (new to the individual). This is why chromosome studies are often performed on the parents when a child is found to have an abnormality.

8.6 Mutations

The mutation is "any heritable change to the DNA sequence." Heritable refers to somatic cell division (the proliferation of cells in tissues) and germline inheritance (from parents to child). Spontaneous or induced gene mutations can result in defective genetic material, some of which can act as the basis for various types of inherited diseases, carrying these mutated changes from parents to offspring. *Not all genetic disorders are inherited. The main difference between congenital and inherited disorders lies in the fact that hereditary diseases have the potential to be carried from one generation to another.* In contrast, a genetic disease can either be hereditary or not, but there will always be a mutational change in the genetic constitution (genome). Genetic disorders are conditions directly attributed to gene abnormalities, such as having an abnormal number of chromosomes in Down syndrome (Trisomy 21) caused by an extra chromosome on the 21st chromosome pair.

8.7 Congenital and Developmental Disorders

Congenital disorders are present at birth. Congenital disorders may be genetic (e.g. Down's syndrome) or may not be genetic (e.g. congenital syphilis). Genetic defects cause 25% of these, and the causes of 75% are not known. The lack of certain genes or their mutations results in abnormal development. Examples include cleft lip and dwarfism. Drugs, X-ray exposure, and alcohol are some of the exogenous causes. Pathogenic teratogens include toxoplasma, rubella, cytomegalovirus, herpes virus, Epstein-Barr virus, varicella virus, *Listeria monocytogenes,* and *Leptospira.* Birth injury may rarely occur due to mechanical trauma during delivery. Not all genetic diseases are congenital. For example, patients with Huntington's disease begin to manifest their disease in the third or fourth decades. Developmental disorders resulting in physical defects are often defined as those originating in the embryo and foetus in the prenatal period. A developmental toxicant is involved in this process. A toxic agent or condition to which the pregnant mother is exposed can cause a developmental defect in the foetus. Developmental defects comprise all structural and functional deficits detected in the implanted embryo, foetus, neonate, infant, or child. The causes of developmental defects include intrinsic and extrinsic causes. Intrinsic causes include genetic defects (mutations), endogenous chromosomal imbalances (e.g. meiotic nondisjunctions), and endogenous metabolism (e.g. phenylketonuria). Extrinsic causes include a variety of environmental inputs such as infection, nutritional deficiencies and excesses, lifestyle factors (e.g. alcohol), and the myriad agents such as pharmaceuticals, synthetic chemicals, solvents, pesticides, fungicides, herbicides, cosmetics, food additives, natural plant and animal toxins and products, and other environmental chemicals encountered by humans. Other environmental factors, such as hyperthermia, ultraviolet irradiation, and X-rays, are also included.

8.8 Summary

Chromosomes represent the genome of an organism that carries genetic information. Genes consist of deoxyribonucleic acid (DNA), which contains the code to synthesise a protein. The genotype or genome is a person's unique combination of genes or genetic makeup. The phenotype is how the genotype manifests in a person. There are four inheritance patterns which include single-gene, sex-linked, mitochondrial, and multifactorial inheritance. Genetic disorders can be caused by a mutation in a single gene (monogenic), multiple genes (polygenic), or by chromosomal (cytogenetic) abnormalities. Monogenic disorders can be autosomal dominant, autosomal recessive, or X-linked. Congenital disorders are present at birth. Congenital disorders may be genetic or not genetic.

Bibliography

Maitra A. Genetic and pediatric diseases. In: Kumar V, Abbas AK, Aster JC, editors. Robbins basic pathology. 10th ed. Philadelphia: Elsevier; 2018. p. 243–95.

National Research Council (US) Committee on Developmental Toxicology. Scientific frontiers in developmental toxicology and risk assessment. Washington (DC): National Academies Press (US); 2000. 2, Developmental defects and their causes. https://www.ncbi.nlm.nih.gov/books/NBK225664/

Simon Herrington C. Muir's textbook of pathology. 15th ed. Clinical Genetics; 2014. p. 31–48.

Tobias E, Connor M, Fergusson-Smith M. Essential Medical Genetics. 6th ed. Oxford: Wiley-Blackwell; 2011.

Infectious and Communicable Diseases: An Overview

9.1 Introduction

An infection, by definition, is the invasion of tissues by pathogens, their multiplication, and the reaction of host tissues to the infectious agent and the toxins they produce. Infectious diseases are caused by infectious agents such as bacteria, viruses, parasites, and fungi and their toxic products. When the host's defence is weak, some non-pathogenic commensal organisms in the body can become pathogenic and cause diseases. Such infections are known as opportunistic infections. One example of opportunistic infections includes oral candidiasis in HIV disease. Many infectious diseases are communicable diseases. Communicable diseases (contagious diseases) are illnesses caused by viruses or bacteria that people spread to one another through contact with bodily fluids, blood products, contaminated surfaces, insect bites, or the air. Some infectious diseases are notifiable. This means legislation requires that each detected case is reported to health departments. Notifiable diseases include blood-borne diseases, gastrointestinal diseases, sexually transmissible infections, vaccine-preventable diseases, vector-borne diseases, and zoonoses. Some examples of notifiable communicable diseases include HIV, hepatitis A, B, and C, measles, COVID-19, salmonella, measles, and blood-borne illnesses. The most common forms of the spread of communicable diseases include faecal-oral, food, sexual intercourse, insect bites, contact with contaminated fomites, droplets, or skin contact. Nosocomial infections, also called hospital-acquired infections, are a subset of infectious diseases acquired in a healthcare facility. To be considered nosocomial, the infection cannot be present at admission; instead, it must develop at least 48 h after admission.

This chapter aims to highlight the mechanisms involved in the causation and mechanisms involved in the pathology of infectious diseases. The description of individual diseases is beyond the scope of this chapter.

9.2 The Concept of Chain of Infection

The chain of infection can be detailed in the following six steps:

1. **The pathogen** is the infectious agent introduced. Some are more infectious than others, and some people are more susceptible to certain microorganisms than others. Infectious agents include bacteria, fungi, viruses, prions, and parasites.
2. **The reservoir** is the source of microorganisms, including humans, plants, animals, the environment, food, or water.
3. **The portal of exit** is the way the microorganism leaves the reservoir to solidify its position as an infection. The portal of exit depends on where the organism is located in the body, which can include the GI tract, respiratory tract, genitourinary tract, blood, skin, mucous membrane, or transplacental (mother to foetus).
4. **The transmission mode** is how the microorganism travels from person to person. There are three types of infection transmission: direct (person-to-person), indirect (vehicle-borne or object-to-person), and airborne (droplets or dust in the air).
5. **The portal of entry** is how a microorganism enters the body. Broken skin, mucous membranes, digestive system, and respiratory system are some examples.
6. **Infection of a susceptible host** is the final step in this cycle. Traits that define a susceptible host include age, receiving immunosuppressive treatment, having an immune deficiency condition, having a chronic disorder of any type, or being a hospitalised patient (Fig. 9.1).

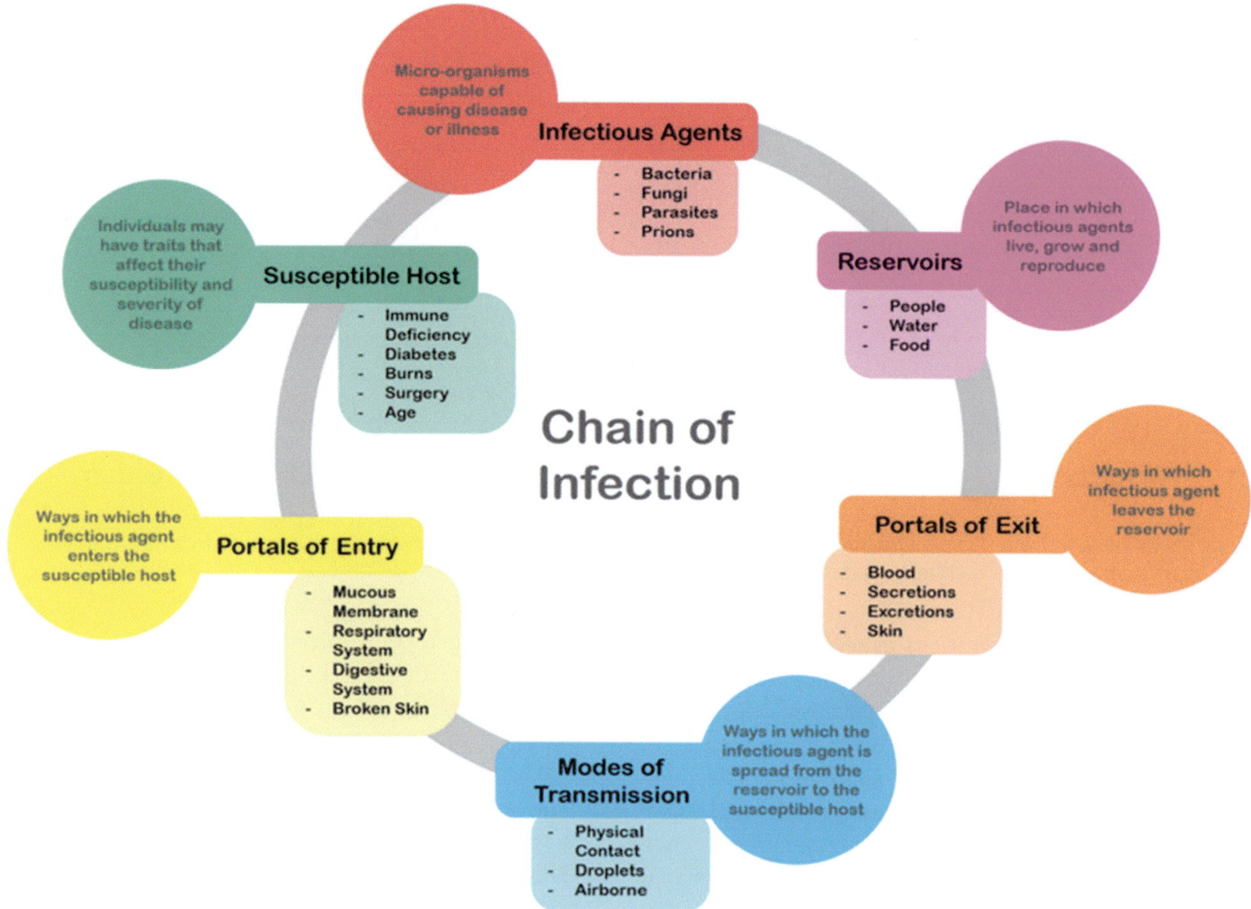

Fig. 9.1 Chain of infection

9.3 Routes and Modes of Entry of Microbes

Routes (portals) of entry of pathogens include skin, mucous membranes, respiratory tract, urogenital tract, and vertical transmission (mother to foetus or new-born child) via placental-foetal transmission, during child delivery, or postnatal transmission in breast milk).

Modes of transmission of infection include direct or indirect contact transmission.

9.3.1 Direct Transmission

1. **Person to Person.** Person-to-person transmission occurs when an infected person contacts or exchanges body fluids with a non-infected person. A mother can also transmit infections to the unborn child via the placenta. A sexually transmitted disease such as gonorrhoea is an example of direct transmission (vertical transmission).

2. **Droplet Transmission.** An infected person's droplets spread during sneezing, speaking, and coughing can transmit infections. The infections can also spread by touching the nose and mouth with hands contaminated with infectious droplets. The droplets are so minute that they travel only a short distance before falling. The people nearby might contract infections. Covid-19 transmission is an example.

3. **Spread by the skin.** There are a few infections, such as chickenpox, conjunctivitis, head lice, ringworm, etc., which spread when the skin of an infected person comes in contact with the skin of the non-infected person.

4. **Spread through body fluids or blood.** A few diseases spread when an infected person's body fluids or blood come in contact with an uninfected person's mucous membrane or bloodstream. Diseases such as hepatitis, HIV, cytomegalovirus infections, etc., spread through semen and vaginal fluids, saliva, breast milk, urine, etc.

9.3.2   Indirect Transmission

1. **Airborne Transmission.** Some infectious agents remain suspended in the air for an extended period. These pathogens might attack the immune system of a person in contact. For example, in a room initially occupied by a patient with measles, a non-infected person is likely to get infected with the disease.
2. **Contaminated Objects.** Using the contaminated household or office objects initially used by a diseased person might render the uninfected individual to acquire infection. Contaminated blood and medical supplies can also spread infections.
3. **Vector-Borne Diseases.** Blood-sucking insects transmit some infectious agents. The insects feed on hosts such as birds, animals, and humans and carry infectious agents. These infections are transmitted to some new host. Malaria and Lyme disease are two vector-borne diseases.
4. **Food and Drinking Water.** Improperly canned and undercooked food is the main source of infections. Water also carries various pathogens from rivers and lakes. It should be boiled or filtered before use. *E. coli* is transmitted through contaminated food which causes various stomach problems. The consumption of improperly canned food causes botulism. Cholera is one example of a water-borne disease that can affect people consuming contaminated water.
5. **Transmission through Animals.** When an infected animal bites or scratches against a person, it transfers the infectious agents to the person. These agents can also be transmitted through animal waste. When diseases are transferred from animals to people, zoonosis occurs. Anthrax (sheep), rabies (dogs), and plague (rodents) are some of the diseases transmitted from animals to humans. Pregnant women and people with weak immune systems are more prone to such infections.
6. **Environmental Factors.** The infectious agents are present in the soil, water, and plants. These agents can be transmitted to people and may cause diseases. For example, Hookworm is transmitted through contaminated soil. Legionnaires' disease is spread by water supplied to condensers and cooling towers.

Infectious diseases result from the interaction of host immune responses and microbial virulence factors. Infectious agents can cause disease by (1) entering cells and directly causing cell death, (2) releasing cytotoxic toxins, (3) releasing tissue-degrading enzymes, (4) damaging blood vessels, (5) causing tissue necrosis due to ischemia, and (6) inducing host inflammatory responses that can cause tissue injury.

9.4   Host Defences against Infection

Physical barrier. The epithelial surfaces of the body serve as an effective physical barrier against most microorganisms. *The epithelial surfaces of the skin or mucous membranes protect against the colonisation of pathogens by preventing pathogen adherence and secreting antimicrobial enzymes and peptides.* For example, the antibacterial enzyme lysozyme is secreted in tears and saliva, and the acid pH of the stomach and the digestive enzymes of the upper gastrointestinal tract creates a substantial chemical barrier to infection.

Most epithelial surfaces are associated with a normal flora of non-pathogenic bacteria that compete with pathogenic microorganisms for nutrients and attachment sites on cells. The normal flora can also produce antimicrobial substances.

Phagocytosis. When microorganisms cross an epithelial barrier and begin to replicate in the host's tissues, they are, in most cases, immediately recognised by the mononuclear phagocytes, or macrophages, that reside in tissues. Cell types such as macrophages or neutrophils are considered "professional phagocytic cells" as they function to eliminate foreign material and pathogens as part of an organism's immune response. Macrophages have a crucial role in host defence. They encounter pathogens in the tissues and are soon reinforced by the recruitment of a large number of neutrophils to sites of infection. *Macrophages and neutrophils recognise pathogens using cell-surface receptors that discriminate between the surface molecules displayed by pathogens and the host.* Macrophages and neutrophils have granules called lysosomes that contain enzymes, proteins, and peptides that can mediate an intracellular antimicrobial response. Phagocytic cells take up microbes and other particles into membrane-bounded organelles called phagosomes. Phagosome undergoes a maturation process, transforming into a phagolysosome (Fig. 9.2). Upon phagocytosis, macrophages and neutrophils also produce various other toxic products that help kill the engulfed microorganism. The most important of these are hydrogen peroxide (H_2O_2), superoxide anion (O_2^-), and nitric oxide (NO), which are directly toxic to bacteria.

Inflammatory and immune responses. *Phagocytosis leads to an inflammatory response. Once the inflammation has begun, the first cells attracted to the site of infection are generally neutrophils. They are followed by monocytes, which differentiate into more tissue macrophages.* In the later stages of inflammation, other leukocytes, such as eosinophils and lymphocytes, enter the infected site. The inflammatory response causes the accumulation of plasma proteins, including the complement components that provide circulating (humoral) innate immunity.

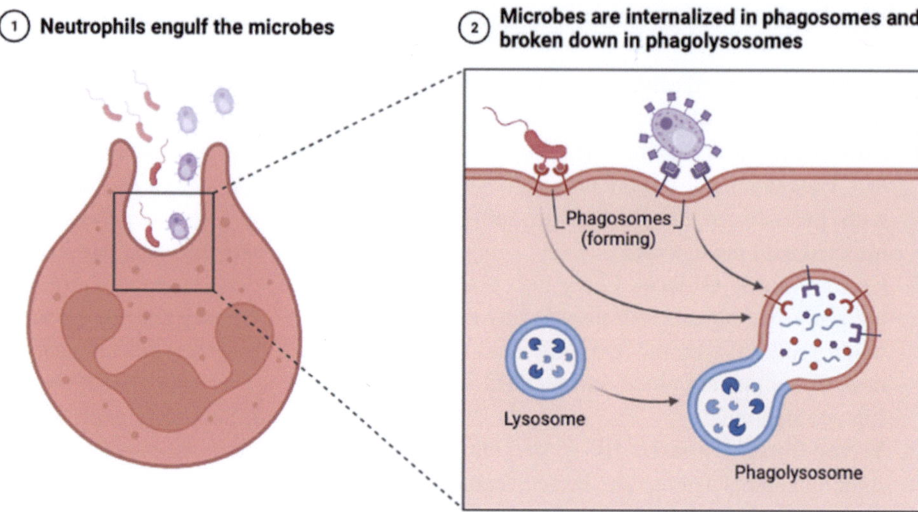

Fig. 9.2 The antimicrobial function of phagocytosis

Innate immunity provides host defence through effector mechanisms that engage the pathogen directly. These mechanisms often succeed in preventing an infection from becoming established. Innate responses often fail to clear the infection. In this case, macrophages and other cells activated in the early innate response help to initiate the development of an adaptive immune response.

9.5 Types of Infectious Agents and Mechanism of Infections

There are five major types of infectious agents: bacteria, viruses, fungi, protozoa, and helminths. In addition, a new class of infectious agents, the prions, has been recognised. Below is a brief description of the general characteristics of each of these agents and examples of some diseases they cause.

9.5.1 Bacteria

Bacteria are unicellular prokaryotic organisms with no organised internal membranous structures such as nuclei, mitochondria, or lysosomes. Their genomes are circular, double-stranded DNA associated with much less protein than eukaryotic genomes. Most bacteria reproduce by growing and dividing into two cells in a process known as binary fission. There are a variety of morphologies among bacteria, but three of the most common are bacillus (rod-shaped), coccus (spherical), or spirillum (helical rods). The energy sources for bacteria vary. Some bacteria are photosynthetic and obtain their energy directly from the sun. Others oxidise inorganic compounds to supply their energy needs. Still, other bacteria generate energy by breaking down organic compounds such as amino acids and sugars in a respiratory process. Some bacteria require oxygen (aerobes), while others cannot tolerate it (anaerobes). Some bacteria can grow either with or without oxygen (facultative anaerobes). Bacteria are frequently divided into two broad classes based on their cell wall structures, which influence their Gram stain reaction (Gram-negative and Gram-positive bacteria). Gram-negative bacteria appear pink, and Gram-positive bacteria purple after the staining procedures.

9.5.1.1 Mechanisms of Bacterial Injury

The ability of bacteria to cause disease depends on their ability to adhere to host cells (adherence or adhesion), invade host cells and tissues, and deliver toxins that can damage host cells and tissues (Fig. 9.3).

Adherence to host cells: Surface molecules called adhesins bind to the specific host cells. This phenomenon is known as tissue tropism. Adherence is also mediated by filamentous bacterial surface proteins called *pili*.

Invasion, cell lysis, and evasion of host defences: Once the cells are invaded, bacteria can kill the host cells by rapid replication and lysis. However, some bacteria permit cellular viability and proliferate within endosomes or cytoplasm, thus evading intracellular defences.

Production of toxins and tissue damage: Toxins produced by bacteria are integral to infectious-disease processes. Bacterial toxins are divided into exotoxins and endotoxins. Exotoxins are proteins produced inside pathogenic bacteria, most commonly Gram-positive bacteria, as part of their growth and metabolism. Exotoxins are then secreted or released into the surrounding medium following lysis. Endotoxins are lipid portions of lipopolysaccharides that are part of Gram-negative bacteria's outer membrane of the cell wall. Endotoxins are liberated when the bacteria die, and the cell wall breaks apart.

In some cases, more than one toxin is produced by a given bacteria. *Staphylococcus aureus* strains, for example, can

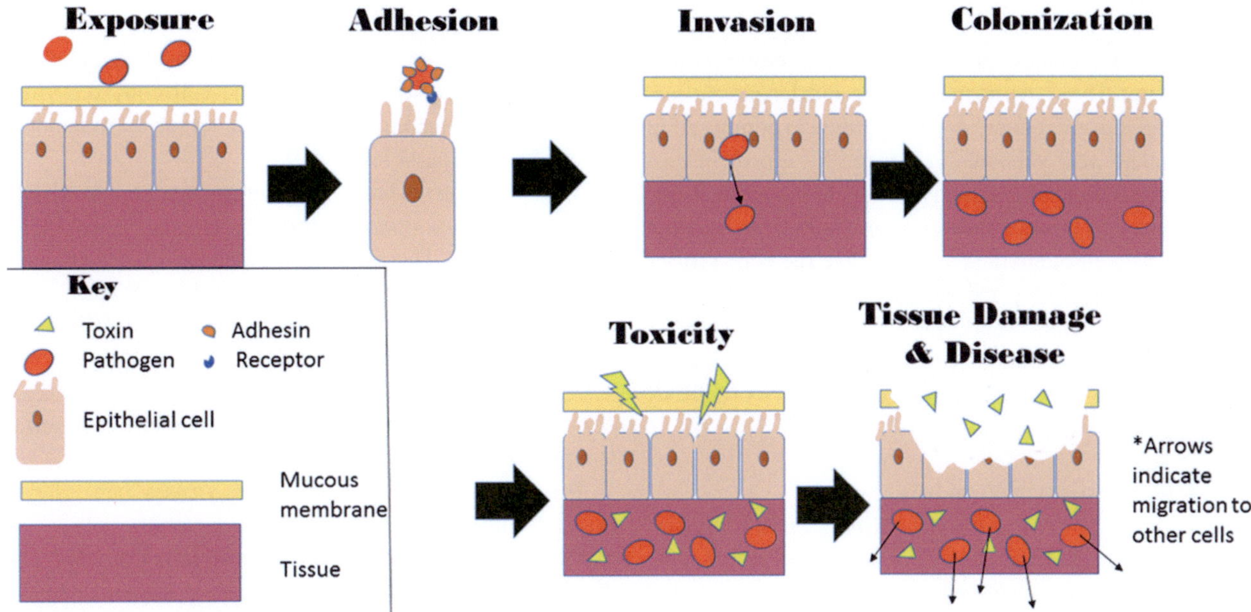

Fig. 9.3 Steps of pathogenic bacterial infection (Wikipedia)

release toxins such as haemolysins, leukotoxins, exfoliative toxins, enterotoxins, and toxic shock syndrome toxin 1 (TSST-1). The causative organisms of diphtheria and pertussis are *Corynebacterium diphtheriae* and *Bordetella pertussis*, which express diphtheria toxin [DT] and pertussis toxin [PT], respectively. Clostridial neurotoxins produced by *Clostridium tetani* (TeNT) and *Clostridium botulinum* (BoNT) are among the most potent poisons.

Infection occurs over many steps, first starting with exposure to the pathogen. Once exposed, the pathogen travels through the mucous membrane and attaches to epithelial cells. This will ultimately give the pathogen a chance to invade further into the skin and grow in numbers or colonise that area. Once there is a high enough number of pathogens that have proliferated, the microbes use quorum sensing to determine when they are enough to spread further to other tissues. The pathogens then release toxins that subsequently cause tissue damage and disease.

9.5.1.2 Examples of Bacterial Diseases

Only a few examples are provided below.

Staphylococcal infections include skin infections, abscesses, endocarditis, osteomyelitis, and pneumonia. Common streptococcal infections are pharyngitis, scarlet fever, pneumonia, rheumatic fever, and glomerulonephritis. Enterococcal infections include cystitis, pyelonephritis, catheter-associated urinary tract infections (UTIs), and endocarditis. Neisserial infections cause Neisseria meningitidis

and Neisseria gonorrhoeae. Spirochetal (*Treponema pallidum*) infection causes the sexually transmitted disease syphilis. Lyme disease, also known as Lyme borreliosis, is a vector-borne disease caused by the Borrelia bacterium, Pertussis, commonly known as whooping cough, is a disease of the respiratory tract caused by the bacterium *Bordetella pertussis*, mycobacterial infections include tuberculosis (*M. tuberculosis*) and leprosy (*M. laprae*), and *Salmonella typhi* causes typhoid.

Orofacial examples of bacterial infections. Oral and maxillofacial infections may be conveniently categorised as odontogenic and non-odontogenic. More than 90% of all infections in the head and neck region can be traced back to an odontogenic origin. Odontogenic infections include dental caries, periodontal disease, and suppurative deep space infections. Non-odontogenic infections include pyogenic infections of the face and neck, infections of the oral mucosa, oropharyngeal candidosis (candidiasis), sialadenitis, and parotitis. The most common bacterial species involved in odontogenic infections are anaerobic Gram-positive cocci, such as *Peptostreptococcus* and *Streptococcus milleri*. Anaerobes generally outnumber aerobes at all sites by a factor of 10:1. While anaerobes are likely the predominant pathogens in most orofacial infections, other pathogens such as *Staphylococcus aureus* and facultative Gram-negative rods, including *Pseudomonas aeruginosa*, may be present in a small but significant proportion of cases, particularly in immunocompromised patients.

9.5.2 Viruses

Viruses are the smallest particles, typically ranging from 0.02 to 0.3 μm. They have no metabolism and depend entirely on living cells to reproduce. A virus particle is composed of a viral nucleic acid genome surrounded by a protein coat called a capsid. In addition, many viruses infect animals and are surrounded by an outer lipid envelope, which they acquire from the host cell membrane as they leave the cell. Viruses are classified principally according to the nature and structure of their genome. There are DNA viruses and RNA viruses; each type may have single or double strands of DNA (a DNA virus) or double- or single-strands of RNA (an RNA virus).

9.5.2.1 Mechanism of Viral Infections

Pathogenic mechanisms of the viral disease include implantation of the virus at the portal of entry, local replication, spread to target organs (disease sites), and spread to sites of shedding the virus into the environment. For the successful initiation of infection, three requirements must be satisfied: (1) An inoculum containing sufficient viable virus to establish an infection, (2) viruses must first reach and interact with susceptible cells capable of supporting virus replication, and (3) the host's innate immunity and pre-existing adaptive immunity must be insufficient to abort the infection immediately. When a virus infects a cell, it forces it to make thousands of more viruses. It makes the cell copy the virus's DNA or RNA, making viral proteins, which all assemble to form new virus particles (Fig. 9.4).

The following six basic overlapping stages are involved in the mechanism of viral infection.

Attachment. The virus first attaches to the host cell at one or several receptor molecules on the cell surface. For example, the human immunodeficiency virus (HIV) infects human T cells because of its surface protein, glycoprotein 120 (gp120), which is essential for virus entry into cells as it plays a vital role in attachment to specific cell surface receptors.

Penetration follows attachment; viruses penetrate the host cell through endocytosis or fusion with the cell.

Uncoating. After entering the host cell, the virus separates from the outer cover. This uncoating happens when the viral capsid is removed and destroyed by viral enzymes or host enzymes, thereby exposing the viral nucleic acid.

Replication of virus particles is when viral messenger RNA is used in the protein synthesis systems to produce viral proteins.

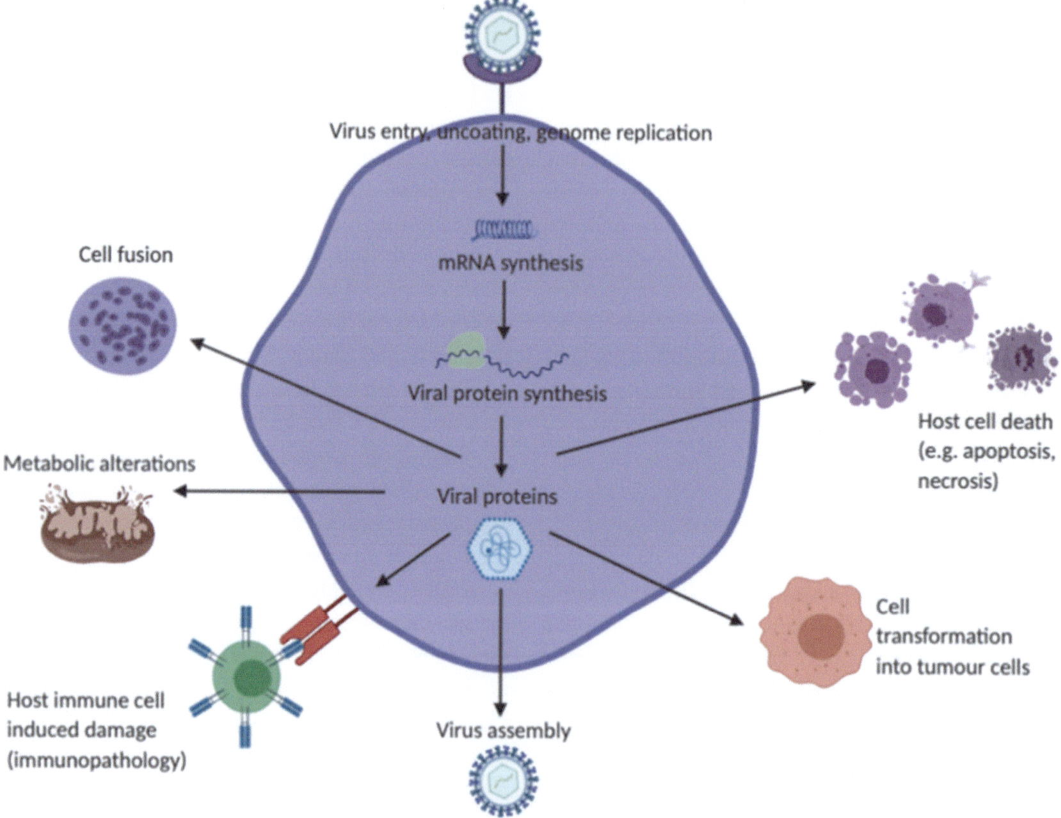

Fig. 9.4 Mechanisms by which viruses cause damage and disease to host cells. (Wikipedia) Credit: By Isabellelyy- CC BY-SA 4.0, https://en.wikipedia.org/w/index.php?curid=63643177

Assembly occurs in the cell when the newly created viral proteins and nucleic acid combine to form hundreds of new virus particles.

Release occurs when the new viruses escape or are released from the cell. Most viruses achieve this by making the cells burst, a process called lysis. Other viruses, such as HIV, are released more gently by a process called budding.

Each step of viral replication involves different enzymes and substrates and offers an opportunity to interfere with the infection process.

Retroviruses use reverse transcription to create a double-stranded DNA copy (a provirus) of their RNA genome, which is inserted into the genome of their host cell. Reverse transcription is accomplished using the enzyme reverse transcriptase, which the virus carries inside its shell. Examples of retroviruses are the human immunodeficiency virus (HIV) and the human T-cell leukaemia virus.

A latent viral infection is a type of persistent viral infection distinguished from a chronic one. Latency is the phase in certain viruses' life cycles in which, after initial infection, the proliferation of virus particles ceases. However, the viral genome is not eradicated. The virus can reactivate and produce large amounts of viral progeny (the lytic part of the viral life cycle) without the host becoming reinfected by the new virus and staying within the host indefinitely. Examples include herpes zoster and labial herpes simplex infections.

Examples of viral diseases: Viruses can cause a wide range of infections involving several organ systems, including the central nervous system, respiratory system, cardiovascular system, gastrointestinal system, genitourinary system, liver, pancreas, salivary glands, skin, and oral and pharyngeal mucosa (Fig. 9.5). Some viruses are oncogenic and predispose to certain cancers. Examples include Human papillomavirus (HPV), which causes cervical carcinoma, penile carcinoma, vaginal carcinoma, anal carcinoma, oropharyngeal carcinoma, and oesophageal carcinoma. Human T-lymphotropic virus 1 causes certain types of human leukaemia and lymphoma. Epstein-Barr virus (EBV): causes nasopharyngeal carcinoma, Burkitt lymphoma, Hodgkin lymphoma, and lymphomas in immunosuppressed organ transplant recipients. Hepatitis B and hepatitis C viruses cause Hepatocellular carcinoma is associated with Kaposi sarcoma (predominantly in HIV disease).

Orofacial examples of viral infections. In most instances, viral infections of the orofacial region give rise to short-term local illnesses. Common infections include

Fig. 9.5 An overview of viral infections (Wikipedia)

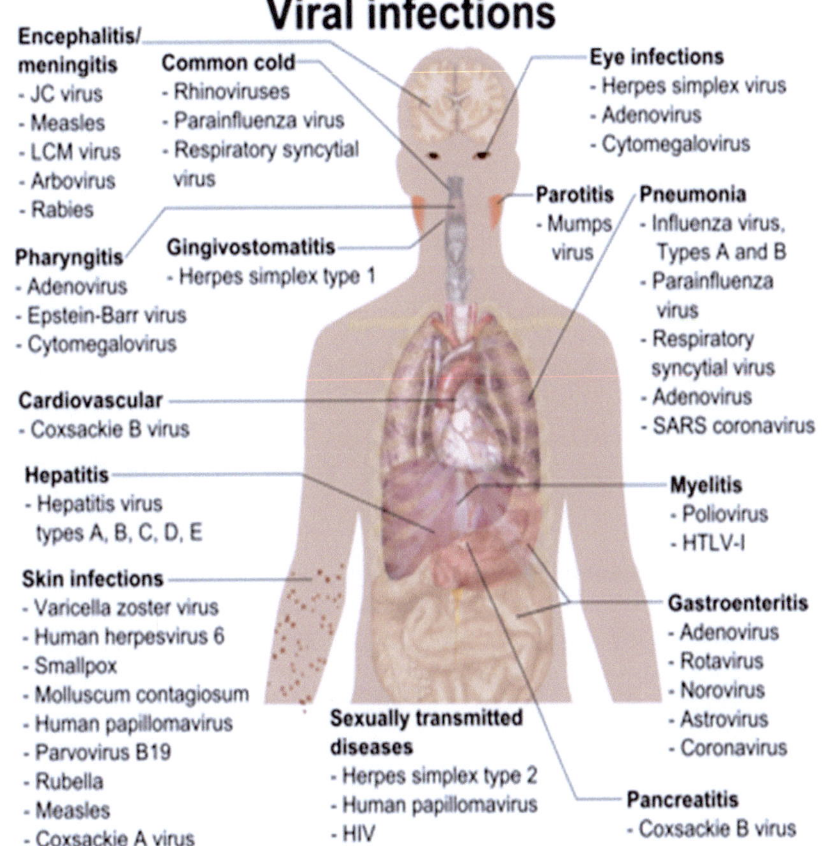

herpetic gingivostomatitis (herpes simplex virus), shingles (varicella zoster), infectious mononucleosis (EBV), cytomegalovirus infection, and mumps. Infections such as Human Immunodeficiency viruses (HIV), Epstein-Barr virus (EBV), and the oncogenic types of Human Papillomavirus (HPV) can cause significant orofacial disease that increases patient morbidity. A detailed description of oral viral infections can be found in oral medicine textbooks.

9.5.3 Fungi

Fungi are eukaryotic, heterotrophic organisms with rigid cellulose- or chitin-based cell walls and reproduce primarily by forming spores. Being eukaryotes, a typical fungal cell contains a true nucleus, mitochondria, and a complex system of internal membranes, including the endoplasmic reticulum and Golgi apparatus. The cell wall comprises polysaccharides, proteins, lipids, and pigments. The fungal cell wall gives shape and form, protects against mechanical injury, and prevents osmotic lysis. Fungal cells have two basic morphological types: true hyphae (multicellular filamentous fungi) and yeasts (unicellular fungi). Most fungi grow as hyphae, cylindrical, thread-like structures 2–10 μm in diameter and up to several centimetres in length. Fungi like moist and slightly acidic environments; they can grow with or without light or oxygen. Fungi are saprophyte heterotrophs using dead or decomposing organic matter as a carbon source. They can reproduce sexually and asexually. Sexual reproduction occurs by the fusion of two haploid nuclei (karyogamy), followed by the meiotic division of the diploid nucleus. Asexual reproduction occurs via the division of nuclei by mitosis. They reproduce asexually by fragmentation, budding, or producing spores.

Pathogenic fungi. Fungi pathogenic to humans include *Candida species (Candida albicans, Candida stellatoidea, Candida tropicalis, Candida pseudotropicalis, Candida krusei, Candida parapsilosis, and Candida guilliermondii), Aspergillus fumigatus, Aspergillus flavus, Cryptococcus neoformans, Histoplasma capsulatum,* and *Pneumocystis jirovecii.*

9.5.3.1 Mechanism of Fungal Infections

Fungal infections can be local or systemic. Local fungal infections typically involve the skin, mouth, and vagina (causing and may occur in normal or immunocompromised hosts. Systemic fungal infections can affect the skin and organs such as the lungs, liver, and brain and typically occur in immunocompromised hosts. Primary fungal infections usually result from the inhalation of fungal spores, which can cause localised pneumonia as the primary manifestation of infection. *Many fungi are opportunists and are generally not pathogenic except in an immunocompromised host. Causes of immunocompromise include AIDS, diabetes mellitus, lymphoma, leukaemia, other haematologic cancers, burns, and therapy with corticosteroids, immunosuppressants, or antimetabolites.*

Since Candidal infection is the most common fungal infection, the following discussion focuses on its mechanism of infection. *Candida albicans* normally exists as harmless commensal yeast on the mucosal surfaces of most of the human population. Only under certain circumstances (imbalance of the normal microbial flora, immunosuppression, damage of tissue barriers) can *C. albicans* cause superficial (oral thrush in 90% of all untreated HIV patients, vaginal thrush in 75% of all women once in their lifetime) or life-threatening systemic infections. Almost all *C. albicans* infections are endogenous infections caused by commensal strains of patients' microflora.

C. albicans selectively adheres to buccal and vaginal epithelial cells in humans, and adherence may play a critical role in the pathogenesis of mucocutaneous candidiasis. It can utilise two mechanisms to invade host cells: induced endocytosis and active penetration. Induced endocytosis usually takes place within 4 h of initial contact of *Candida* with the cells of the epithelium. For induced endocytosis, the fungus expresses specialised proteins on the cell surface that mediate binding to host ligands, thereby triggering the engulfment of the fungal cell into the host cell. The general steps in tissue invasion by *C. albicans* include (1) Adhesion to the epithelial cells, (2) Colonisation, (3) Epithelial penetration/invasion by hyphae, (4) Vascular dissemination, and (5) Endothelial colonisation/penetration.

Adherence/colonisation: As soon as the host's environment is optimal for invasion, *Candida* species express adhesins, which help them adhere to the epithelium of mucosal membranes, such as the oral cavity and vaginal tract, as well as the plastics used for catheterisation.

Invasion/epithelial penetration: Alternative proteins (invasins) are expressed once the *Candida* has adhered. Enzymes, such as Secreted Aspartyl Proteases (SAPs), help to break down the host cell membrane. Another contributing factor to the invasion of tissue is the dimorphic switch from yeast form to hyphal form.

Endothelial colonisation/dissemination: Once the *Candida* has penetrated the epithelial basement membrane, they are exposed to the bloodstream, where they are disseminated throughout the body. Disseminated candidiasis only occurs when *Candida* escapes the immune system, penetrates vascular tissues, and enters the blood. Different genes are upregulated for *Candida* to survive and propagate in the blood. The presence of *Candida* in the blood leads to a condition called candidemia. From the blood, the yeast is disseminated to various vital organs in the body, where it causes systemic infections. Disseminated candidiasis is highly facilitated by extracellular hydrolytic enzymes, adhesins, phenotypic switching, and cytolytic proteins. *Candida* in the blood can also give rise to candiduria as the organism can gain access to the upper urinary tract (antegrade infection) (Fig. 9.6).

9.5.3.2 Examples of Fungal Diseases

Fungal infections are often classified as either primary or opportunistic. Primary infections can develop in immunocompetent hosts, whereas opportunistic infections develop mainly in immunocompromised patients, including those with AIDS, chemotherapy, or organ recipients. Some opportunistic fungal infections are serious. Examples include cryptococcal meningitis (caused by *C. neoformans*) and aspergillosis (lung infection caused by *Aspergillus* species). Cryptococcal meningitis is one of the leading causes of death in HIV patients and is a severe problem for other immunocompromised populations. Fungal spores in the soil generally cause community-acquired fungal infections. People inhale the spores when the soil is disrupted, resulting in diseases such as blastomycosis, histoplasmosis, and coccidioidomycosis (valley fever). Bloodstream Candidal infection (Candidemia) can occur as a hospital-acquired (nosocomial) fungal infection.

Orofacial examples of fungal infections. This opportunistic pathogen causes oral candidiasis (thrush), usually in immunosuppressed individuals, such as patients with HIV/AIDS or undergoing chemotherapy. Patients with diabetes who wear dentures, use steroid inhalers, or have chronic xerostomia (dry mouth) are also at risk of developing oral candidiasis. In addition, antibiotic therapy can decrease the number of bacteria in the oral cavity that competes with *C. albicans* for available nutrients, leading to oral candidiasis.

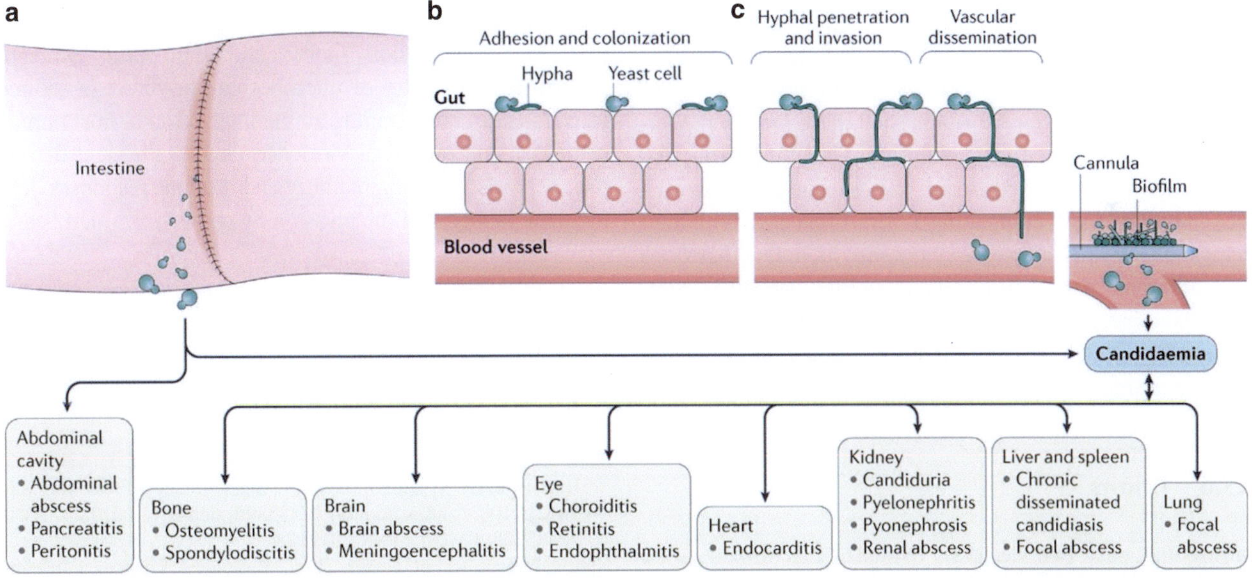

Fig. 9.6 Pathogenesis of invasive candidiasis. *Candida* spp. can be detected on the mucosal surfaces of ~50–70% of healthy humans. (**a**) When breaches in the intestinal barriers occur, for example, after gastrointestinal surgery, *Candida* spp. can directly disseminate to the abdominal cavity and invade the bloodstream (candidaemia). (**b**) Under normal conditions, the fungus behaves as a commensal organism without causing disease. (**c**) Impairment of immune response, among other factors, can promote fungal overgrowth in the gut and candidaemia, leading to deep-seated opportunistic infections in various organs (invasive candidiasis). Source: Pappas, P., Lionakis, M., Arendrup, M. et al. Invasive candidiasis. Nat Rev Dis Primers 4, 18,026 (2018). https://doi.org/10.1038/nrdp.2018.26. Publisher: Springer Nature. Copyright © 2018, Macmillan Publishers Limited

9.5.4 Protozoa

Protozoa are unicellular, heterotrophic eukaryotes that include the familiar amoeba and paramecium. Because protozoa do not have cell walls, they can perform various rapid and flexible movements. *Protozoa can be acquired through contaminated food or water or by biting an infected arthropod such as a mosquito.* Diarrheal disease in the United States can be caused by two common protozoan parasites, *Giardia lamblia* and *Cryptosporidium parvum*. Malaria, a tropical illness that causes 300 million to 500 million cases of the disease annually, is caused by several species of the protozoan *Plasmodium*.

9.5.5 Helminths

Helminths are simple, invertebrate animals, some of which are infectious parasites. They are multicellular and have differentiated tissues. *Many helminths have complex reproductive cycles that include multiple stages, many, or all of which require a host.* Examples include *Schistosoma* and Trichinosis. Schistosoma **is** a flatworm that causes the mild disease swimmer's itch in the United States; another species of *Schistosoma* causes the much more serious schistosomiasis, which is endemic in Africa and Latin America. *Schistosoma* eggs hatch in freshwater, and the resulting larvae infect snails. When the snails shed these larvae, the larvae attach to and penetrate human skin. They feed, grow, and mate in the human bloodstream; the damage to human tissues caused by the accumulating *Schistosoma* eggs with their sharp spines results in disease symptoms, including diarrhoea and abdominal pain. Liver and spleen involvement is common. Trichinosis is a disease caused by the roundworm *Trichinella spiralis*. This infectious agent is typically ingested in improperly cooked pork from infected pigs.

9.5.6 Prions

During the past two decades, evidence has linked some degenerative disorders of the central nervous system to infectious particles that consist only of protein. These "proteinaceous infectious particles" have been named prions.

Examples of diseases caused by prions include Creutzfeldt-Jakob disease (CJD) in humans), scrapie in sheep, and bovine spongiform encephalopathy ("mad cow disease" in cattle). These frequently result in brain tissue that is riddled with holes. While some prion diseases are inherited (e.g. familial CJD), others are apparently due to infection by eating infected tissue or through medical procedures such as transplants. Prion diseases are fatal.

9.6 Summary

Invasion of tissues by pathogens, their multiplication, and the reaction of host tissues to the infectious agent and the toxins they produce are essential elements of infectious diseases. Diseases caused by microbes can be infectious, communicable, or opportunistic. Infections depend on the invasion of tissues by pathogens, their multiplication, and the reaction of host tissues to the infectious agent and the toxins they produce. Communicable diseases, also known as contagious diseases, are illnesses caused by viruses or bacteria that people spread to one another. When non-pathogenic commensal organisms in the body become pathogenic and cause diseases, the infection is called opportunistic infection. The chain of infection involves the pathogen, the reservoir, the portal of exit, the transmission mode, and the portal of entry. Transmission of entry of microbes can be direct or indirect. Infectious diseases result from the interaction of host immune responses and microbial virulence factors. Physical barriers, phagocytosis, and inflammatory and immune responses determine the outcome of the invasion by pathogenic microbes.

Bibliography

McAdam AJ, Frank KM. General pathology of infectious diseases. In: Kumar V, Abbas AK, Aster JC, editors. Robbins basic pathology. 10th ed. Philadelphia: Elsevier; 2018. p. 341–58.

Horn F, Heinekamp T, Kniemeyer O, Pollmächer J, Valiante V, Brakhage AA. Systems biology of fungal infection. Front Microbiol. 2012;3:108. https://doi.org/10.3389/fmicb.2012.00108. PMID: 22485108; PMCID: PMC3317178

National Institutes of Health (US). Biological sciences curriculum study. Bethesda (MD): National Institutes of Health (US); 2007.

Ryan KJ, Ray CG. Chapter 7 viral pathogenesis. In: Sherris medical microbiology. 6th ed. New York: Mc Graw Hill Medical; 2014.

10.1 Introduction

There are continuous advances in our current understanding of the immune system and how it functions to protect the body from infection. Given the complex nature of this subject, it is beyond the scope of this chapter to provide an in-depth review of all aspects of immunology. Instead, this chapter aims to provide a basic introduction to the main components and function of the immune system and its role in both health and disease.

10.2 The Immune System: Innate and Adaptive Immunity.

The immune system refers to a collection of cells, chemicals, and processes that function to protect the skin, respiratory passages, intestinal tract, and other areas from foreign antigens, such as microbes (organisms such as bacteria, fungi, and parasites), viruses, cancer cells, and toxins.

10.2.1 Innate Immunity

Innate immunity represents the first line of defence against an intruding pathogen. It is an antigen-independent (non-specific) defence mechanism used by the host immediately or within hours of encountering an antigen. The innate immune response has no immunologic memory and, therefore, cannot recognise or "memorise" the same pathogen should the body be exposed to it in the future. Adaptive immunity, on the other hand, is antigen-dependent and antigen-specific and, therefore, involves a lag time between exposure to the antigen and maximal response. The hallmark of adaptive immunity is the capacity for memory which enables the host to mount a more rapid and efficient immune response upon subsequent exposure to the antigen. Innate and adaptive immunities are not mutually exclusive mechanisms of host defence but complementary, with defects in either system resulting in host vulnerability or inappropriate responses.

Innate immunity comprises four types of defensive barriers: anatomic (skin and mucous membrane), physiologic (temperature, low pH, and chemical mediators), endocytic and phagocytic, and inflammatory. Table 10.1 summarises the non-specific host-defence mechanisms for each of these barriers. Cells and processes that are critical for effective innate immunity to pathogens that evade anatomic barriers have been widely studied. Innate immunity to pathogens relies on pattern recognition receptors (PRRs) which allow a limited range of immune cells to detect and respond rapidly to a wide range of pathogens that share common structures, known as pathogen-associated molecular patterns (PAMPs). Examples include bacterial cell wall components such as lipopolysaccharides (LPS) and double-stranded ribonucleic acid (RNA) produced during viral infection.

An essential function of innate immunity is the rapid recruitment of immune cells to sites of infection and inflammation through the production of cytokines and chemokines (small proteins involved in cell-cell communication and recruitment). Cytokine production during innate immunity mobilises many defence mechanisms throughout the body while also activating local cellular responses to infection or injury. Key inflammatory cytokines released during the early response to bacterial infection are tumour necrosis factor (TNF), interleukin 1 (IL-1), and interleukin 6 (IL-6). These cytokines are critical for initiating cell recruitment and local inflammation, which is essential for the clearance of many pathogens. They also contribute to the development of fever. Dysregulated production of such inflammatory cytokines is often associated with inflammatory or autoimmune disease, making them important therapeutic targets.

The complement system is a biochemical cascade that identifies and opsonises (coats) bacteria and other pathogens. It renders pathogens susceptible to phagocytosis, a process by which immune cells engulf microbes and remove cell debris, and also kill some pathogens and infected cells

S. R. Prabhu, *Textbook of General Pathology for Dental Students*, https://doi.org/10.1007/978-3-031-31244-1_10

Table 10.1 Summary of non-specific host-defence mechanisms for barriers to innate immunity

Barrier	Mechanism
Anatomic	
Skin	• Mechanical barrier retards the entry of microbes • Acidic environment (pH 3–5) retards the growth of microbes
Mucous membrane	• Normal flora compete with microbes for attachment sites • Mucous entraps foreign microbes • Cilia propel microbes out of the body
Physiologic	
Temperature	• Body temperature/fever response inhibits the growth of some pathogens
Low pH	• Acidic pH of the stomach kills most undigested microbes
Chemical mediators	• Lysozyme cleaves bacterial cell wall • Interferon induces antiviral defences in uninfected cells • Complement lyses microbes or facilitates phagocytosis
Phagocytic/endocytic barriers	
	• Various cells internalise (endocytosis) and break down foreign macromolecules • Specialized cells (blood monocytes, neutrophils, tissue macrophages) internalise (phagocytose), kill, and digest whole organisms
Inflammatory barriers	
	• Tissue damage and infection induce leakage of vascular fluid containing serum protein with antibacterial activity, leading to an influx of phagocytic cells into the affected area

directly. The phagocytic action of the innate immune response promotes the clearance of dead cells or antibody complexes and removes foreign substances present in organs, tissues, blood, and lymph. It can also activate the adaptive immune response through the mobilisation and activation of antigen-presenting cells (APCs).

Numerous cells are involved in the innate immune response, such as phagocytes (macrophages and neutrophils), dendritic cells, mast cells, basophils, eosinophils, natural killer (NK) cells, and innate lymphoid cells (Table 10.1). Phagocytes are subdivided into two main cell types: neutrophils and macrophages. These cells share a similar function: to engulf (phagocytose) microbes and kill them through multiple bactericidal pathways. In addition to their phagocytic properties, neutrophils contain granules and enzyme pathways that assist in the elimination of pathogenic microbes. Unlike neutrophils (which are short-lived cells), macrophages are long-lived cells that not only play a role in phagocytosis but are also involved in antigen presentation to T cells (Table 10.2).

Dendritic cells also phagocytose and function as APCs, initiating the acquired immune response and acting as impor-

tant messengers between innate and adaptive immunities. Mast cells and basophils share many salient features, and both are instrumental in initiating acute inflammatory responses, such as those seen in allergies and asthma. Mast cells also have essential functions as immune "sentinel cells" and are early producers of cytokines in response to infection or injury. Unlike mast cells, which generally reside in the connective tissue surrounding blood vessels and are particularly common at mucosal surfaces, basophils reside in circulation. Eosinophils are granulocytes that possess phagocytic properties and play an important role in destroying parasites that are often too large to be phagocytosed.

Along with mast cells and basophils, they also control mechanisms associated with allergy and asthma. Natural killer (NK) cells play a major role in rejecting tumours and destroying cells infected by viruses. Destruction of infected cells is achieved through the release of perforins and granzymes (proteins that cause the lysis of target cells) from NK-cell granules which induce apoptosis (programmed cell death). NK cells are also an important source of another cytokine, interferon-gamma (IFN-γ), which helps to mobilise APCs and promote the development of effective anti-viral immunity. Innate lymphoid cells (ILCs) play a more regulatory role. Depending on their type (i.e. ILC-1, ILC-2, ILC-3), they selectively produce cytokines such as IL-4, IFN-γ, and IL-17 that help to direct the appropriate immune response to specific pathogens and contribute to immune regulation in that tissue.

The main characteristics and functions of the cells involved in the innate immune response are summarised in Table 10.2.

10.2.2 Adaptive Immunity

The development of adaptive immunity is aided by the actions of the innate immune system and is critical when innate immunity is ineffective in eliminating infectious agents. The primary functions of the adaptive immune response include recognition of specific "non-self" antigens, distinguishing them from "self" antigens; the generation of pathogen-specific immunologic effector pathways that eliminate specific pathogens or pathogen-infected cells; and the development of an immunologic memory that can quickly eliminate a specific pathogen should subsequent infections occur. Adaptive immune responses are the basis for effective immunisation against infectious diseases. *The cells of the adaptive immune system include antigen-specific T cells, which are activated to proliferate through the action of APCs, and B cells which differentiate into plasma cells to produce antibodies.* (Fig. 10.1).

Table 10.2 Characteristics and function of cells involved in innate immunity (Turvey and Broide 2010; Murphy et al. 2007; Stone et al. 2010)

Cell	Image	% in adults	Nucleus	Functions	Lifetime	Main targets
Macrophage[a]		Varies	Varies	• Phagocytosis • Antigen presentation to T cells	Month—years	• Various
Neutrophil		40–75%	Multi-lobed	• Phagocytosis • Degranulation (discharge of contents of a cell)	6 h—few days	• Bacteria • Fungi
Eosinophil		1–6%	Bi-lobed	• Degranulation • Release of enzymes, growth factors, cytokines	8–12 days (circulate for 4-5 h)	• Parasites • Various allergic tissues
Basophil		<1%	Bi- or tri-lobed	• Degranulation • Release of histamine, enzymes, cytokines	Lifetime uncertain; likely a few hours—few days	• Various allergic tissues
Mast cell		Common in tissues	Central, single-lobed	• Degranulation • Release of histamine, enzymes, cytokines	Months to years	• Parasites • Various allergic tissues
Lymphocytes (T cells)		20–40%	Deeply staining, eccentric	T helper (Th) cells (CD4+): immune response mediators Cytotoxic T cells (CD8+): cell destruction	Weeks to years	• Th cells: intracelluar bacteria • Cytotoxic T cells: virus infected and tumour cells • Natural killer cells: virus-infected and tumour cells
Monocyte		2–6%	Kidney shaped	Differentiate into macrophages and dendritic cells to elicit an immune response	Hours—days	• Various
Natural killer (NK) cell		15% (varies) of circulating lymphocytes and tissues	Single-lobed	• Tumour rejection • Destruction of infected cells • Release of perforin and granzymes which induce apoptosis	7–10 days	• Viruses • Tumour cells

[a]Dust cells (within pulmonary alveolus), histiocytes (connective tissue), Kupffer cells (liver), microglial cells (neural tissue), epithelioid cells (granulomas), osteoclasts (bone), mesangial cells (kidney)

10.2.3 T Cells and Antigen Presenting Cells(APCs)

T cells are derived from haematopoietic stem cells in the bone marrow and, following migration, mature in the thymus. These cells express a series of unique antigen-binding receptors on their membrane, known as the T-cell receptor (TCR). Each T cell expresses a single type of TCR and can rapidly proliferate and differentiate if it receives the appropriate signals. As previously mentioned, T cells require the action of APCs (usually dendritic cells, but also macrophages, B cells, fibroblasts, and epithelial cells) to recognise a specific antigen.

The surfaces of APCs express a group of proteins known as the major histocompatibility complex (MHC). MHCs are classified as either class I (also termed human leukocyte antigen [HLA] A, B, and C), which are found on all nucleated cells, or class II (also termed HLA DP, DQ, and DR), which are found only on certain cells of the immune system, including macrophages, dendritic cells, and B cells. Class I MHC molecules present endogenous (intracellular) peptides, while class II molecules on APCs present exogenous (extracellular) peptides in T cells. The MHC protein displays fragments of antigens (peptides) when a cell is infected with an intracellular pathogen, such as a virus, or has phagocytosed foreign proteins or organisms.

T cells have a wide range of unique TCRs which can bind to specific foreign peptides. During the development of the immune system, T cells that would react to antigens normally found in our body are largely eliminated. T cells are activated when they encounter an APC that has digested an antigen and displays the correct antigen fragments (peptides) bound to MHC molecules. The opportunities for the right T cells to be in contact with an APC carrying the appropriate

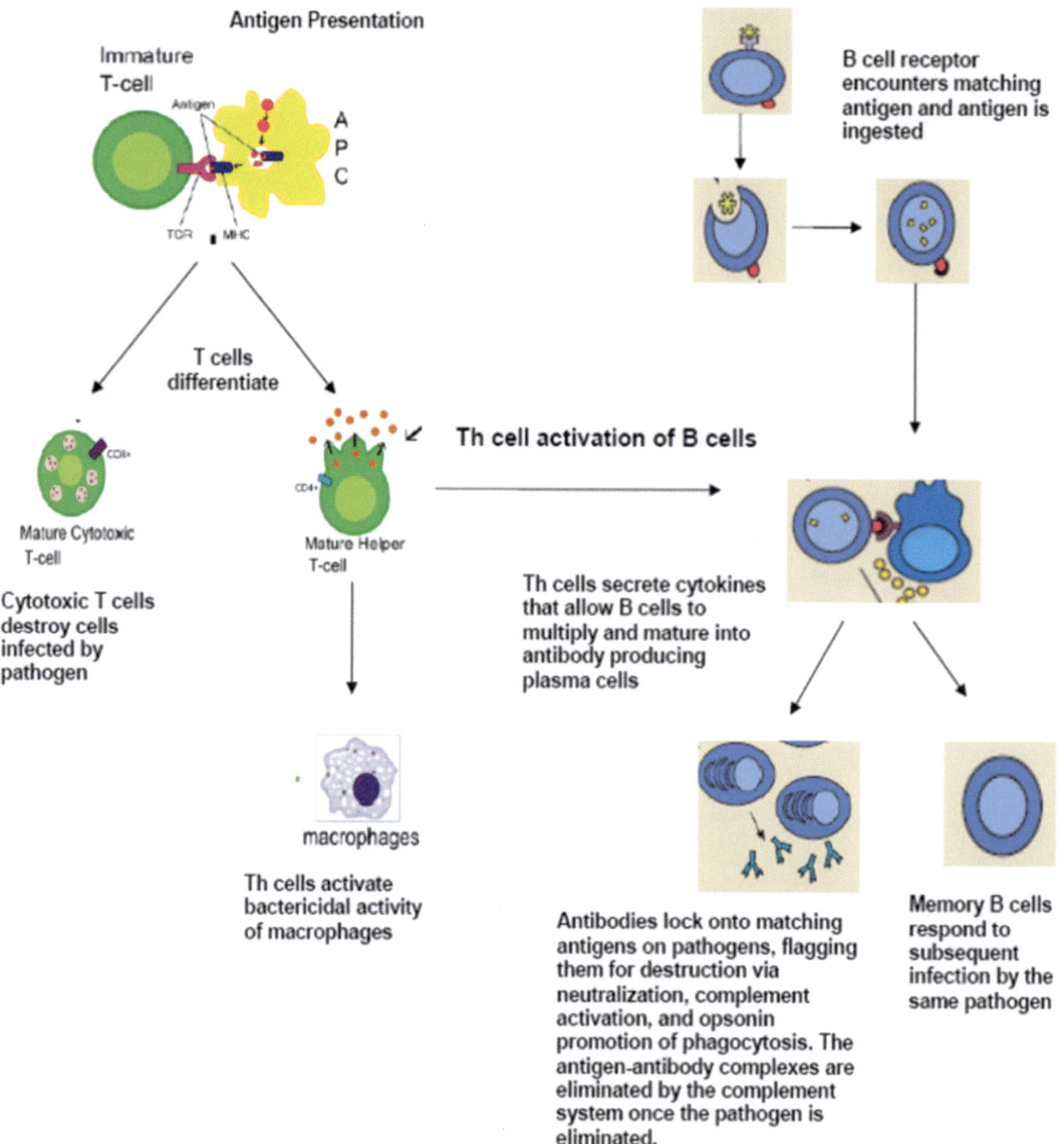

Fig. 10.1 Adaptive immunity: T-cell and B-cell activation and function. *APC* antigen-presenting cell, *TCR* T-cell receptor, *MHC* major histocompatibility complex. CD4+ Th cells are important in establishing and maximising the immune response. These cells have no cytotoxic or phagocytic activity and cannot directly kill infected cells or clear pathogens. However, they "mediate" the immune response by directing other cells to perform these tasks and regulate the type of immune response that develops. Th cells are activated through TCR recognition of antigens bound to class II MHC molecules. Once activated, Th cells release cytokines that influence the activity of many cell types, including the APCs that activate them (figure adapted from images available at: http://en.wikipedia.org/wiki/Image:B_cell_activation.png and http://commons.wikimedia.org/wiki/Image:Antigen_presentation.svg)

peptide MHC complex are increased by the circulation of T cells throughout the body (via the lymphatic system and bloodstream) and their accumulation (together with APCs) in lymph nodes. The MHC-antigen complex activates the TCR, and the T cell secretes cytokines which further control the immune response. This antigen presentation process stimulates T cells to differentiate primarily into either cytotoxic T cells (CD8+ cells) or T-helper (Th) cells (CD4+ cells) (Fig. 10.1). CD8+ cytotoxic T cells are primarily involved in the destruction of cells infected by foreign agents, such as viruses, and the killing of tumour cells expressing appropriate antigens. They are activated by the interaction of their TCR with peptides bound to MHC class I molecules. Clonal expansion of cytotoxic T cells produces effector cells which release substances that induce apoptosis of target cells. Upon resolution of the infection, most effector cells die and are cleared by phagocytes. However, a few of these cells are retained as memory cells that can quickly differentiate into effector cells upon subsequent encounters with the same antigen.

Several types of Th cell responses can be induced by an APC, with Th1, Th2, and Th17 being the most frequent. The Th1 response is characterised by the production of IFN-γ, which activates the bactericidal activities of macrophages and enhances anti-viral immunity and immunity to other intracellular pathogens. Th1-derived cytokines also contribute to the differentiation of B cells to make opsonising antibodies that enhance the efficiency of phagocytes. An inappropriate Th1 response is associated with certain autoimmune diseases.

The Th2 response is characterised by the release of cytokines (IL-4, 5, and 13) which are involved in the development of immunoglobulin E (IgE) antibody-producing B cells, as well as the development and recruitment of mast cells and eosinophils that are essential for effective responses against many parasites. In addition, they enhance the production of certain forms of IgG that aid in combating bacterial infection. As mentioned earlier, mast cells and eosinophils are instrumental in initiating acute inflammatory responses, such as those in allergies and asthma. IgE antibodies are also associated with allergic reactions (see Table 10.3). Therefore, an imbalance of Th2 cytokine production is associated with developing atopic (allergic) conditions. Th17 cells have been more recently described. They are characterised by the production of cytokines of the IL-17 family and are associated with ongoing inflammatory responses, particularly in chronic infection and disease. Like cytotoxic T cells, most Th cells will die upon resolution of infection, with a few remaining as Th memory cells.

A subset of the CD4+ T cell, known as the regulatory T cell (T reg), also plays a role in the immune response. T reg cells limit and suppress immune responses and, thereby, may function to control aberrant responses to self-antigens and the development of autoimmune disease. T-reg cells may also help resolve normal immune responses as pathogens or antigens are eliminated. These cells also play a critical role in developing "immune tolerance" to certain foreign antigens, such as those found in food.

10.2.4 B Cells

B cells arise from haematopoietic stem cells in the bone marrow and, following maturation, leave the marrow expressing a unique antigen-binding receptor on its membrane. Unlike T cells, B cells can recognise antigens directly, without needing APCs, through unique antibodies expressed on their cell surface. The principal function of B cells is the production of antibodies against foreign antigens, which requires further differentiation. Under certain circumstances, B cells can also act as APCs.

When activated by foreign antigens to which they have an appropriate antigen-specific receptor, B cells undergo proliferation and differentiate into antibody-secreting plasma cells or memory B cells. Memory B cells are "long-lived" survivors of past infection and continue to express antigen-binding receptors. These cells can be called upon to respond quickly by producing antibodies and eliminating an antigen upon re-exposure. On the other hand, plasma cells are relatively short-lived cells that often undergo apoptosis when the inciting agent that induced the immune response is eliminated. However, these cells produce large amounts of antibodies that enter the circulation and tissues providing effective protection against pathogens.

Given their function in antibody production, B cells play a major role in the humoral or antibody-mediated immune response (as opposed to the cell-mediated immune response, which is governed primarily by T cells).

Table 10.3 Major functions of human Ig antibodies (Schroeder and Cavacini 2010)

Ig antibody	Function
IgM	• First immunoglobulin (Ig) expressed during B cell development (primary response; early antibody) • Opsonizing (coating) antigen for destruction • Complement fixation
IgG	• Main Ig during a secondary immune response • Only antibodies capable of crossing the placental barrier • Neutralization of toxins and viruses • Opsonizing (coating) antigen for destruction • Complement fixation
IgD	• Function unclear; appears to be involved in homeostasis
IgA	• Mucosal response; protects mucosal surfaces from toxins, viruses, and bacteria through either direct neutralisation or prevention of binding to the mucosal surface
IgE	• Associated with hypersensitivity and allergic reactions • Plays a role in the immune response to parasites

10.3 Antibody-Mediated versus Cell-Mediated Immunity

Antibody-mediated immunity is the branch of the acquired immune system mediated by B-cell antibody production. The antibody-production pathway begins when the B cell's antigen-binding receptor recognizes and binds to the antigen in its native form. Local Th cells secrete cytokines that help the B cell multiply and direct the type of antibody that will be subsequently produced. Some cytokines, such as IL-6, help B-cells to mature into antibody-secreting plasma cells. The secreted antibodies bind to antigens on the surface of pathogens, flagging them for destruction through complement activation, opsonin promotion of phagocytosis, and pathogen elimination by immune effector cells. Upon elimination of the pathogen, the antigen-antibody complexes are cleared by the complement cascade.

Five major types of antibodies are produced by B cells: IgA, IgD, IgE, IgG, and IgM. IgG antibodies can be further subdivided into structurally distinct subclasses with differing abilities to fix complement, act as opsonins, etc. The major classes of antibodies have substantially different biological functions and recognise and neutralise specific pathogens. Table 10.3 summarises the various functions of the five Ig antibodies.

Antibodies play an important role in containing virus proliferation during the acute phase of infection. However, they are not generally capable of eliminating a virus once the infection has occurred. Once an infection is established, cell-mediated immune mechanisms are most important in host defence against most intracellular pathogens.

Cell-mediated immunity does not involve antibodies but instead protects an organism through the following:

1. The activation of antigen-specific cytotoxic T cells that induce apoptosis of cells displaying foreign antigens or derived peptides on their surface, such as virus-infected cells, cells with intracellular bacteria, and cancer cells displaying tumour antigens.
2. The activation of macrophages and NK cells, enabling them to destroy intracellular pathogens; and.
3. The stimulation of cytokine (such as IFNγ) production further mediates the effective immune response.

Cell-mediated immunity is directed primarily at microbes that survive in phagocytes and those that infect non-phagocytic cells. This type of immunity is most effective in eliminating virus-infected cells and cancer cells but can also participate in defending against fungi, protozoa, cancers, and intracellular bacteria. Cell-mediated immunity also plays a major role in transplant rejection.

10.4   Passive vs. Active Immunisation

Acquired immunity is attained through either passive or active immunisation. Passive immunisation refers to the transfer of active humoral immunity, in the form of "ready-made" antibodies, from one individual to another. It can occur naturally by transplacental transfer of maternal antibodies to the developing foetus, or it can be induced artificially by injecting a recipient with exogenous antibodies that are usually manufactured for this purpose and targeted to a specific pathogen or toxin. The latter is used when there is a high risk of infection and insufficient time for the body to develop its immune response or to reduce the symptoms of chronic or immunosuppressive diseases.

Active immunisation refers to producing antibodies against a specific antigen or pathogen after exposure to the antigen. It can be acquired through either natural infection with a microbe or through administering a vaccine consisting of attenuated (weakened) pathogens, inactivated organisms,

specific proteins, or carbohydrates known to induce immunity. Effective active immunisation often requires "adjuvants," which improve the ability of the immune system to respond to antigen injection.

10.5   Immunopathology

As mentioned earlier, defects or malfunctions in the innate or adaptive immune response can provoke illness or disease. Such disorders are generally caused by an overactive immune response (known as hypersensitivity reactions), an inappropriate reaction to self (known as autoimmunity), or ineffective immune responses (known as immunodeficiency).

10.5.1   Hypersensitivity Reactions

Hypersensitivity reactions refer to undesirable responses produced by the normal immune system. There are four types of hypersensitivity reactions:

Type I: immediate hypersensitivity
Type II: cytotoxic or antibody-dependent hypersensitivity
Type III: immune complex disease
Type IV: delayed-type hypersensitivity

Type I hypersensitivity is the most common type of hypersensitivity reaction. It is an allergic reaction provoked by re-exposure to a specific type of antigen, referred to as an allergen. Unlike the normal immune response, the type I hypersensitivity response is characterised by the secretion of IgE by plasma cells. IgE antibodies bind to receptors on the surface of tissue mast cells and blood basophils, causing them to be "sensitised." Later exposure to the same allergen cross-links the bound IgE on sensitised cells resulting in degranulation and the secretion of active mediators such as histamine, leukotrienes, and prostaglandins that cause vasodilation and smooth-muscle contraction of the surrounding tissue. Common environmental allergens inducing IgE-mediated allergies include pet (e.g. cat, dog, horse) epithelium, pollen, house dust mites, and moulds. Food allergens are also a common cause of type I hypersensitivity reactions; however, these types of reactions are more frequently seen in children than adults. Treatment of type I reactions generally involves trigger avoidance and, in the case of inhaled allergens, pharmacological intervention with broncholdilators, antihistamines, and anti-inflammatory agents. Some types of allergic diseases can be treated with immunotherapy. Severe cases of type 1 hypersensitivity (anaphylaxis) may require immediate treatment with epinephrine.

Type II hypersensitivity reactions are rare and take 2 to 24 h to develop. These reactions occur when IgG and IgM antibodies bind to the patient's cell-surface molecules, form-

Table 10.4 Types of hypersensitivity reactions

Type	Alternate name	Examples	Mediators
I	Allergy (immediate)	• Atopy – Anaphylaxis – Asthma – Allergic rhinitis – Angioedema – Food allergy	IgE
II	Cytotoxic, antibody dependent	• Erythroblastosis fetalis • Goodpasture syndrome • Autoimmune anaemias, thrombocytopenias	IgG, IgM
III	Immune complex disease	• Systemic lupus erythematosus • Serum sickness • Reactive arthritis • Arthus reaction	Aggregation of antigens IgG, IgM Complement proteins
IV	Delayed-type hypersensitivity, cell mediated, antibody independent	• Contact dermatitis • Tuberculosis • Chronic transplant rejection	T cells, monocytes, macrophages

ing complexes that activate the complement system. This, in turn, leads to opsonisation, red blood cell agglutination (the process of agglutinating or "clumping together"), cell lysis, and death. Some examples of type II hypersensitivity reactions include erythroblastosis fetalis, Goodpasture syndrome, and autoimmune anaemias.

Type III hypersensitivity reactions occur when IgG and IgM antibodies bind to soluble proteins (rather than cell surface molecules as in type II hypersensitivity reactions), forming immune complexes that can deposit in tissues, leading to complement activation, inflammation, the neutrophil influx, and mast cell degranulation. This type of reaction can take days, or even weeks, to develop, and treatment generally involves anti-inflammatory agents and corticosteroids. Examples of type III hypersensitivity reactions include systemic lupus erythematosus (SLE), serum sickness, and reactive arthritis.

Unlike the other types of hypersensitivity reactions, type IV reactions are cell mediated and antibody independent. They are the second most common type of hypersensitivity reaction and usually take two or more days to develop. These reactions are caused by the overstimulation of T cells and monocytes/macrophages, leading to the release of cytokines that cause inflammation, cell death, and tissue damage. These reactions are generally easily resolvable through trigger avoidance and topical corticosteroids. An example of this is the skin response to poison ivy. A brief summary of the four types of hypersensitivity reactions is provided in Table 10.4.

10.5.2 Autoimmunity

Autoimmunity involves the loss of normal immune homeostasis such that the organism produces an abnormal response to its tissue. *The hallmark of autoimmunity is the presence of self-reactive T cells, auto-antibodies, and inflammation.* Examples of autoimmune diseases include Celiac disease, type 1 diabetes mellitus, Addison's disease, and Graves' disease.

10.5.3 Immunodeficiency

Immunodeficiency is a state in which the immune system's ability to fight infectious disease is compromised or absent. Immunodeficiency disorders may result from a primary genetic defect (primary immunodeficiency—see Primary Immunodeficiency article in this supplement) which can affect either innate or acquired immune function through inhibition of selected immune cells or pathways, or it may be acquired from a secondary cause (secondary immunodeficiency), such as viral or bacterial infections, malnutrition, autoimmunity, or treatment with drugs that induce immunosuppression. Certain diseases, such as leukaemia and multiple myeloma, can also directly or indirectly impair the immune system. Immunodeficiency is the hallmark of acquired immunodeficiency syndrome (AIDS), caused by the human immunodeficiency virus (HIV). HIV directly infects Th cells and indirectly impairs other immune system responses.

10.6 Inflammation

Poorly regulated inflammatory responses and tissue damage from inflammation are often immunopathological features. Defects in immune regulation are associated with many chronic inflammatory diseases, including rheumatoid arthritis, psoriasis, inflammatory bowel disease, and asthma. Classical features of inflammation are heat, redness, swelling, and pain. Inflammation can be part of the normal host response to infection and a necessary process to rid the body of pathogens. It may become uncontrolled and lead to chronic inflammatory disease. The overproduction of inflammatory cytokines (such as TNF, IL-1, and IL-6) and the recruitment of inflammatory cells (such as neutrophils and monocytes) through the function of chemokines are important drivers of the inflammatory process.

Additional mediators produced by recruited and activated immune cells induce changes in vascular permeability and pain sensitivity.

10.7   Conclusions and Summary

Innate immunity is the first immunological, non-specific mechanism for fighting against infections. This immune response is rapid, occurring minutes or hours after aggression, and is mediated by numerous cells, including phagocytes, mast cells, basophils, and eosinophils, as well as the complement system. Adaptive immunity develops with innate immunity to eliminate infectious agents; it relies on the tightly regulated interplay among T cells, APCs, and B cells. A critical feature of adaptive immunity is the development of immunologic memory or the ability of the system to learn or record its experiences with various pathogens, leading to effective and rapid immune responses upon subsequent exposure to the same or similar pathogens. A brief overview of the defining features of innate and adaptive immunities is presented in Table 10.5

Table 10.5 Overview of the defining features of innate and adaptive immunities

	Innate immune system	Adaptive immune system
Cells	Haematopoietic cells: • Macrophages • Dendritic cells • Mast cells • Neutrophils • Basophils • Eosinophils • NK cells • T cells non-haematopoietic cells • Epithelial cells (skin, airways, gastrointestinal tract)	Haematopoietic cells: • T cells • B cells
Molecules	• Cytokines • Complement • Proteins and glycoprotein	• Antibodies (Ig) • Cytokines
Response time	• Immediate	• Delayed by hours to days
Immunologic memory	• None: responses are the same with each exposure.	• Responsiveness enhanced by repeated antigen exposure

There is a great deal of synergy between the adaptive immune system and its innate counterpart, and defects in either system can lead to immunopathological disorders, including autoimmune diseases, immunodeficiencies, and hypersensitivity reactions. The remainder of this supplement will focus on the appropriate diagnosis, treatment, and management of some more prominent disorders, particularly those associated with hypersensitivity reactions.

Acknowledgement This chapter is reproduced from Marshall, J.S., Warrington, R., Watson, W. et al. An introduction to immunology and immunopathology. Allergy Asthma Clin Immunol 14 (Suppl 2), 49 (2018). https://doi.org/10.1186/s13223-018-0278-1 (Creative Commons Attribution 4.0 International License). BMC. Part of Springer Nature. (A full list of bibliography can be accessed at https://doi.org/10.1186/s13223-018-0278-1)

Bibliography

Bonilla FA, Oettgen HC. Adaptive immunity. J Allergy Clin Immunol. 2010;125(Suppl. 2):S33–40.

Castro C, Gourley M. Diagnostic testing and interpretation of tests for autoimmunity. J Allergy Clin Immunol. 2010;125(Suppl. 2):S238–47.

Chinen J, Shearer WT. Secondary immunodeficiencies, including HIV infection. J Allergy Clin Immunol. 2010;125(Suppl. 2):S195–203.

Gell PGH, Coombs RRA. Clinical aspects of immunology. 1st ed. Oxford: Blackwell; 1963.

Murphy KM, Travers P, Walport M. Janeway's immunobiology. 7th ed. New York: Garland Science; 2007.

Notarangelo LD. Primary immunodeficiencies. J Allergy Clin Immunol. 2010;125(Suppl. 2):S182–94.

Rajan TV. The Gell-Coombs classification of hypersensitivity reactions: a re-interpretation. Trends Immunol. 2003;24:376–9.

Schroeder HW, Cavacini L. Structure and function of immunoglobulins. J Allergy Clin Immunol. 2010;125(Suppl. 2):S41–52.

Stone KD, Prussin C, Metcalfe DD. IgE, mast cells, basophils, and eosinophils. J Allergy Clin Immunol. 2010;125(Suppl. 2):S73–80.

Turvey SE, Broide DH. Innate immunity. J Allergy Clin Immunol. 2010;125(Suppl. 2):S24–32.

11.1 Introduction

Neoplasia is the uncontrolled growth of abnormal new cells that are not under physiological control. Neoplasm is the abnormal tissue that grows by cellular proliferation more rapidly than normal and continues to grow after the stimuli that initiated the new growth cease. Neoplasm may be either benign or malignant. When the abnormal growth forms a mass, it is usually called a tumour. Before the development of molecular biology, the neoplasm was defined as *"an abnormal mass of tissue, the growth of which exceeds and is uncoordinated with that of normal tissue and persists in the same excessive manner when the stimulus evoking the change is removed"* (Willis 1952). Neoplasia can also be defined as "a disorder of cell growth triggered by a series of acquired mutations affecting a single cell and its clonal progeny." This means neoplasm arises from a single cell with a genetic mutation. This chapter deals briefly with the basics of neoplasia and carcinogenesis. For detailed information, the reader should refer to the resources listed in the bibliography.

11.2 Classification of Neoplasms

Neoplasm is often synonymous with the term tumour. These terms are often used interchangeably. The term tumour is used originally as a sign of inflammation characterised by swelling. A tumour refers to a lump (swelling), whereas a neoplasm refers to new growth, which can present as a swelling or ulcer. The term "cancer" implies malignancy. "Carcinoma" is the term used for a malignant neoplasm arising from the epithelial tissues, and the word "sarcoma" is used for malignant neoplasms arising from connective tissues. Neoplasms are classified according to their clinical behaviour and cell of origin. Behavioural classification divides neoplasms into two types: Benign and malignant.

11.2.1 Benign Neoplasms

Benign neoplasms are non-invasive, localised, slow-growing, non-metastasizing, and encapsulated neoplasms with close histological resemblance to normal tissue/cell of origin. These neoplasms are amenable to local surgical removal; most are usually not lethal. A suffix-"oma" usually designates benign neoplasms to the cell type from which the neoplasms arise. The exception to this rule is melanoma and lymphoma, which are malignant neoplasms. Major categories of benign neoplasms include the following:

- **Benign neoplasms of the epithelial tissue:**
  - Stratified squamous cell of the epithelium: Squamous cell papilloma
  - Basal cell of the epithelium: Basal cell papilloma
  - Glandular or secretary epithelium: Adenoma
- **Benign neoplasms of the connective tissue/mesenchymal tissue:**
  - Fibrous tissue origin: Fibroma
  - Adipose tissue: Lipoma
  - Bone: Osteoma
  - Cartilage: Chondroma
  - Smooth muscle: Leiomyoma
  - Striated muscle: Rhabdomyoma
  - Blood vessels: Angioma
  - Mesothelium: Benign mesothelioma

11.2.2 Malignant Neoplasms

Malignant neoplasms are invasive, locally destructive, non-encapsulated, rapidly growing, and capable of metastasising to distant sites. Histologically, these neoplasms exhibit variable resemblance to the parent tissue. Malignant neoplasms are also classified based on the cell/tissue of origin. Major categories in this classification include those arising from epithelial cells, connective tissue cells, and lymphoid and hematogenous organs. Some examples are given below:

- **Malignant neoplasms of the epithelial tissue:**
  - Stratified squamous cell of the epithelium: Squamous cell carcinoma
  - Basal cell of the epithelium: Basal cell carcinoma
  - Glandular or secretary epithelium: Adenocarcinoma
- **Malignant neoplasms of the connective tissue/mesenchymal tissue**
  - Fibrous tissue origin: Fibrosarcoma
  - Adipose tissue: Liposarcoma
  - Bone: Osteosarcoma
  - Cartilage: Chondrosarcoma
  - Smooth muscle: Leiomyosarcoma
  - Striated muscle: Rhabdomyosarcoma
  - Blood vessels: Angiosarcoma
  - Mesothelium: Malignant mesothelioma
- **Malignant neoplasms from other tissues**
  - Lymphoid tissue: Lymphoma (Hodgkin's or non-Hodgkin's lymphoma)
  - Haematopoietic tissue: Leukaemia
  - Melanocytes: Malignant melanoma

Benign and malignant tumours can be found in the same organs, derived from the same cell types, reach the same size, are induced by the same agents or hereditary mutations, and occur spontaneously.

11.3   Other Tumour Terminologies

Embryonal neoplasms. Some neoplasms bear close histological resemblance to the embryonic form of the tissue or organ from which they arise. Almost exclusively, these occur in children under 5 years of age. These neoplasms are designated by the suffix- *"blastoma."* Some examples include hepatoblastoma, medulloblastoma, nephroblastoma, neuroblastoma, and retinoblastoma.

Neoplasms with a combination of cell types. Neoplasms with two or more cell types are called "mixed tumours." Pleomorphic adenoma of the parotid gland and fibroadenoma of the female breast are mixed tumours. In pleomorphic adenoma, microscopically, a mixture of epithelial components dispersed in a fibromyxoid stroma (sometimes with cartilage or bone) can be seen. In the fibroadenoma of the female breast, a mixture of ductal elements embedded in fibrous tissue is frequently seen.

Germ cell tumours: Teratomas. Neoplasms with more than one cell type arising from more than one germ layer are called teratomas. Examples include ovarian and testicular teratomas. Ovarian teratomas are almost always benign, whereas testicular teratomas are predominantly malignant.

Eponymously named neoplasms. Some neoplasms are known by persons who first recognised or described them. Examples include (1) Hodgkin's lymphoma (a malignant lymphoma histologically characterised by the presence of Reed-Sternberg cells, (2) Burkitt's lymphoma (a B-cell lymphoma associated with Epstein-Barr virus commonly occurs in African children), (3) Kaposi's sarcoma (a malignant neoplasm derived from endothelial cells associated with Human herpes viruseight8 commonly occurs in AIDS), (4) Ewing's sarcoma (a malignant neoplasm of bone, and (5) Pindborg tumour (a benign jaw tumour, also called a calcifying epithelial odontogenic tumour (CEOT).

Inconsistencies in terminology. In the terminology of neoplasms, some inconsistencies exist. Neoplasms such as *lymphoma, mesothelioma,* and *melanoma* are malignant neoplasms, and the suffix- *"oma" is traditionally used for* these neoplasms.

11.4   Non-Neoplastic Tumour-like Lesions

Often non-neoplastic tumour-like lesions clinically mimic benign or malignant lesions. These include hamartomas and Choristomas.

Hamartomas and Choristomas. *Hamartoma and Choristomas are lesions characterised by non-neoplastic, mass-forming malformations.* They lack the autonomy of neoplastic features. Hamartoma is an overgrowth of mature tissues that usually occurs in an expected area or organ but with disorganisation. Some examples include fibrous hamartoma in infancy, neurocritical hamartoma, folliculosebaceous cystic hamartoma, and meningothelial hamartoma. *Choristomas are a mass of normal tissue in an abnormal location.* Examples include osseous choristoma and gastric tissue located in the distal ilium in the Meckel diverticulum. Since cancer is a major cause of mortality, the discussion below mainly focuses on malignant neoplasms.

11.5   Epidemiology of Cancer

The global burden and regional variations of cancer

Cancer is a significant public health issue throughout the world. It is a leading cause of death worldwide. Breast, lung, colon, rectum, and prostate cancers are most common in the United States. *Around one-third of deaths from cancer are due to tobacco use, high body mass index, alcohol consumption, low fruit and vegetable intake, and lack of physical activity.* Cancer-causing infections, such as human papillomavirus (HPV) and hepatitis, are responsible for approximately 30% of cancer cases in low- and lower-middle income countries. The most common cancers vary between countries. Oral cancer is common in the Indian subcontinent and is the sixth most common cancer.

Cancer epidemiology provides estimates of the number of new cancer diagnoses (incidence), the burden of cancer (prevalence), the number of deaths due to cancer (mortality), and the rate of death among individuals diagnosed with cancer (case–fatality rate). Worldwide, an estimated 19.3 million new cancer cases (18.1 million excluding nonmelanoma skin cancer) and almost 10.0 million cancer deaths (9.9 million excluding nonmelanoma skin cancer) occurred in 2020. Lung, prostate, and colorectal cancers are common in males and Breast, colorectal, lung, and cervical cancers are common in females. Globally, considerable geographic differences in the burden of cancer exist. Most often, regional differences in cancer incidence rates are due to environmental aetiologic causes. Examples include hepatocellular carcinoma in Africa due to the high prevalence of hepatitis B infection and exposure to carcinogenic aflatoxins in ground nuts. In India, oral cancer is prevalent due to the widespread practice of chewing betel-quid and areca-nut. Melanoma is a common skin cancer among fair-skinned people in sunny parts of Australia due to exposure to ultraviolet radiation. The risk of colon cancer is significant in populations with high consumption of a diet rich in meat.

11.6 Aetiology of Cancer

Carcinogens are agents capable of initiating the development of malignant tumours by inducing cellular genetic changes. The transformation of a normal cell to a malignant cell is thought to be due to successive and cumulative exposures to carcinogens and other factors over decades. Most human cancers result from exposure to environmental (or exogenous) carcinogens. Other carcinogens that cause malignant transformation include a broad group of factors from within the body, termed endogenous factors. *According to the mechanism of carcinogenesis, carcinogens can be grouped into genotoxic carcinogens, non-genotoxic (epigenetic) carcinogens, procarcinogens, and co-carcinogens.*

Genotoxic carcinogens bind directly to DNA, causing irreversible damage to the genome. Polycyclic aromatic hydrocarbons (PAHs) of tobacco fall into this category. Some carcinogens do not directly cause DNA damage but could participate in the promotion of growth. These are known as non-genotoxic carcinogens or epigenetic carcinogens. Hormones fall into this group. Agents that are not carcinogenic but turn into carcinogenic substances in the body are known as procarcinogens. An example includes nitrates taken in the diet, which change into carcinogenic nitrosamines. Co-carcinogens are substances that promote the activity of other carcinogens in causing cancer, but they are not carcinogenic on their own. Most cancers are related to environmental, lifestyle, or behavioural exposures, and only a minority are due to inherited genetic mutations.

Potential carcinogens can be categorised into chemical, physical, and biological. Other substances, outside of these groups such as asbestos and nickel, are also considered as carcinogens.

11.6.1 Chemical Carcinogens

Numerous chemicals are known to cause cancer in humans. Many of these chemicals carry out their effects only on specific organs (Table 11.1). *Chemical carcinogens act directly*

Table 11.1 Chemical carcinogens, their source, and tumours induced

Examples of chemical carcinogens			
Chemical agent	Source	Tumour-induced	Comments
Polycyclic aromatic hydrocarbons (PAH) E.g. 3,4-benzpyrene)	Tobacco smoke Tobacco chewing Fossil fuels	Lungs Oral and pharyngeal mucosa Oral mucosa Lungs	PAHs are indirect acting carcinogens PAHs are procarcinogens requiring metabolic conversion to form ultimate carcinogens at the site of contact by hydroxylating enzymes in tissues. These can cause cancers at distant sites such as the bladder if absorbed
Aromatic amines (E.g. beta-naphthylamine	Dye and rubber industry	Bladder cancer	These agents have no local effect Require conversion in the liver into the active carcinogenic metabolite
Nitrosamines (E.g. nitrates)	Food additives Contaminated drinking water by fertilisers	Intestinal cancers	Not themselves carcinogenic Animal experiments indicate that these agents are converted into carcinogenic metabolites by commensal bacteria in the gut
Azo-dyes E.g. 2-acetylaminofluorine	Butter yellow (margarine)	Bladder and liver cancers	Derivatives of aromatic amines Currently restricted use for human consumption Evidence comes from laboratory animal studies
Alkylating agents (E.g.cyclophosphamide)	Chemotherapeutic agent for a variety of cancers They are also used as an immunosuppressive agent	Leukaemia	Small risk in humans
Other examples Nickel sulphate Arsenic sulphate Vinyl chloride	Ore Pesticides Contaminated drinking water PVC manufacture	Nasal and lung cancers Lung, bladder, and skin cancers Skin cancer Liver (angiosarcoma)	Only the inhalation route is associated with cancer Only the inorganic form of arsenic is carcinogenic to humans Exposed industrial workers primarily through inhalation

or indirectly. Directly acting-chemical carcinogens do not require metabolic conversion, whereas those acting indirectly require metabolic conversion into active carcinogens (ultimate carcinogens). The basic biological action of a chemical leading to cancer is an attack on DNA to produce a change that is not repaired by the body's DNA repair mechanisms, which are then passed from cell to cell during cell division. When an interaction between a chemical carcinogen and DNA results in a mutation, the chemical is said to be a mutagen. Many chemicals are only tumour initiators. Those capable of only initiation are known as incomplete carcinogens. Many chemicals can be initiators as well as promoters. These are known as complete carcinogens. Targets of chemical carcinogens include protooncogenes and tumour suppressor genes. The major effect of tumour promoters is the stimulation of cell proliferation. Some of the most potent promoting agents are hormones, which stimulate the replication of cells in target organs.

11.6.1.1   Mechanisms of Chemical Carcinogenesis.

Most chemical carcinogens are mutagenic. Chemical carcinogenesis is a multistep process. DNA damage starts chemical carcinogenesis. Cancer originates in a single cell and develops through the clonal proliferation of its progeny. A chemical carcinogen causes a genetic error by modifying the molecular structure of DNA, which can lead to a mutation during DNA synthesis. *Chemical carcinogenesis can be divided into three steps: tumour initiation, tumour promotion, and tumour progression,* as discussed below.

The initiation stage involves the alteration, change, or mutation of genes. This change can be induced by exposure to a carcinogenic agent. Genetic alterations can result in the dysregulation of biochemical signalling pathways associated

with cellular proliferation, survival, and differentiation. Several factors, including the rate and type of carcinogenic metabolism and the response of the DNA repair function, can influence these events.

The promotion stage is a relatively lengthy and reversible process. Within this stage, actively proliferating preneoplastic cells accumulate. Progression is the phase between a premalignant (potentially malignant) lesion and the development of invasive cancer (Fig. 11.1).

Progression is the final stage of neoplastic transformation, where genetic and phenotypic changes and cell proliferation occur. This involves a rapid increase in the tumour size, where the cells may undergo further mutations with invasive and metastatic potential.

11.6.2   Physical Carcinogens

Physical carcinogens include various agents: electromagnetic radiation of different kinds, low and high temperatures, mechanical trauma, and solid and gel materials. *Radiant (radiation) energy is the most important of the physical carcinogenic agents.* Radiation may originate from ultraviolet rays, X-rays, radioactive isotopes, or atomic energy sources. Cell phones emit radiofrequency energy, a form of non-ionizing electromagnetic radiation, which can be absorbed by tissues closest to where the phone is held. Studies thus far have not shown a consistent link between cell phone use and cancers of the brain, nerves, or other tissues of the head or neck.

Ultraviolet (UV) radiation from sunlight (non-ionizing radiation) is a major causal factor of skin cancers. Fair-skinned people are more vulnerable due to the lack of melanocytes which generally have a protective role against

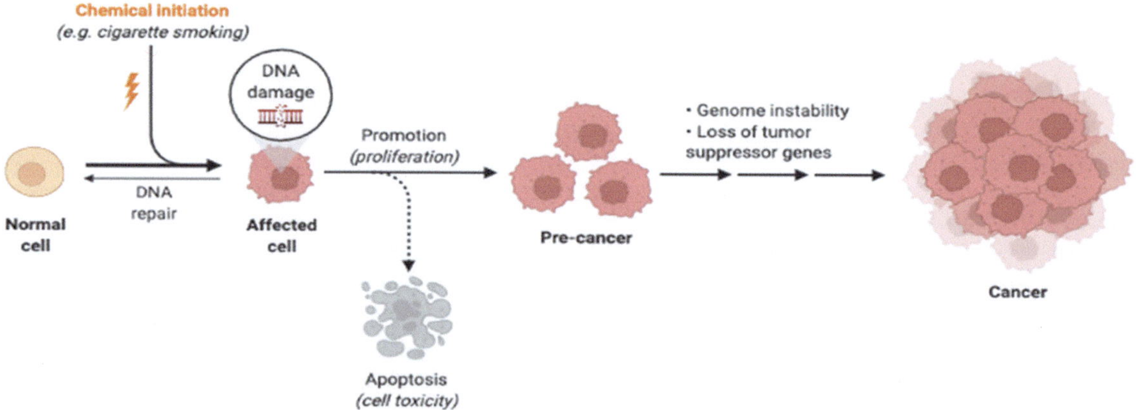

Fig. 11.1   Chemical carcinogenesis (Source: BioRender.com. Licensee: The University of Queensland, Brisbane, Australia)

ultraviolet-induced damage. Melanoma, basal cell carcinoma, and squamous cell carcinoma of the skin are common in sunny climates of Australia. UV radiation from sunlight causes DNA damage to the skin, thus causing cellular mutations, which may lead to the malignant transformation of cells.

Ionising radiation in high doses is carcinogenic. X-rays used for diagnostic purposes are safe if properly used. High doses of X-rays are used to treat malignant neoplasms (radiation therapy). Such radiation exposure carries an absolute risk of developing secondary cancers after a long latent period. However, the benefits of radiation therapy for cancer outweigh the risk of secondary cancers.

Radioactive substances from the environment pose a risk for carcinogenesis. Ionising radiation is emitted by radioactive substances (radionuclides), such as uranium, radon, and plutonium. The risk of developing carcinoma of the lungs has been reported in miners exposed to radioactive uranium. The thyroid gland is susceptible to cancer after exposure to radioactive iodine, because radioactive iodine concentrates in the thyroid gland. The thyroid, breast, bone, and hematopoietic tissue are particularly vulnerable to radiation damage.

11.6.2.1 Mechanism of Physical Carcinogenesis

Radiation increases the risk of developing cancer. It has been shown that ionising radiation can, by itself, induce a type of genomic instability in cells, which enhances the rate at which mutations and other genetic changes arise in the descendants of the irradiated cell after many generations of replication. It has long been known that radiation can induce a broad spectrum of DNA lesions, including damage to nucleotide bases, cross-linking, and DNA single- and double-strand breaks (DSBs). Misrepaired DSBs are the principal lesions of importance in the induction of both chromosomal abnormalities and gene mutations. Genetic alterations can also occur in cells that receive no direct radiation exposure. Damage signals are transmitted from neighbouring irradiated cells. This is called the Bystander Effect. The probability of cancer occurrence increases with effective radiation dose, but the severity of the cancer is independent of dose.

Radiation deposits enough energy in organic tissue to cause ionisation. This tends to break molecular bonds and thus alter the molecular structure of the irradiated molecules. Less energetic radiation, such as visible light, only causes excitation, not ionisation, which is usually dissipated as heat with relatively little chemical damage. Ultraviolet light is usually categorised as non-ionizing, but it is actually in an intermediate range that produces some ionization and chemical damage. Hence, the carcinogenic mechanism of ultraviolet radiation is similar to that of ionizing radiation.

11.6.3 Viral Carcinogens (Oncogenic Viruses)

Some oncogenic viruses are briefly discussed below.

Human papillomavirus (HPV): More than 100 types of human papillomaviruses (HPV) have been identified. HPVs are non-enveloped DNA viruses that infect epithelial cells to cause warts in the skin, condylomas in mucous membranes, and malignancies of the cervix, vulva, anal canal, and oropharyngeal cancers. Cofactors such as smoking, oral contraceptives, and immunological and hormonal status may play a role in the progression of HPV-associated malignancy. Cervical cancer is the third most common cancer in women worldwide. *Cervical cancer is a sexually transmitted disease associated with high-risk HPV types, including HPV16, −18, −31, −33, and − 45, found in approximately 90% of all cervical cancers.*

Epstein Barr virus (EBV): EBV contains a double-stranded DNA genome that codes for immediate-early, early, and late gene products. The B lymphocyte is the preferential target cell of EBV. *There is a strong association between EBV infection and Burkitt's lymphoma (BL), undifferentiated nasopharyngeal carcinoma (NPC), Hodgkin's disease, T-cell lymphoma, and some gastric carcinomas.* Burkitt's lymphoma is the most common childhood cancer in equatorial Africa. EBV infection, climatic factors, and the high incidence of *Plasmodium falciparum* malaria predispose children in these areas to Burkitt's lymphoma of the maxillofacial region. EBV is etiologically associated with nasopharyngeal carcinoma. Nasopharyngeal carcinoma is a relatively rare disease in Europe and North America but is almost endemic among Southeast Asian populations, particularly those of southern China. Hodgkin's disease is a lymphoma characterised by a malignant population of mononuclear B and multinuclear Reed-Sternberg cells set within a background of reactive non-malignant lymphocytes. EBV is associated with its development. Gastric carcinoma is caused by EBV in approximately 10% of all cases and is associated with the lymphoepithelial subtype of stomach cancer.

Hepatitis B virus (HBV): HBV is an enveloped DNA-containing virus. Hepatitis B is widespread throughout Asia, Africa, and South America. Transmission of HBV is through blood and sexual contact. Vertical transmission from the mother to child during the birthing process is common in some Asian countries. HBV has been reported to chronically infect more than 80% of individuals with liver cancer. *HBV likely causes cancer by a combination of virus-specific and host-related factors, and 90% of hepatocellular carcinoma (HCC) cases develop in a cirrhotic liver.* After 20–30 years of chronic infection, 20–30% of patients develop liver cirrhosis. Hepatocarcinogenesis is a complex multistep process involving the genetic and epigenetic alteration, activation of cellular oncogenes, inactivation of tumour suppressors, and dysregulation of multiple signal transduction pathways.

Hepatitis C virus (HCV): The Hepatitis C virus (HCV) is a retrovirus. It is blood-borne and is spread through transfusions, intravenous drug use, tattoo parlours, multiple uses of needles for vaccination, and sexual contact. The acute phase of hepatitis C is often mild and undiagnosed in adults and children. *HCV establishes persistent viral infections and chronic disease in 60–80% of these patients leading to cirrhosis and hepatocellular carcinoma (HCC).* Once the virus has infected the liver, inflammatory agents such as reactive oxygen species (ROS) and cell death signals promote a higher mutation rate and liver scarring. Chronic liver inflammation caused by HCV infection is considered an important carcinogenic factor.

Kaposi sarcoma-associated herpesvirus (KSAHV): Kaposi Sarcoma-Associated Herpesvirus (KSHV) or Human herpesvirus 8 (HHV-8) is a large, enveloped double-stranded DNA virus. KSAHV was identified as the pathogen responsible for several malignancies, including Kaposi sarcoma (KS), body cavity-based or primary effusion lymphoma, and multicentric Castleman disease. *KS is a vascular tumour of endothelial cells that affects older men in Mediterranean and African populations (endemic KS).* However, with the onset of AIDS, a more aggressive and often lethal form of KS appeared. The Kaposi Sarcoma-Associated Herpesvirus (KSHV) infects the spindle cells of the skin, which are probably derived from lymphatic endothelial cells. Angiogenesis causes a proliferation of small red patches over the entire body, including oral mucosa.

The human T-lymphotropic virus type 1 is known by the acronym HTLV-1 or human T-cell leukaemia type 1. The virus can cause adult T-cell leukaemia/lymphoma (ATL).

Merkel cell polyomavirus (MCPyv) is the most recently discovered human oncogenic virus and is associated with Merkel cell carcinoma (MCC), an aggressive malignancy of the dermis.

11.6.3.1　Mechanism of Viral Carcinogenesis.

Many human tumours are known to be aetiologically associated with DNA and RNA viruses. These oncogenic viruses infect but do not kill their host cell. Instead, they establish long-term persistent infections that, after many years, may produce cancer. DNA virus genomes integrate directly into the host genome (Fig. 11.2). In contrast, before integration, RNA virus genomes must undergo reverse transcription into DNA and insert into the host genome using a viral enzyme called integrase. DNA tumour viruses usually cause malignant transformation by inhibiting the normal function (growth control) of tumour suppressor genes, whereas retroviruses usually deregulate signal transduction pathways.

Certain viruses derived from different taxonomic groups can induce cancer development. They tend to use one of the following mechanisms to stimulate the proliferation of their host cells:

– Insertion of a strong promoter in the vicinity of a host cell proto-oncogene
– Expression of proteins that neutralise host cell tumour suppressor proteins.
– Expression of proteins that prevent or delay apoptosis.

Viral Carcinogenesis

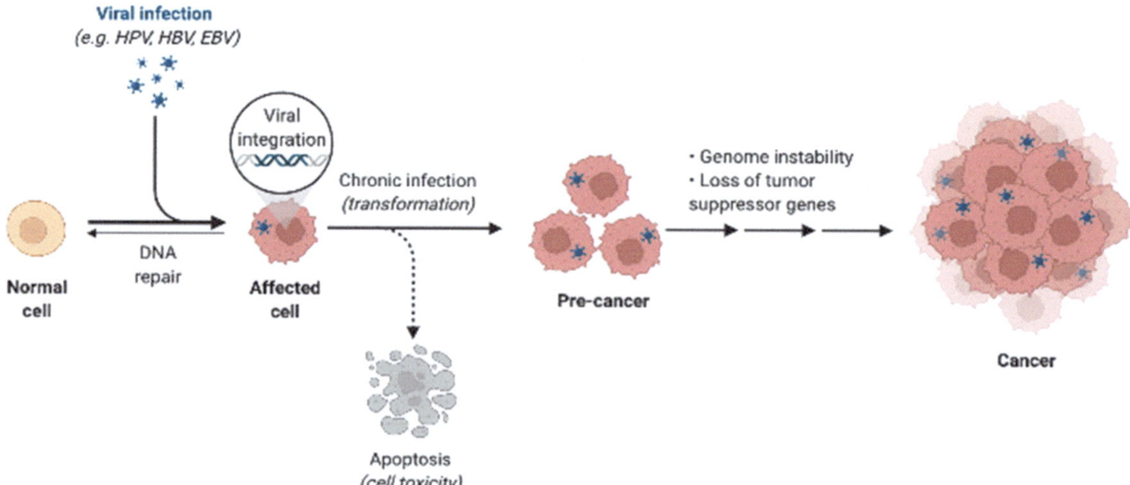

Fig. 11.2 Viral carcinogenesis. (Source: BioRender.com. Licensee: The University of Queensland, Brisbane, Australia)

Characteristics of viral carcinogenesis include the following:

— Tumour viruses often establish persistent infections in the human host.
— Host factors are important determinants of virus-induced carcinogenesis.
— Viruses are rarely complete carcinogens; they require additional factors to activate carcinogenesis fully.

In viral carcinogenesis, normal cellular genes (proto-oncogenes) can be transformed into oncogenes by four basic mechanisms: point mutation, gene amplification, chromosomal rearrangement, and insertion of the viral genome. These events are briefly discussed below:

Point mutation is a genetic alteration caused by substituting a single nucleotide for another nucleotide and is also called a point variant. Point mutations have been identified in several human tumours carrying a *ras* gene.

Gene amplification refers to an increase in the number of copies of a gene in a genome. Cancer cells sometimes produce multiple copies of a gene in response to signals from other cells. Amplification of proto-oncogenes can contribute to tumorigenesis and tumour progression.

Chromosomal rearrangements can cause cancer if they mutate a tumour suppressor gene or activate an oncogene. These facilitate cancer development, progression, and metastasis. Chromosomal rearrangements can be simple, involving a single balanced fusion that preserves the proper complement of genetic information, or complex with one or more fusions that disrupt this balance. A translocation involving *c-myc* (a proto-oncogene) is critical to developing most cases of Burkitt's lymphoma (BL). In the human genome, *c-myc* is located on chromosome 8. A piece of chromosome 8 is translocated next to chromosome 14 in BL.

Insertion of the viral genome. Most DNA oncogenic viruses frequently encode oncogenes that transform infected cells, targeting *p53* and *pRB*. In addition, the integration of viral DNA into the human genome also plays a vital role in promoting tumour development for several viruses, including HBV and HPV.

11.6.4 Bacteria, Fungi, and Parasites as Carcinogens

Helicobacter pylori, a major cause of gastritis and peptic ulcers, has been implicated in developing gastric lymphomas. A fungal toxin called aflatoxin produced by the fungus *Aspergillus flavus* has been identified as an essential carcinogenic agent for hepatocellular carcinomas, particularly in Africa. Parasites such as *Schistosoma haematobium* are strongly implicated in the high incidence of bladder cancers in Egypt. Liver flukes *Clonorchis Sinensis* and *Opisthorchis viverrini* have been reported to be associated with adenocarcinoma of the bile duct in parts of the Middle East.

11.7 Role of Host Factors in Carcinogenesis

In addition to the above-listed carcinogenic agents, host factors can influence cancer risk. These include race, age, diet, gender, inherited factors, premalignant lesions, and hormones.

Race and ethnicity: Determining the specific role of race and ethnicity in the causation of cancer is complicated, because racial factors are often mixed with other factors such as diet, place of residence, socioeconomic status, cultural practices, and habits. However, some reports indicate that a considerable proportion of the risk of developing prostate and breast cancer can be attributed to heritable factors. For example, a higher risk exists for prostate cancer in men of African ancestry than in men of European origin. Skin cancer is uncommon in the black race because of the protective role of melanin in their skin.

Age: Advancing age is the most important risk factor for cancer overall and many individual cancer types. The incidence rates for cancer overall climb steadily as age increases. For example, the median age at diagnosis is 62 years for breast cancer, 67 years for colorectal cancer, 71 years for lung cancer, and 66 years for prostate cancer.

Diet: Obesity and alcohol increase the risk of several types of cancer; these are the most important nutritional factors contributing to the total burden of cancer worldwide. For colorectal cancer, processed meat and red meat increases the risk; dietary fibre, dairy products, and calcium likely reduce the risk. Foods containing mutagens can cause cancer; certain salted fish cause nasopharyngeal cancer, and foods contaminated with aflatoxin cause liver cancer. Fruits and vegetables are not linked to cancer risk, although very low intakes might increase the risk for aerodigestive and some other cancers.

Gender: Gender plays a vital role in the incidence, disease prognosis, and mortality of various cancers. Gender differences influence cancer susceptibility at the genetic/molecular levels. Sex hormones also negatively or positively affect the development of multiple cancers. Breast cancer, for example, is 200 times more common in women than in men due to the more significant mammary tissue and hormonal influences.

Inherited factors: Some individuals Inherit characteristics that put them at a higher risk category for developing cancers. Examples include familial breast cancer (due to mutated BRCA1 gene on chromosome 17), UV-exposure-related skin cancer (basal cell carcinoma) in individuals with xeroderma pigmentosum due to deficiency of DNA repair system, and retinoblastoma in children.

Premalignant/potentially malignant lesions: *Premalignant lesions (potentially malignant lesions) are identifiable local abnormal lesions. These are associated with an increased risk for development of cancer.* Examples: chronic ulcerative colitis increases the risk for colorectal cancers; cervical cancer is often preceded by epithelial dysplasia of the cervix; and oral leukoplakia can transform into squamous cell carcinoma of the oral mucosa.

Hormones. Excessive hormonal stimulation of cell proliferation increases the risk of mutation and subsequent proliferation of clones of mutated cells. Therefore, hormones can act as potent carcinogens and are considered a "complete carcinogen," because they both initiate and promote the development of cancers. Hormones have been implicated in the genesis of breast, prostate, uterine, ovarian, testicular, thyroid, and bone cancers. Increased exposure to oestrogen and progesterone hormones in females has been demonstrated to increase the risk of breast cancer. The early onset of menstruation, late first pregnancy, obesity, late menopause, and the use of oral contraceptives increase the exposure of breast tissue to oestrogen, stimulating increased proliferation. Similarly, the male sex hormone testosterone has been implicated in developing prostate cancer.

11.8   Clinical Effects of Neoplasms

The average time between when the initial genetic and cellular changes leading to the development of cancer occur and the emergence of symptoms related to a tumour is estimated to be as long as 15–20 years. The clinical effects of benign and malignant neoplasms can cause local and systemic problems for the host. Some local effects include impingement on the adjacent structures. Effects on hormonal and metabolic activity may lead to paraneoplastic syndromes. Bleeding, ulceration, infection, and infarction are common signs of malignant neoplasms. Wasting (cancer cachexia) is common in many malignant diseases.

Local effects: The tumour's location is essential for both benign and malignant tumours. For example, an adenoma of the pituitary gland can compress and destroy the normal gland and cause hypopituitarism. Even a small biliary duct carcinoma in the common bile duct may induce biliary duct obstruction with a fatal outcome.

Hormonal effects: Adenoma and carcinoma of the beta cells of the islets of the pancreas can cause hyperinsulinism.

Paraneoplastic syndromes: Paraneoplastic syndromes are rare disorders triggered by an altered immune system response to a neoplasm. They are clinical syndromes involving nonmetastatic systemic effects accompanying the malignant disease. These syndromes are collections of symptoms that result from substances produced by the tumour and occur remotely from cancer itself. The symptoms may be endocrine, neuromuscular, musculoskeletal, cardiovascular, cutaneous, hematologic, gastrointestinal, renal, or miscellaneous.

Cancer cachexia is a wasting syndrome characterised by weight loss, anorexia, asthenia, anaemia, and skeletal muscle and fat loss. It is estimated to occur in up to 80% of people with advanced cancer, depending on different factors.

11.9   Cancer Staging

Cancer staging is the process of determining how much cancer is in the body and where it is located.

Four different types of cancer staging are used:

Clinical staging determines how much cancer there is based on physical examination, and imaging tests, of affected areas.

Pathological staging can be determined when a patient has surgery to remove a tumour. Pathological staging combines the results of both the clinical staging with the surgical results.

Post-therapy or post-neoadjuvant therapy staging determines how much cancer remains after a patient is treated with systemic therapy (chemotherapy or hormones) and/or radiation therapy prior to surgery or where no surgery is performed. This can be assessed by clinical staging guidelines after the therapy. It may also be assessed by pathological staging guidelines after surgery following the therapy.

Recurrence or retreatment staging is used to determine the extent of the disease if cancer comes back after treatment. Recurrence or retreatment staging helps determine the best treatment options for cancer that has returned.

Clinical staging of cancer is a method used to find out the stage of cancer (amount or spread of cancer in the body) using tests that are done before surgery. This is done before any treatment begins. Cancer's stage can also be used to help predict the course it will likely take, as well as how likely it is that treatment will be successful. The TNM system is the most widely used cancer staging system.

TNM Staging System. In this system, the **T** refers to the size and extent of the main tumour. The main tumour is usually called the primary tumour. The **N** refers to the number of nearby lymph nodes where cancer may have spread, and the **M** refers to whether the cancer has metastasised to other parts of the body.

In the TNM system, there will be numbers after each letter that give more details about cancer; for example, T1N0MX or T3N1M0. The following explains what letters and numbers mean.

11.9.1 Primary Tumour (T)

TX: The main tumour cannot be measured.

T0: The main tumour cannot be found.

T1, T2, T3, T4: Refers to the size and/or extent of the main tumor. The higher the number after the T, the larger the tumour or the more it has grown into nearby tissues. T's may be further divided to provide more detail, such as T3a and T3b.

11.9.2 Regional Lymph Nodes (N)

NX: Cancer in nearby lymph nodes cannot be measured.

N0: There is no cancer in nearby lymph nodes.

N1, N2, N3: Refers to the number and location of lymph nodes that contain cancer. The higher the number after the N, the more lymph nodes that contain cancer.

11.9.3 Distant Metastasis (M)

MX: Metastasis cannot be measured.

M0: Cancer has not spread to other parts of the body.

M1: Cancer has spread to other parts of the body.

Because each cancer type has its own classification system, letters and numbers do not always mean the same thing for every kind of cancer. Once the T, N, and M are determined, they are combined and an overall stage of 0, I, II, III, and IV are assigned. Sometimes these stages are subdivided as well, using letters such as IIIA and IIIB. *Stage I cancers are the least advanced and often have a better prognosis. Higher-stage cancers are often more advanced but, in many cases, can still be treated successfully.*

11.10 Spread of Cancer: Metastasis

The development of secondary tumours in a part of the body that is far from the original primary cancer site is termed "metastasis." Cancer cells can break away from the mass (or tumour) and travel via the bloodstream or lymphatic system to different parts of the body. These cells can settle in other parts of the body to form secondary cancer or metastasis. For many types of cancer, it is also called stage IV cancer. Metastatic cancer cells have features like that of primary cancer and not like the cells in the place where the metastatic cancer is found. Metastatic cancer also has the same name as primary cancer. For example, breast cancer that spreads to the lung is called metastatic breast cancer, not lung cancer. It is treated as stage IV breast cancer, not as lung cancer. Sometimes when people are diagnosed with metastatic cancer, it is not clear where it started. This type of cancer is called cancer of unknown primary origin, or CUP. Metastatic cancer does not always cause symptoms. Some common signs of metastatic cancer include pain and fractures when cancer has spread to the bone, headache, seizures, or dizziness when cancer has spread to the brain, shortness of breath when cancer has spread to the lung and jaundice or swelling in the abdomen when cancer has spread to the liver.

To successfully colonise a secondary site, a cancer cell must complete a sequential series of steps before it becomes a clinically detectable lesion. These steps typically include invasion, intravasation, circulation, extravasation, and colonisation (Fig. 11.3). The initial steps of metastasis require the proliferation of the primary tumour and invasion through adjacent tissues and basement membranes. This process continues until the tumour invades blood vessels or lymphatic channels when individual tumour cells detach from the pri-

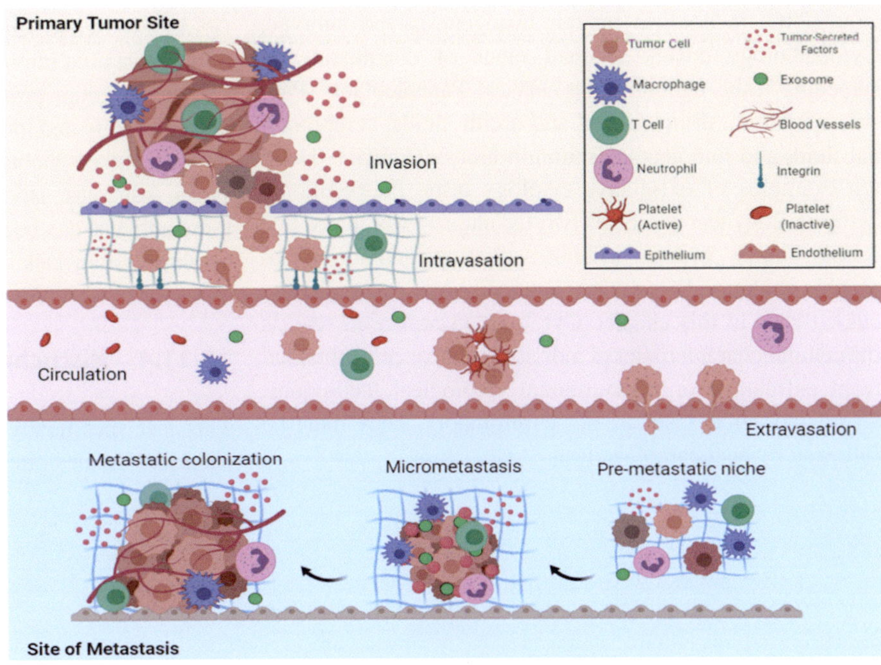

Fig. 11.3 Overview of the metastatic cascade: The five key steps of metastasis include invasion, intravasation, circulation, extravasation, and colonisation. (Source: Fares, J., Fares, M.Y., Khachfe, H.H. et al. Molecular principles of metastasis: a hallmark of cancer revisited. Sig Transduct Target Ther 5, 28 (2020). https://doi.org/10.1038/s41392-020-0134-x. (Springer: Creative Commons Attribution 4.0 International license)

mary tumour mass and are carried via the blood or lymph to a distant target organ. Subsequently, tumour cells arrest in small vessels within the distant organ, extravasate into the surrounding tissue, and proliferate at the secondary site. All these steps must be performed while tumour cells avoid and survive apoptotic signals and host immune responses.

11.11 Cancer Diagnosis: Investigations

Biopsy to confirm the diagnosis and tissue of origin is almost always required when cancer is suspected. This is carried out in the clinic or in a hospital setting, and the formalin-fixed tissue sample is sent to the pathology laboratory for processing, sectioning, and staining before the pathologist makes a diagnosis. The choice of biopsy site is usually determined by ease of access and degree of invasiveness. A fine needle or core biopsy may reveal the cancer type if lymphadenopathy is present. Core biopsies or lymph node excision are recommended for diagnosing lymphomas, because preservation of nodal architecture is essential for accurate histologic diagnosis. Sometimes an open biopsy is needed. Other biopsy routes include bronchoscopy or mediastinoscopy for easily accessible mediastinal or central pulmonary tumours, percutaneous liver biopsy if liver lesions are present, and CT- or ultrasound-guided biopsy of lung or soft tissue masses.

11.11.1 Histopathology and Cytopathology

Historically, histopathology and cytopathology have been the main tools utilised to diagnose cancer. Cancer diagnosis using these techniques is based on microscopic examination of haematoxylin and eosin (H&E) stained slides. The evaluation of tumours is also carried out using immunocytochemistry (IHC) to confirm tumour histogenesis and subtype. Cytopathology covers a broad range of diagnostic and screening tests, including the cervical Papanicolaou (Pap) smear, sputum, urine, pleural and ascitic fluids, cerebrospinal fluid, and fine needle aspiration biopsy (FNAB). These are examples of exfoliative cytology tests. Interventional cytopathology test combines two techniques, which are fine needle biopsy, with or without aspiration, and ultrasonographic guidance. Some other cancer diagnostic tests are discussed later in this chapter. Cytologic examination reveals the cellular characteristics of individual cancer cells obtained from exfoliative or interventional cytological techniques. Cytopathological tests are not confirmatory. They must be followed by histopathology tests.

11.11.2 Histological Grading of Cancer

The cancer grading is a histologic measure of cell anaplasia (reversion of differentiation) in the sampled tumour tissue. It is based on the resemblance of the tumour to the tissue of origin. Grading in cancer is distinguished from staging, which measures the extent to which cancer has spread.

Systems for describing tumour grade can differ depending on the type of cancer. But most tumours are graded as X, 1, 2, 3, or 4.

Grade X: Grade cannot be assessed (undetermined grade)
Grade 1: Well-differentiated (low grade)
Grade 2: Moderately differentiated (intermediate grade)
Grade 3: Poorly differentiated (high grade)
Grade 4: Undifferentiated (high grade)

In grade 1 (low-grade), cancer cells look more like normal cells and tend to grow and spread more slowly than high-grade cancer cells. Grading systems are different for each type of cancer. The cancer grading system is used to help plan treatment and determine prognosis.

11.11.3 Tumour Marker Tests

Tumour markers are substances made by cancer cells or normal cells in response to cancer in the body. Some tumour markers are specific to one type of cancer. Others can be found in various kinds of cancers. Because tumour markers can also appear in certain noncancerous conditions, tumour marker tests are not usually used to diagnose cancer or screen people at low risk of the disease. These tests are most often done on people already diagnosed with cancer. *Tumour markers can help determine if cancer has spread, whether treatment is working, or if cancer has returned after treatment.* Some examples include the following: the prostate serum antigen (PSA) test used to screen for prostatic adenocarcinoma is one of the most used tumour marker tests. PSA levels may also be elevated in benign prostatic hyperplasia. Hence, this test shows low specificity and low sensitivity for cancer screening. Other tumour markers include carcinoembryonic antigen (CEA) for colon, pancreas, stomach, and breast carcinoma. Because these antigens can be produced in various non-carcinomatous conditions, they lack specificity and sensitivity.

11.11.4 Histochemistry

This test specifically stains constituents of cells and biochemical tissues: mucins, lipids, nucleic acids, amyloid, microorganisms, and other proteins. This test is helpful for the classification of leukaemia and salivary gland neoplasms.

11.11.5 Immunohistochemistry (IHC)

IHC tests detect the expression of distinct protein patterns in different tumours. IHC is commonly used to detect breast, lung, gastrointestinal, and prostate cancers.

11.11.6 Flow Cytometry

This laboratory method measures the number of cells, the percentage of live cells, and certain characteristics of cells, such as size and shape, in blood, bone marrow, or another tissue sample. The presence of tumour markers on the cell's surface, such as antigens, is also measured. The cells are stained with a light-sensitive dye, placed in a fluid, and then passed one at a time through a beam of light. The measurements are based on how the stained cells react to the light beam. Flow cytometry is used in basic research and to help diagnose and manage certain diseases, including cancer.

11.11.7 Molecular Diagnosis

This laboratory method uses a tissue, blood, or other body fluid sample to check for certain genes, proteins, or other molecules that may be a sign of a disease or condition, such as cancer. Molecular testing can also check for changes in a gene or chromosome that may increase a person's risk of developing cancer or other diseases. Molecular testing may be done with other procedures, such as biopsies, to help diagnose some types of cancer. It may also allow planning treatment, determining how well the treatment works, making a prognosis, or predicting whether cancer will come back or spread to other body parts. These tests are also called biomarker testing and molecular profiling. *Molecular tests comprising chromosomal analysis, polymerase chain reaction (PCR), fluorescent in situ hybridisation (FISH), and cell surface antigen testing help to delineate the origin of metastatic cancers*, particularly for cancers of unknown primary source, and may help select therapy.

11.11.8 Imaging Tests

Cancers usually display several structural, physiologic, and molecular changes and common acquired biological capabilities that can be evaluated with imaging. Diagnosis of cancer frequently requires imaging studies that, in many cases, use small amounts of radiation. *Procedures such as X-rays, computed tomography (CT), magnetic resonance imaging (MRI), positron emission tomography (PET), and single-photon emission computed tomography (SPECT) are important in clinical decision making, including therapy and follow-up.* Diagnostic imaging can be divided into two broad categories: (1) those methods that define very precisely anatomical details and (2) those that produce functional or molecular images. The first method (using CT and MRI) can provide exquisite details on lesion location, size, morphology, and structural changes to surrounding tissues but only delivers limited information as to the tumour's functioning. The second method (using PET and SPECT) can give insight into the tumour physiology down to the molecular level but cannot provide anatomical details.

Imaging can be used to determine if a person has any suspicious areas or abnormalities that might be cancerous. Mammograms are an example of a familiar imaging tool used to screen for breast cancer. Screening for cancer is usually recommended for people who are at increased risk (due to their family history, lifestyle, or age) for developing a particular type of cancer.

Imaging can be used to find out where a cancer is located in the body, if it has spread, and how much is present. Used in this way, imaging can help determine what stage (how advanced) the cancer is, and if the cancer is in, around, or near important organs and blood vessels. When a biopsy is necessary, imaging may be used to help guide doctors to the tumour and take a sample of it (Example: breast cancer biopsy guided by ultrasound or MRI).

Imaging can help guide the delivery of cancer treatments in numerous ways. Imaging can help make cancer treatments less invasive by narrowly focusing treatments on the tumours. For instance, ultrasound, MRI, or CT scans may be used to determine exact tumour locations so that therapy procedures can be focused on the tumour, minimising damage to surrounding tissue.

Imaging can be used to see if a tumour is shrinking or if the tumour has changed and is using less of the body's resources than before treatment. For example, in some current cancer treatment trials, X-rays, MRIs, and CT scans are done at intervals to see if a treatment is working and if the tumour is shrinking. PET and other molecular imaging and nuclear medicine techniques are used to monitor the ways the tumour uses the body's resources. Magnetic resonance spectroscopy is used to study chemical changes in the tumour.

Imaging can be used to see if a previously treated cancer has returned or if the cancer is spreading to other locations.

11.11.9 Diagnostic Surgery: Sentinel Node Mapping

This technique illustrates how imaging can reduce the need for extensive diagnostic surgery. In this procedure, called sentinel node mapping, only the sentinel node (the first lymph node to which breast cancer is likely to spread) is removed rather than all the lymph nodes. In order to identify the sentinel node, the radiologists inject a relatively non-toxic radioactive substance and see which lymph node it reaches first. This lymph node is the sentinel node and is surgically removed.

11.12 Carcinogenesis

11.12.1 Host Defence Against Cancer

An essential function in protecting against cancer is surveillance and identifying foreign or non-self-substances. The immune system, which recognises foreign microorganisms as "non-self" and mounts a response to destroy these disease-causing agents, plays a similar role in protecting the body from malignancy. *The damaged DNA in cancer cells frequently directs the mutated cell to produce abnormal proteins known as tumour antigens.* These abnormal tumour proteins mark cancer cells as "non-self." The immune system likely encounters and eliminates cancer cells daily. However, cancer cells possess mechanisms that allow them to escape the immune responses that ordinarily prevent the development of malignant tumours. Interaction between the tumour and host is necessary for the host's defence against cancer. Immune responses can also help to eliminate abnormal cells of the body that develop into cancer. Tumour antigens can be recognised by T cells as well as by antibodies. The immune system can identify and destroy nascent tumour cells in a cancer immunosurveillance process, which functions as an essential defence against cancer. Most tumours are immunogenic, but the immunity they evoke is either too weak to reject rapidly growing tumours, or cancer induces a suppressor effect on the host immune system. Several immunocyte populations are active in the natural cellular defence against tumours. These include macrophages, Natural Killer Cells, Cytotoxic cells, chemokines, and lymphokines.

11.12.2 Stages of Cancer Development

Percival Pott, a London physician, identified the first link between cancer and environmental agents when he noted a high incidence of scrotal cancer among chimney sweeps. He hypothesised that it was caused by exposure to coals and tars. This observation resulted in proposing the two-stage model of cancer development by agents (1) initiators and (2) promoters. The initial experimental studies of carcinogenesis were conducted in animals. Subsequently, chemicals were tested for their ability to cause cancer in animals. The model used was mouse skin carcinogenesis. In this system, researchers painted test chemicals on the skin and observed the growth of tumours. Researchers found that applying a DNA-reactive substance only resulted in tumour formation when the animals were further treated with another non-reactive substance. Since these initial experiments, the compound that reacted with DNA and somehow changed the genetic makeup of the cell is called a mutagen, and those mutagens which predisposed cells to develop tumours are called initiators. The non-reactive compounds that stimulate tumour development are called promoters. Approximately 70% of known mutagens are also carcinogens: cancer-causing compounds. A compound that acts as both an initiator and a promoter is referred to as a "complete carcinogen," because tumour development can occur without the application of another compound.

Initiation. Initiation is the first step in the two-stage model of cancer development. Since initiation is the result of permanent genetic change, daughter cells produced from the division of the mutated cell will also carry the mutation. In studies of mouse skin carcinogenesis, a linear relationship has been observed between the dose of initiator and the quantity of tumours that can be produced; thus, any exposure to the initiator increases risk and this risk increases indefinitely with higher levels of exposure.

Promotion. Once a cell has been mutated by an initiator, it is susceptible to the effects of promoters. These compounds promote the proliferation of the cell, giving rise to a large number of daughter cells containing the mutation created by the initiator. Unlike initiators, promoters do not covalently bind to DNA or macromolecules within the cell. There are two general categories of promoters: (1) specific promoters that interact with receptors on or in target cells of defined tissues, and (2) nonspecific promoters that alter gene expression without the presence of a known receptor. Promoters are often specific for a particular tissue or species due to their interaction with receptors that are present in different amounts in different tissue types. Very low doses of promoters will not lead to tumour development, and extremely high doses will not produce more risk than moderate levels of exposure.

Progression. In mice, repeated applications of promoters on initiator-exposed skin produce benign papillomas. Most of these papillomas regress after treatment is stopped, but some progress to cancer. The frequency of progression suggests that the papillomas that progress to cancer have acquired an additional, spontaneous mutation. The term progression refers to the stepwise transformation of a benign lesion to a neoplasm and to malignancy. Progression is associated with a karyotypic change, since virtually all tumours that advance have the wrong number of chromosomes (aneuploid). This karyotypic change is coupled with an increased growth rate, invasiveness, metastasis, and an alteration in biochemistry and morphology. As described above, the growth of a tumour from a single genetically altered cell is a stepwise progression.

11.12.3 Molecular and Genetic Basis of Cancer

Cancer is a disease of uncontrolled growth and proliferation whereby cells have escaped the body's normal growth control mechanisms and have gained the ability to divide indefinitely. *Carcinogenesis is a multi-step process requiring many genetic changes over time. These genetic alterations involve the activation of proto-oncogenes to oncogenes and the deregulation of tumour suppressor genes and DNA repair genes.* The process is characterised by cellular, genetic, and epigenetic changes and abnormal cell division.

According to the somatic mutation theory, carcinogens cause mutations in DNA that lead to cancer. Cancer development is based on the accumulation of somatic mutations over a lifetime. Germline mutations are typically not involved, but in rare cases of inherited cancer predisposition, they may contribute to disease progression. Mutations can occur whether the active carcinogenic agent (mutagen) is chemical, ionising radiation, or an oncogenic virus. Chemical mutagens comprise a group of chemicals that modify DNA through various mechanisms, such as alkylation or deamination of DNA bases or through intercalation between base pairs and the formation of DNA adducts (e.g. aromatic hydrocarbons). Oxidative damage may also affect DNA integrity. X-rays and radioactive radiation induce DNA double-strand breaks, whereas UV radiation forms pyrimidine dimers by cross-linking adjacent pyrimidine bases. Viral carcinogenesis involves several proteins produced by oncogenic viruses that can interact with p53, pRb, and other proteins that control cell growth and division, thus increasing the probability of a cell being pushed into repeated cycles of division.

According to the mutational hypothesis, one or more point mutations are responsible for initial and critical steps in the neoplastic process. Errors in the DNA sequence interrupt the genetic codes that govern the structure and function of the affected cell. A proliferating cell with DNA damage divides to give rise to two daughter cells, each capable of dividing, eventually resulting in a population of clones with similar genetic errors and malignant properties.

Transforming normal, healthy cells into cancer cells is directly attributable to genetic damage causing DNA abnormalities that alter cell growth, proliferation, and survival.

These abnormal genetic changes are termed mutations. A mutation is characterised by a change in the DNA sequence of an organism. Mutations can result from errors in DNA replication during cell division, exposure to mutagens, or a viral infection. Mutations may be acquired by the action of chemicals, radiation, or viruses or may be inherited. Mutations may include point mutation, deletion, translocation, insertion, and inversion. A point mutation occurs in a genome when a single base pair is added, deleted, or changed from a DNA sequence of an organism's genome. In several neoplasms, point mutations occur carrying a mutated *ras* gene. A deletion is a type of mutation that involves the loss of one or more nucleotides from a segment of DNA. A deletion can involve the loss of any number of nucleotides, from a single nucleotide to an entire piece of chromosome. In translocation, a segment from one chromosome is transferred to a nonhomologous chromosome or a new site on the same chromosome. Depending on the chromosome breakpoints, a translocation can result in the disruption of normal gene function. These molecular rearrangements, in many cases, are considered to be the primary cause of various cancers. Translocations are common in leukaemias and lymphomas and have been less commonly identified in cancers of solid tissues.

An example would be an exchange between chromosomes 9 and 22 seen in over 90% of patients with chronic myelogenous leukaemia (CML). The exchange leads to the formation of a shortened form of chromosome 22 called the Philadelphia chromosome. Insertion is a type of mutation that involves the addition of one or more nucleotides into a segment of DNA. An insertion can involve adding any number of nucleotides, from a single nucleotide to an entire piece of a chromosome. An inversion in a chromosome occurs when a segment breaks off and reattaches within the same chromosome but in reverse orientation. DNA may or may not be lost in the process. This rearrangement can lead to abnormal gene expression by activating an oncogene or deactivating a tumour suppressor gene.

11.12.4 Hallmarks of Carcinogenesis

The hallmarks of cancer comprise six major biological capabilities acquired during the multistep development of human neoplastic disease. They include sustaining proliferative signalling, evading growth suppressors, activating invasion and metastasis, enabling replicative immortality, inducing angiogenesis, and resisting cell death (Fig. 11.4). Emerging additional features include deregulating cellular metabolism and evading the immune system.

Sustaining proliferative signalling. All normal cells require stimulation by growth factors to undergo proliferation (paracrine signalling). *Cancer cells do not need stimula-*

Fig. 11.4 Hallmarks of cancer. Most cancer cells acquire the above six properties during development by mutations in the relevant genes. (Source: Douglas Hanahan and Robert Weinberg) Hanahan, D. & Weinberg, R. A. The hallmarks of cancer. Cell 100, 57–70 (2000). Source: Hanahan D, Weinberg RA. *Hallmarks of cancer: the next generation.* Cell 2011 Mar 4;144(5):646–74 Available from: http://www.ncbi.nlm. nih.gov/pubmed/21376230

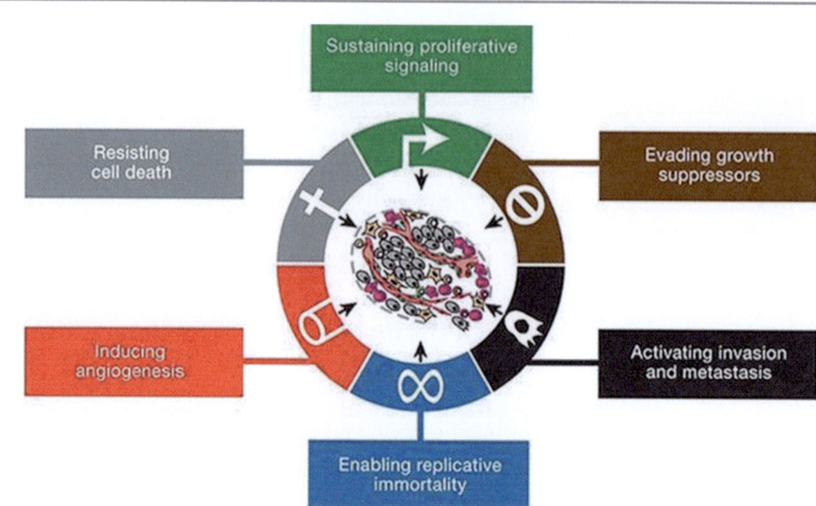

tion from external growth factors to multiply. They can produce signals themselves (autocrine signalling). Tumour cells can proliferate without external stimuli, usually due to oncogene activation.

Evading growth suppressors. *Tumour suppressor genes control cell division.* These genes encode proteins that inhibit cellular proliferation. These genes take information from the cell to ensure that it is ready to divide and will halt division when the DNA is damaged. In cancer, these tumour suppressor proteins are altered so that they don't effectively prevent cell division; In addition, normal cells will also stop dividing when they touch other cells, a process known as contact inhibition. Cancer cells do not have contact inhibition properties. As a result of which, they continue to divide. Cancer cells are generally resistant to growth-preventing signals from their neighbours.

Activating invasion and metastasis. *Cancer cells bypass the mechanism of apoptosis (programmed cell death) by altering the mechanisms that detect cellular damage.* This means that proper signalling cannot occur. Thus, apoptosis cannot be activated. Cancer cells may have defects in the proteins involved in apoptosis, preventing appropriate apoptosis.

Enabling replicative immortality. Non-cancer cells die after a certain number of divisions. They have a limited number of divisions before the cells cannot divide (senescence) or die (crisis). Cancer cells escape this limit and are capable of indefinite growth and division, gaining the status of immortality. But those immortal cells have damaged chromosomes, which can become cancerous. The cause of these barriers is primarily due to the DNA at the end of chromosomes, known as telomeres. Telomeric DNA shortens with every cell division until it becomes so short that it activates

senescence, so the cell stops dividing. Cancer cells bypass this barrier by manipulating enzymes (telomerase) to increase the length of telomeres. Thus, cancer cells can divide indefinitely without initiating senescence.

Inducing angiogenesis. Angiogenesis is the process by which new blood vessels are formed. Cancer cells appear to be able to initiate this process, ensuring that cancer cells receive a continual supply of oxygen and other nutrients. To do this, the cancer cells acquire the ability to produce new vasculature by activating the angiogenic switch. Thus, they control non-cancerous cells in the tumour that can form blood vessels by reducing the production of factors that inhibit blood vessel production and increasing the production of factors that promote blood vessel formation.

Resisting cell death. Cancer cells can break away from their site of origin to invade surrounding tissue and spread (metastasise) to distant body parts. The ability of cancer cells to invade neighbouring tissues dictates whether the tumour is benign or malignant. This multi-step process starts with a local invasion of the cells into the surrounding tissues, invades blood vessels or the lymphatic system, exits this system, and divides into new tissue.

Deregulated metabolism. Most cancer cells use alternative metabolic pathways to generate energy. Cancer cells upregulate glycolysis and lactic acid fermentation in the cytosol, preventing mitochondria from completing normal aerobic respiration. Instead of entirely oxidising glucose to produce as much ATP as possible, cancer cells would convert pyruvate into the building blocks for more cells.

Evading the immune system. Despite cancer cells causing increased inflammation and angiogenesis, they also appear to be able to avoid interaction with the body's immune system via a loss of interleukin-33.

11.12.5 Role of Tumour Suppressor Genes, Cellular Proto-Oncogenes, and Growth Factors in Carcinogenesis

Tumour Suppressor Genes. Tumour suppressor genes encode proteins that are receptors for secreted hormones. Their function includes (1) inhibition of cell proliferation, (2) negatively regulating cell cycle entry or progression and of growth signalling pathways (e.g. APC or PTEN), (3) checkpoint-control of proteins that arrest the cell cycle if DNA is damaged or chromosomes are abnormal, and (4) promotion of apoptosis DNA repair enzymes. *The transformation of a normal cell to a cancer cell is accompanied by the loss of function of one or more tumour suppressor genes.* Both gene copies must be defective to promote tumour development. The first tumour suppressor gene to be identified was by studies of retinoblastoma, a rare childhood eye tumour. The retinoblastoma (Rb) protein controls the cell cycle transition from G1 to S Phase. Rb protein binds regulatory transcription factor E2F, which is required to synthesise DNA replication enzymes. When Rb is bound to E2F, transcription/replication is blocked. The presence of growth factors (via the *Ras* pathway) activates cyclin-dependent kinase 4/6. Active CDK4/6- phosphorylates and inhibits Rb, taking the brakes off E2F, and transition to the S phase occurs.

Disruption/deletion of the Rb gene leads to uncontrolled cell proliferation. The second tumour suppressor gene to have been identified is p 53, which is frequently inactivated in various human cancers, including leukaemias, lymphomas, sarcomas, brain tumours, and carcinomas of many tissues, including breast, colon, and lung. In total, mutations of *p53* may play a role in up to 50% of all cancers, making it the most common target of genetic alterations in human malignancies. Two other tumour suppressor genes (*APC* and *MADR2*) are frequently deleted or mutated in colon cancers. Inherited mutations of two tumour suppressor genes, *BRCA1* and *BRCA2*, are responsible for hereditary breast cancer cases, accounting for 5–10% of the total breast cancer incidence.

Cellular proto-oncogenes and oncogenes. *Proto-oncogenes are physiologic regulators of cell proliferation and differentiation, while oncogenes are characterised by the ability to promote cell growth without normal mitogenic signals.* Their products, oncoproteins, resemble the normal products of proto-oncogenes, except that oncoproteins are devoid of important regulatory elements. Their production in the transformed cells becomes constitutive, not dependent on growth factors or other external signals. Genes that promote autonomous cell growth in cancer cells are called oncogenes. Proto-oncogenes can be converted to oncogenes by several mechanisms, including point mutation and gene amplification resulting in the overproduction of growth factors, flood-ing of the cell with replication signals, uncontrolled stimulation in the intermediary pathways, or cell growth by elevated levels of transcription factors. The *RAS* oncogene is the most frequently mutated in human cancer.

Growth factors and their receptors. Growth factors (GFs) play an important physiological role in the normal process of growth control aimed at maintaining tissue homeostasis. They transmit growth signals from one cell to another. Specific growth factor receptors (GFRs) sense these signals on the cell surface. GFRs transfer the growth signal via signalling pathways to activate target molecules that promote proliferation.

Steps that characterise normal cell proliferation include the binding of a GF to its specific receptor on the cell membrane, transient and limited activation of the GFR, which activates several signal-transducing proteins (e.g. Ras) on the inner leaflet of the plasma membrane, transmission of the signal-by-signal transduction molecules, either to cytosolic targets or to the nucleus where they activate the transcription of specific genes, and entry of the cell into the cell cycle, ultimately resulting in cell division. This pathway is often derailed in cancer and allows wayward cells to generate internal signals that stimulate proliferation and become independent of their environments. Cancer cells can induce their growth stimulatory signals when mutations in the GFR gene occur, which facilitates activation in the absence of GFs or when overproduction of GFs results in an autocrine signalling loop.

Other elements of cell signalling. An alternative strategy by which cancer cells can become GF-independent involves constitutive activation of internal signalling components. For example, the *Ras* protein in normal cells is switched off. It does not signal unless a GFR becomes activated. Through a series of intermediaries, it can activate the *Ras* protein, converting it from its quiescent state to an active, signal-emitting state. After that, the *Ras* protein can release further downstream signals capable of inducing proliferation. In cancer cells, this signalling pathway is deregulated.

11.13 Summary

Neoplasia refers to new abnormal growth. Neoplasms are commonly referred to as tumours. These are classified as benign and malignant (cancer). Cancer is a significant public health issue throughout the world. It is a leading cause of death worldwide. Breast, lung, colon, rectum, and prostate cancers are the most common. Causes of cancer can be broadly grouped as chemical, physical, and viral agents. These agents cause cellular mutations and cause abnormal proliferation of cells. Cancer development is a multistep process. The hallmarks of cancer comprise six major biological capabilities. They include sustaining proliferative signalling, evading growth suppressors, activating invasion and metastasis, enabling replicative immortality, inducing angiogenesis, resisting cell death, and evading the immune system. Clinical staging is helpful in determining the size and location of solid tumours. Biopsy, imaging studies, and molecular tests are used to diagnose cancer.

Bibliography

Cancer Council Australia Oncology Education Committee. Cancer biology: molecular and genetic basis. https://wiki.cancer.org.au/oncologyformedicalstudents_mw/index.php?oldid=1641, 2022 [cited 2022 Aug 26].

Ivan Damjanov. Neoplasia. Pathology for the health professions. (4th Ed). Elsevier 2012. 67–90.

EdCAN (n.d.).https://www.edcan.org.au/edcan-learning-resources/supporting-resources/biology-of-cancer/defining-cancer/carcinogenesis

Hanahan D, Weinberg RA. hallmarks of cancer: the next generation. Cell. 2011;144(5):646–74.

Kumar V, Abbas AK, Aster JC. Neoplasia. In: Robbins basic pathology. 10th ed. Philadelphia: Elsevier; 2018. p. 190–237.

Mori M. Host defense against tumor. JMA J. 2020;3(3):284–5.

Nakamura N. A hypothesis: radiation carcinogenesis may result from tissue injuries and subsequent recovery processes which can act as tumour promoters and lead to an earlier onset of cancer. Br J Radiol. 2020;93:20190843. https://doi.org/10.1259/bjr.20190843.

Roberts F, Macduff E. Neoplasia. In: Roberts F, Macduff E, editors. Pathology Illustrated. 8th ed. Edinburgh: Elsevier; 2017. p. 155–201.

https://wiki.cancer.org.au/oncologyformedicalstudents/Cancer_biology:_Molecular_and_genetic_basis. In: Sabesan S, Olver I, editors. Sydney: Cancer Council Australia. https://wiki.cancer.org.au/oncologyformedicalstudents/Clinical_Oncology_for_Medical_Students. Original Source: Alison MR. Cancer. Encyclopedia of Life Sciences, 2001. Reproduced with permission from John Wiley & Sons.

Strayer DS, Rubin E. Neoplasia. In: Strayer DS, editor. Rubin's pathology-clinicopathologic foundations of medicine. 7th ed. Philadelphia: Wolters Kluwer; 2015. p. 169–242.

Sung H, Ferlay J, Siegel RL, Laversanne M, Soerjomataram I, Jemal A, Bray F. Global cancer statistics 2020: GLOBOCAN estimates of incidence and mortality worldwide for 36 cancers in 185 countries. CA Cancer J Clin. 2021;71(3):209–49. https://doi.org/10.3322/caac.21660. Epub 2021 Feb 4. PMID: 33538338.

Underwood JCE. Carcinogenesis and Neoplasia. In: Underwood JCE, Cross SS, editors. General and systematic pathology. Churchill Livingstone; 2009. p. 221–58.

12

Environmental and Nutritional Pathology

12.1 Introduction

Humans are constantly exposed to hazardous pollutants in the environment, which include the air, water, soil, diet, and workplace. The term ambient environment encompasses various outdoor, indoor, and occupational settings. Other environmental factors include the "personal environment," which comprises tobacco use, alcohol consumption, therapeutic and "recreational" drug consumption, and diet. Environmental disease refers to disorders caused by exposure to chemical or physical agents in the ambient, workplace, and personal environments, including conditions of nutritional origin.

This chapter first deals with the health effects of climate change, followed by the mechanisms of toxicity of chemical and physical agents, and addresses specific environmental disorders, including those of nutritional origin.

12.2 Environmental Pollution

Environmental pollution exposure remains a significant source of health risks worldwide. Pollution introduces substances harmful to humans and other living organisms into the environment. Pollution remains responsible for approximately nine million deaths annually, corresponding to one in six deaths worldwide. *Pollution includes contamination of air by fine particulate matter, ozone; oxides of sulphur and nitrogen; freshwater pollution; contamination of the ocean by mercury, nitrogen, phosphorus, plastic, and petroleum waste; and poisoning of the land by lead, mercury, pesticides, industrial chemicals, electronic waste, and radioactive waste.* Environmental pollutants have various adverse health effects from early life. Some harmful essential impacts are perinatal disorders, infant mortality, respiratory disorders, allergy, malignancies, cardiovascular disorders, increase in oxidative stress, endothelial dysfunction, mental disorders, and various other harmful effects. More than 90% of pollution-related deaths occur in low-income and middle-income countries.

Air pollution is a mix of hazardous substances from both human-made and natural sources. It is the contamination of the indoor or outdoor environment by any chemical, physical, or biological agent that modifies the natural characteristics of the atmosphere. A pollutant is a substance introduced to the environment with undesired or adverse effects.

Sources of air pollutants include motor vehicle emissions, the products of burning fuels, including woodsmoke, and industrial emissions, such as gases produced by oil and coal refineries and materials such as paints and adhesives in new buildings. Environmental dust is an important air pollutant. Exposure to smoke from bushfires can worsen asthma and other respiratory conditions; cause coughing and shortness of breath; and irritate the eyes, nose, and throat.

12.3 Effects of Tobacco, Alcohol, and Substance Abuse

Smoking is the most preventable cause of human death. Tobacco smoke contains more than 2000 compounds. Among these are nicotine, which is responsible for tobacco addiction, and potent carcinogens—mainly polycyclic aromatic hydrocarbons, nitrosamines, and aromatic amines. Approximately 90% of lung cancers occur in smokers. Smoking is also associated with an increased risk of cancers of the oral cavity, larynx, oesophagus, stomach, bladder, and kidney, as well as some forms of leukaemia. Cessation of smoking reduces the risk of lung cancer. Smokeless tobacco use is an important cause of oral cancers. *Tobacco interacts with alcohol in multiplying the risk of oral, laryngeal, and oesophageal cancer and increases the risk of lung cancers from occupational exposures to asbestos, uranium, and other agents.* Tobacco consumption is a significant risk factor for the development of atherosclerosis and myocardial infarction, peripheral vascular disease, and cerebrovascular disease. In the lungs, in addition to cancer, it predisposes to emphysema, chronic bronchitis, and chronic obstructive disease (COPD). Maternal smoking increases the risk of abortion, premature birth, and intrauterine growth retardation.

S. R. Prabhu, *Textbook of General Pathology for Dental Students*, https://doi.org/10.1007/978-3-031-31244-1_12

Acute alcohol abuse causes drowsiness at blood levels of approximately 200 mg/dL. Stupor and coma develop at higher levels. Alcohol is oxidised to acetaldehyde in the liver primarily by alcohol dehydrogenase and, to a lesser extent, by the cytochrome P-450 system and by catalase. Acetaldehyde is converted to acetate in mitochondria and is used in the respiratory chain. Alcohol oxidation by alcohol dehydrogenase depletes NAD, leading to fat accumulation in the liver and metabolic acidosis. The main effects of chronic alcoholism are fatty liver, alcoholic hepatitis, and cirrhosis, which leads to portal hypertension and increases the risk of developing hepatocellular carcinoma. Chronic alcoholism can cause bleeding from gastritis and gastric ulcers, peripheral neuropathy associated with thiamine deficiency, and alcoholic cardiomyopathy, which increases the risk of developing acute and chronic pancreatitis. Chronic alcoholism is a significant risk factor for oral cavity, larynx, and oesophageal cancers. The risk is significantly increased by concurrent smoking or the use of smokeless tobacco.

The common substances of abuse include sedative-hypnotics (barbiturates, ethanol), psychomotor stimulants (cocaine, amphetamine, ecstasy), opioid narcotics (heroin, methadone, oxycodone), hallucinogens (LSD, mescaline), and cannabinoids (marijuana, hashish). They have diverse effects on various organs. The exact cause of substance abuse is unclear, but there are two predominant theories: a genetic predisposition or a habit learned from others. If addiction develops, drug abuse manifests itself as a chronic debilitating disease. Overdose of acetaminophen, for example, may cause centrilobular liver necrosis, leading to liver failure.

12.4   Effects of Radiation

Ionising radiation may injure cells directly or indirectly by generating free radicals from water or molecular oxygen. Ionising radiation damages DNA; therefore, rapidly dividing cells such as germ cells and those in the bone marrow and GI tract are susceptible to radiation injury. DNA damage that is not adequately repaired may result in mutations, predisposing affected cells to neoplastic transformation. Ionising radiation may cause vascular damage and sclerosis, resulting in ischemic necrosis of parenchymal cells and their replacement by fibrous tissue.

Non-ionizing radiation, such as ultraviolet radiation (UV) from sun exposure, can cause both beneficial and harmful effects. Exposure to UV stimulates the endogenous production of vitamin D in the skin. Excessive exposure to UV carries health risks. UV radiation (UV) is classified as a "complete carcinogen," because it is a mutagen and has the properties of both a tumour initiator and a tumour promoter. *UV can damage DNA and cause skin cancers such as basal cell carcinoma, squamous cell carcinoma, and malignant melanoma.*

12.5   Nutrition and Malnutrition.

Nutrition is the science of food and its relationship to health. Carbohydrates, protein, and fat (macronutrients) are required by the body in relatively large amounts, whereas vitamins and some trace minerals (micronutrients) are needed in minute amounts. Macronutrients constitute the bulk of the diet and supply energy. Carbohydrates, proteins (including essential amino acids), fats (including essential fatty acids), macrominerals (sodium, chloride, potassium, calcium, phosphate, and magnesium), and water are macronutrients. Carbohydrates, fats, and proteins are interchangeable as sources of energy: fats yield 9 kcal/g (37.8 kJ/g); proteins and carbohydrates yield 4 kcal/g (16.8 kJ/g).

Carbohydrates, proteins, and fats are digested in the intestine, where they are broken down into their basic units: Carbohydrates into sugars, proteins into amino acids, and fats into fatty acids and glycerol. The body uses these basic units to build substances it needs for growth, maintenance, and activity. Fibre is a complex carbohydrate. Dietary fibre can be soluble or insoluble. Insoluble fibre increases gastrointestinal motility and increases faecal bulk. Insoluble fibre is thought to accelerate the elimination of cancer-causing substances produced by bacteria in the large intestine. Proteins are complex organic molecules that contain carbon, hydrogen, oxygen, and nitrogen. Proteins are required for tissue maintenance, replacement, function, and growth. Specific proteins act as enzymes, make up certain hormones, and play an important role in maintaining fluid balance. If the body is not getting enough calories from dietary sources or tissue stores (particularly of fat), protein may be used for energy. Dietary proteins are broken down into peptides and amino acids. Fats are broken down into fatty acids and glycerol. Fats are required for tissue growth and hormone production. Saturated fatty acids, common in animal fats, tend to be solid at room temperature. Except for palm and coconut oils, fats derived from plants tend to be liquid at room temperature; these fats contain high levels of monounsaturated fatty acids or polyunsaturated fatty acids (PUFAs). Water is considered a macronutrient, because it is required in amounts of about 2500 mL/day. Needs vary with fever, physical activity, and changes in climate and humidity. The adequate intake for total water is 2.7 L for women and 3.7 L for men.

Vitamins and minerals are essential nutrients. That is, they cannot be made by the body from other substances in the diet. Thus, vitamins and minerals must be consumed in the diet. Vitamins are classified as water soluble(8 members of the B Complex vitamins) and Vitamin C) and fat soluble (A,D,E and K). Only vitamins A, D, E, K and B12 are stored in the body. Some minerals are required in fairly large quantities (about 1 or 2 g a day) and are considered macronutrients. They include calcium, chloride, magnesium, phosphorus (occurring mainly as phosphate in the body), potassium, and sodium. Minerals required in small amounts (trace minerals) are considered micronutrients. They include chromium, copper, fluoride, iodine, iron, manganese, molybdenum, selenium, and zinc. Some vitamins (such as vitamins C and E) and minerals (such as selenium) act as antioxidants. Antioxidants protect cells against damage by free radicals, which are by-products of the normal activity of cells. Free radicals readily participate in chemical reactions—some useful to the body and some not—and are thought to contribute to such disorders as heart and blood vessel disorders and cancer.

Malnutrition refers to deficiencies, excesses, or imbalances in a person's energy and nutrient intake. The term malnutrition covers three broad groups of conditions. One is "undernutrition"—which includes stunting (low height for age), wasting (low weight for height), underweight (low weight for age), and micronutrient deficiencies or insufficiencies (a lack of essential vitamins and minerals). The third group is the overweight, obesity, and diet-related noncommunicable diseases (such as heart disease, stroke, diabetes, and cancer).

12.5.1 Nutritional Deficiencies

A healthy diet provides sufficient energy, in the form of carbohydrates, proteins, and fats for the body's daily metabolic needs. Amino acids and fatty acids are used as building blocks for the synthesis of structural and functional proteins and lipids, and vitamins and minerals, which function as coenzymes or hormones in vital metabolic pathways or, as in the case of calcium and phosphate, as important structural components. Deficiencies in essential nutrients can lead to stunted growth, poor immune function, and classical conditions such as scurvy, osteoporosis, depression, and xerophthalmia.

12.5.1.1 Caloric and Protein Deficit

Marasmus and Kwashiorkor are the two nutrient deficiencies prevalent, particularly in less developed countries. *Marasmus is a result of severe malnutrition in children due to caloric deficit. It is associated with muscle atrophy and general failure of growth.* Kwashiorkor is severe childhood malnutrition resulting from a diet that is very low in protein but high in carbohydrates. Kwashiorkor is associated with growth failure, muscle wasting, and specific changes, including oedema, anaemia, changes in skin and hair pigment, and excessive fat storage in the liver. The liver in kwashiorkor, but not in marasmus, is enlarged and fatty. *Protein malnutrition produces alterations in the bone marrow that lead to cellular depletion.* The bone marrow in kwashiorkor and marasmus may be hypoplastic, mainly due to decreased cell precursors. This, in turn, results in anaemia with significant reticulocyte reduction and leukopenia.

12.5.1.2 Vitamin Deficiencies

Vitamins are a group of organic compounds essential for normal physiological functioning. The body does not synthesise endogenously and must be sequestered in small quantities from the diet. The body needs them in small amounts (micronutrients). In total, humans require adequate amounts of 13 vitamins: four fat-soluble vitamins (A, D, E, K) and nine water-soluble vitamins, which comprise vitamin C and the eight B vitamins: thiamine (B1), riboflavin (B2), niacin (B3), pantothenic acid (B5), pyridoxamine (B6), biotin (B7), folate (B9), and Cobalamin(B12). A deficiency of folic acid, vitamin B12, Vitamin B6, Vitamin B3, Vitamin C, and Vitamin E mimics radiation in damaging DNA by causing single- and double-strand breaks, oxidative lesions, or both. One or more of the B vitamins are involved in every aspect of the essential catabolic process of generating energy within cells, and deficiency in any one B vitamin will have negative consequences for this process. Deficiencies of specific vitamins are found throughout the world.

Vitamin A is necessary for normal embryonic development and postnatal tissue homeostasis and affects cell proliferation, differentiation, and apoptosis. Retinoic acid, the main biologically active form of vitamin A, influences the expression of collagens, laminins, entactin, fibronectin, elastin, and proteoglycans, which are the major components of the extracellular matrix. As cell behaviour, differentiation and apoptosis are influenced by the extracellular matrix, its modifications potentially compromise organ function and may lead to disease. *Vitamin A deficiency causes night blindness, squamous metaplasia, and infection vulnerability.*

The B vitamins comprise a group of water-soluble vitamins that perform essential, closely interrelated roles in cellular functioning, acting as co-enzymes in many catabolic and anabolic enzymatic reactions. These include thiamine (B1), riboflavin (B2), niacin (B3), pantothenic acid (B5), vitamin B6, folate (B9), and vitamin B12). *Vitamin B deficiencies cause beriberi, pellagra, and pernicious anaemia.*

Vitamin C (ascorbic acid) is a well-known antioxidant. It plays a central role in regenerating vitamin E and constitutes a strong line of defence in retarding free radical-induced cellular damage. *Scurvy is a pathological condition caused by severe vitamin C deficiency.*

Vitamin D deficiency is the most common nutritional deficiency in the world. Vitamin D is an essential nutrient for maintaining skeletal muscle and bone health. Vitamin D is responsible for the absorption of calcium and phosphate from the intestinal tract. It is one of the key controllers of systemic inflammation, oxidative stress, mitochondrial respiratory function, and, thus, the human ageing process. Hypovitaminosis D impairs mitochondrial functions and enhances oxidative stress and systemic inflammation. *The deficiency of vitamin D causes rickets in children and osteomalacia in adults.*

Vitamin E (α-Tocopherol) is a vital lipid peroxidation antioxidant in cell membranes. Vitamin E protects cell membranes from the damaging effects of free radicals. Vitamin E possesses anti-cancer properties and has also been found to reduce risk factors for arterial clotting by platelet aggregation and cholesterol. *Vitamin E deficiency can lead to neurological problems, such as difficulty coordinating movements (ataxia) and speech (dysarthria), loss of reflexes in the legs (lower limb areflexia), and a loss of sensation in the extremities (peripheral neuropathy).*

12.5.1.3 Deficiency of Other Essential Micronutrients

Iron is an essential micronutrient that facilitates cell proliferation and growth. It participates in various metabolic processes, including oxygen transport, deoxyribonucleic acid (DNA) synthesis, and electron transport. Dietary iron occurs in two forms: haem and non-haem. The primary sources of haem iron are haemoglobin and myoglobin from the consumption of meat, poultry, and fish, whereas non-haem iron is obtained from cereals, pulses, legumes, fruits, and vegetables. Iron deficiency is the most common nutritional deficiency in the world. The primary causes of iron deficiency include low intake of bioavailable iron, increased iron requirements due to rapid growth, pregnancy, menstruation, and excess blood loss caused by pathologic infections, such as hookworm and whipworm, causing gastrointestinal blood loss. *When iron stores are depleted, and insufficient iron is available for erythropoiesis, haemoglobin synthesis in erythrocyte precursors becomes impaired, and hematologic signs of iron deficiency anaemia appear.*

Zinc is involved in many aspects of cellular metabolism. The richest food sources of zinc include meat, fish, and seafood. It is required for the catalytic activity of hundreds of enzymes. It enhances immune function, protein synthesis, wound healing, cell signalling, and division. Zinc also supports healthy growth and development during pregnancy, infancy, childhood, and adolescence and is involved in the sense of taste. Zinc deficiency is associated with poor growth and development and impaired immune response. Zinc deficiency can also affect the skin, bones, digestive, reproductive, and central nervous systems.

12.5.2 Nutrient Excesses

Excessive nutrients can, over time, lead to unwanted weight gain, affect metabolic processes, and increase the risk of nutritional toxicities. Chronic nutrient overload disturbs metabolic homeostasis. The overflux of intracellular metabolites burdens the organelles within the cell, fuels the pathways favouring energy storage and biosynthesis, and inhibits energy-consuming pathways. Glycolysis is elevated to accelerate nutrient oxidation, but the process is not equipped to degrade nutrients completely.

12.5.2.1 Excesses of Carbohydrates, Proteins, and Fats

Carbohydrates, proteins, and fats all contribute calories to the diet, with carbohydrates providing primary fuel source. However, once the energy needs are met, excess carbohydrates can convert to fatty acids for storage in the adipose tissue. The dietary proteins and fats supply amino acids and fatty acids to the body, and, once the requirements for these nutrients are met, the excess can also convert to fat tissues.

12.5.2.2 Overweight and Obesity

Overweight and obesity refer to excess body weight. It mainly occurs because of an imbalance between energy intake (from the diet) and energy expenditure (through physical activities and bodily functions). The body stores the excess energy as fat. *Of all nutrients, excessive fat intake plays the most crucial role in the pathogenesis of overweight and obesity.* They have a relatively high energy value (per gram). Obese individuals cannot adequately burn fat during excessive supply, and the body responds by storing fat.

Body mass index (BMI) is often used to diagnose overweight and obesity. BMI is an internationally recognised standard for classifying overweight and obesity in adults. BMI is calculated by dividing a person's weight in kilograms by the square of their height in metres. A BMI of 25.0–29.9 is classified as overweight but not obese, while a BMI of 30.0 or over is classified as obese. A BMI of greater than 35.0 is classified as severely obese. Waist circumference for adults is a good indicator of total body fat and is a better predictor of certain chronic conditions than BMI, such as cardiovascular risk and type 2 diabetes (NHMRC 2013). A waist circumference above 80 cm for women and above 94 cm for men is associated with an increased risk of chronic conditions. A waist circumference above 88 cm for women and above 102 cm for men is associated with a substantially increased risk of chronic diseases (WHO 2000).

Obesity is associated with an increased incidence of several important diseases, such as hypertension, coronary heart disease, stroke, diabetes, and cancer. Excess cholesterol predisposes to atherosclerosis.

12.5.2.3 Hypervitaminosis

Although vitamins are essential for human health, they are each associated with adverse effects if consumed in excess. Hypervitaminosis occurs when the storage levels of vitamins are abnormally high. Hypervitaminosis can lead to toxic symptoms and diverse health effects. With few exceptions, like some vitamins from B-complex, hypervitaminosis usually occurs with the fat-soluble vitamins A and D, which are stored in the liver and fatty tissues of the body. These vitamins build up and remain longer in the body than water-soluble vitamins. Conditions include toxicity of hypervitaminosis A, D, and Vitamin B (B3 and B6).

Hypervitaminosis A is a lipid-soluble compound of the retinoic acid family that is mainly stored in the hepatic stellate (Ito) cells. It is essential for normal vision, the immune system, and reproduction. Hypervitaminosis A refers to the toxic effects of ingesting too much preformed vitamin A (retinyl esters, retinol and retinal). Vitamin A. Vitamers A, retinol (A1) or retinal (A2), and retonic acid all have vitamin A functions essential for maintaining epithelial cells. *An excess of vitamin A active compounds results in an enlargement of the liver and spleen, skin lesions, epithelial keratinisation, hyperplasia of head cartilage, and abnormal bone formation, including fusion of vertebrae.* Hypercalcemia can also occur due to the administration of vitamin A and its analogues (cis-retinoic acid).

Hypervitaminosis D: Vitamin D is a crucial prohormone vital in maintaining healthy bones and calcium levels. Hypervitaminosis D is a product of excessive vitamin D intake in children and adults. Although vitamin D increases intestinal absorption of calcium, the dominant mechanism of hypercalcaemia is excessive bone resorption. *Vitamin D toxicity, confusion, apathy, recurrent vomiting, abdominal pain, polyuria, polydipsia, and dehydration are the most often noted clinical symptoms.*

Vitamin B6 Excess (Vitamin B6 Toxicity). The body uses vitamin B6 in numerous enzymatic reactions, including neurotransmitter production, amino acid metabolism, glucose metabolism, lipid metabolism, haemoglobin synthesis and function, and gene expression. The most common symptoms associated with vitamin B6 (excess) toxicity are similar to those with vitamin B6 deficiency. *A patient with vitamin B 6 excess will experience peripheral sensory neuropathy.*

Vitamin B3 Excess(Vitamin B3 toxicity) Vitamin B3 is one of the 8 B vitamins. It is also known as niacin (nicotinic acid) and has 2 other forms, niacinamide (nicotinamide) and inositol hexanicotinate. Niacin, in its forms of nicotinic acid and nicotinamide, is mainly metabolised in the liver. Niacin, in its forms of nicotinic acid and nicotinamide, is mainly metabolised in the liver. It is used for the prevention and treatment of niacin deficiency. Before statin drugs became available, nicotinic acid was used to treat hypercholesterolemia and hypertriglyceridemia. *At higher doses, niacin toxicity can cause severe reactions, including hypotension,*

hepatotoxicity, and multiple organ failure. Niacin-associated hepatotoxicity is generally related to ingestions of around 3 g per day.

12.5.2.4 Iron Excess (Iron Toxicity)

Iron is found in many over-the-counter (OTC) multivitamins. Iron toxicity from intentional or accidental ingestion is common. Ingestion of less than 20 mg/kg of elemental iron is non-toxic. Ingestion of 20 mg/kg to 60 mg/kg results in moderate symptoms. Ingestion of more than 60 mg/kg can result in severe toxicity and lead to severe morbidity and mortality. Severe overdose causes impaired oxidative phosphorylation and mitochondrial dysfunction, which can result in cellular death. The liver is one of the organs most affected by cellular iron toxicity, but other organs such as the heart, kidneys, lungs, and the hematologic systems also may be impaired. *With chronic iron overload, the deposit of iron into the heart may cause death due to myocardial siderosis.*

12.6 Summary

Environmental and nutritional disorders pose significant public health issues. Air pollution, environmental radiation, tobacco, alcohol, substance abuse, protein and calorie deficit and excess, and vitamin deficiencies and excesses cause diseases in many parts of the world.

Bibliography

Bhupathiraju SN and Hu F 2023. Carbohydrates, proteins and fats https://www.merckmanuals.com/.../carbohydrates,-proteins,-and-fats.

Boffetta P, Hecht S, Gray N, et al. Smokeless tobacco and cancer. Lancet Oncol. 2009;9:667.

Hayes DP. Adverse effects of nutritional inadequacy and excess: a hormetic model. Am J Clin Nutr. 2008;88(2):578S–81S. https://doi.org/10.1093/ajcn.88.2.578S.

Hollick MF. Vitamin D deficiency. N Engl J Med. 2007;357:266.

Kumar V, Abbas AK, Aster JC. Chapter 8. Environmental and nutritional diseases. In: Robbins basic pathology. 10th ed. Philadelphia: Elsevier; 2018. p. 299–338.

Overweight and Obesity. Australian Institute of Health and Welfare. 2022. https://www.aihw.gov.au/reports/australias-health/overweight-and-obesity.

Strayer DS, Rubin E. Environmental and nutritional pathology. In: Strayer DS, editor. Rubin's pathology-Clinicopathologic foundations of medicine. 7th ed. Philadelphia: Wolters Kluwer; 2015. p. 327–66.

WHO (World Health Organization) (2000) Obesity: Preventing and managing the global epidemic.

Yuen H-W, Becker W. Iron Toixicity. Treasure Island (FL): StatPearls Publishing; 2023. https://www.ncbi.nlm.nih.gov/books/NBK459224/.

Hemodynamic Disorders

13

13.1 Introduction

Hemodynamic is the general term used to refer to the study of blood flow. The vascular system is a closed circuit. The intact circulatory system is essential for the normal function and metabolism of organs of the body. Hemodynamic disorders are characterised by disturbances in perfusion that result in cellular injury. These include hyperemia and congestion, haemorrhage, thrombosis, embolism, infarction, oedema, and shock.

13.2 Hyperemia and Congestion

Hyperemia refers to active engorgement of vascular beds with a normal or decreased outflow of blood. *Hyperemia is a dynamic process resulting from an increased inflow of blood into tissue because of arteriolar vasodilation.* This commonly occurs in exercising a skeletal muscle or acute inflammation. Affected tissue becomes red as there is engorgement with oxygenated blood. Neurogenic reflexes and the release of vasoactive substances, such as histamine and prostaglandins, mediate the change to promote the delivery of inflammatory mediators to the site. Tissues with hyperemic vessels are bright red and warm, and there is engorgement of the arterioles and capillaries.

Congestion is an abnormal collection of fluid, often blood, causing engorgement in an organ. *Congestion is a passive process resulting from the impaired outflow of blood from tissue.* Irregularities in intravascular pressures, coagulation, vessel structure, and other anatomic changes can obstruct flow and lead to congestion. Venous congestion produces a state of passive hyperemia, where accumulated blood in the venous system leads to cyanosis and, ultimately, ischemia of the skin and tissues. This occurs systemically in cardiac failure or locally in isolated venous obstruction. The affected tissue appears blue-red due to the accumulation of deoxygenated blood. In long-standing congestion (also called chronic passive congestion states), poorly oxygenated blood causes hypoxia, which can result in parenchyma cell degeneration or cell death.

13.3 Haemorrhage

Haemorrhage is the extravasation of blood (bleeding) outside the blood vessel. Haemorrhages can occur when a blood vessel ruptures or when blood leaves through intact blood vessels.

Clinically haemorrhage can manifest in different forms. Extravasated blood enclosed within a tissue, or a cavity, is known as a hematoma; minute 1–2 mm haemorrhages occurring in the skin, mucosal membrane, or serosal surface are called petechiae; slightly larger than 3 mm haemorrhage occurring in the skin is referred to as purpura and larger than 1–2 cm subcutaneous hematoma is called ecchymosis (bruises).

Presentation of haemorrhage varies by anatomic location. Sites of haemorrhage include bleeding from the nose (epistaxis), blood in the vomit (hematemesis), blood in the sputum (hemoptysis), bleeding from the uterus (menorrhagia), blood in stools (melena), blood in the urine (haematuria), blood in the thoracic cavity (haemothorax), and bleeding within the skull (intracranial bleeding).

Causes of external haemorrhage include physical trauma (lacerations, incisions, contusions), infections, septicemia, necrosis, ulcers in skin or mucosa, and neoplasms. Endogenous factors that cause haemorrhage include inadequate blood clotting due to qualitative and quantitative defects of platelets, missing or low levels of prothrombin, fibrinogen, and other clotting factor precursors, and insufficient vitamin K leading to clotting factor deficiency. A detailed discussion of these is beyond the scope of this chapter.

The effects of haemorrhage depend on the location, rate, and amount of blood loss. In a healthy adult, there is an aver-

S. R. Prabhu, *Textbook of General Pathology for Dental Students*, https://doi.org/10.1007/978-3-031-31244-1_13

age of 4.5–5.5 L (or 70–90 mL/kg) of blood circulating at any given time. Most adults can tolerate losing up to 14% of their blood volume without physical symptoms or deviations in their vital signs. If more than 20% of the total blood volume is rapidly lost from the body, it may lead to hypovolemic shock and death. Chronic loss of blood leads to anaemia.

13.4   Haemostasis

Haemostasis is the physiologic response to vascular injury resulting in a platelet-fibrin clot that prevents haemorrhage at the site of an injury. There are two main components of haemostasis: Primary and secondary. *Primary haemostasis refers to platelet aggregation and platelet plug formation.* Platelets are activated and adhere to the injury site and each other, plugging the injury. *Secondary haemostasis refers to the deposition of insoluble fibrin, forming a mesh incorporated into and around the platelet plug.* The proteolytic coagulation cascade generates this. This mesh strengthens and stabilises the blood clot. Both primary and secondary processes happen simultaneously. Blood clot seals the injured area and control and prevents further bleeding while tissue regeneration occurs. Once the injury starts to heal, the plug slowly remodels, and it dissolves with the restoration of normal tissue at the site of the damage.

The mechanism of haemostasis includes several events. The normal haemostatic system limits blood loss by highly regulated interactions among vessel wall components, circulating platelets, and plasma proteins. Haemostasis may be categorised into primary (platelet plug formation), secondary (formation of a stabilised fibrin clot through the coagulation cascade), and tertiary (formation of plasmin for the breakdown of fibrin via fibrinolysis) concurrent processes.

Soon after the trauma to the blood vessels, a vascular spasm occurs, resulting in vasoconstriction. The extracellular matrix (ECM) and collagen at the site of the endothelial injury become exposed to the blood components. The ECM immediately releases cytokines and inflammatory markers. This facilitates the adhesion and aggregation of platelets at the site of endothelial injury, forming a platelet plug and sealing the defect. The interaction mediates this process between various receptors and proteins. These include tyrosine kinase receptors, glycoprotein receptors, other G-protein receptors, and the von Willebrand Factor (vWF). The adhered and aggregated platelets release their cytoplasmic granules, including ADP, thromboxane A2, serotonin, and multiple other activation factors. A primary platelet plug forms at the damaged endothelial surface with these mechanisms involved. The plug is temporary and is removed as wound healing occurs.

13.5   Disorders of haemostasis

Disorders of haemostasis may lead to bleeding (hypercoagulation) disorders such as haemophilia, von Willebrand disease, intrinsic platelet disorders, or thromboembolic disorders.

Clotting disorders are usually recognised clinically by excessive haemorrhage. They may be hereditary or acquired. *Hereditary bleeding disorders occur due to the absence or deficiency of specific clotting proteins.* Haemophilia A, B, and von Willebrand disease are the three most common hereditary bleeding disorders.

Haemophilia A is an X-linked recessive genetic heredity disorder characterised by Factor VIII deficiency. Haemophilia B, also known as Christmas disease, is an X-linked genetic coagulopathy characterised by Factor IX deficiency. Females may be asymptomatic carriers of the haemophilia gene or may be found to have a partial lack of the specific factors involved. Von Willebrand disease is an autosomal-dominant trait with no predilection for sex. Individuals with moderate-to-severe haemophilia may exhibit mucosal or gingival bleeding, easy bruising, and hematoma formation. Those with mild haemophilia may only present bleeding after a traumatic injury or surgery. Von Willebrand disease can exhibit clinical signs and symptoms starting in childhood with a history of easy bruising and bleeding.

The platelet-related haemostatic disease includes thrombocytopenia. This refers to a reduced platelet number (the normal range is 140,000–400,000/μL). When the platelet count drops below 30,000–40,000/μL, bleeding may result.

The causes of thrombocytopenia include pregnancy (gestational thrombocytopenia), drugs that cause immune-mediated platelet destruction (commonly, heparin, trimethoprim/sulfamethoxazole), and rarely vaccinations (e.g. influenza, shingles, measles, mumps, and rubella, A COVID-19), drugs that cause dose-dependent bone marrow suppression (e.g. chemotherapeutic agents, ethanol), systemic infection and Immune disorders (immune thrombocytopenia).

13.6   Laboratory diagnosis of haemostatic disorders

Bleeding Time is the traditional initial test for detecting and evaluating primary haemostasis. The bleeding time (BT) assesses the function of the platelets and blood vessel integrity. BT is the time a standardised skin wound takes to stop bleeding. The normal range is 2.5–9.5 min. Bleeding times can be delayed in patients with vWF deficiency or medications that interfere with platelet function (e.g. NSAIDs, aspirin, and valproic acid). Routine laboratory analysis for clotting disorders also starts with platelet count, prothrombin time (PT), partial thromboplastin time (aPTT), and the international normalised ratio (INR); the normal platelet count ranges from 150,000 to 500,000/mL. Prothrombin time (PT) (normal = 11.5 to 14 s) represents the function of coagulation factors II, V, VII, and X. These are vitamin-K-dependent factors. Patients taking warfarin will affect the PT and INR as it interferes with the synthesis of vitamin-K-dependent factors. The INR (normal = 0.8 to 1.2) is a ratio used to estimate the percent of functional clotting factors. For example, an INR of 2 to 3 correlates approximately with 10% of active clotting factors. For normal coagulation, it is necessary to have at least 30% of the clotting factors. Haemophiliacs will have an elevated aPTT and a normal PT/INR, bleeding time, and platelet count. The aPTT, a measure of the intrinsic pathway, will be elevated due to low Factor VIII levels. In von Willebrand disease, bleeding time increases and vWF levels decrease.

13.7 Thrombosis

Thrombosis is the formation of a thrombus (plural: thrombi) which refers to a blood clot that forms within a vein, artery, or in the heart when blood platelets, proteins, and cells stick together. A thrombus may block the flow of blood.

Thrombi form only in living persons. *Platelets and clotting factors are involved in the pathogenesis of thrombus.* Three factors predispose to thrombus formation: damage to the endothelial lining of the vessel wall, arterial or venous blood stasis, and a hypercoagulable state. These factors are collectively called Virchow's triad. Any one of these can form a thrombus.

Endothelial injury is the most important factor in thrombus formation. A monolayer of endothelial cells constitutes the inner cellular lining of the blood vessels. The endothelium is a major player in controlling blood fluidity, platelet aggregation, and vascular tone. Alterations in normal blood flow, such as turbulence or stasis, promote thrombus formation. One example of an endothelial injury promoting thrombosis is an ulcerated atherosclerotic plaque. This irregularity on the endothelial surface exposes the subendothelial extracellular matrix and causes local blood flow turbulence.

13.8 Arterial or Venous Blood Stasis and Turbulence

The cellular elements in normal blood flow centrally in the vessel lumen (laminar flow). Cells are separated from the vascular endothelium by a clear zone of plasma. Stasis and turbulence of blood flow disrupt the laminar flow and bring platelets into contact with the endothelium. *Aneurysms (aortic and arterial dilations) cause local turbulence; a dilated atrium in the presence of atrial fibrillation is a site of significant stasis that may provoke thrombus development.* Additional conditions associated with stasis include sickle cell anaemia and polycythaemia, which may predispose a patient to thrombosis.

13.9 Hypercoagulable State

Hypercoagulability refers to any alteration of the coagulation pathway that places the patient at risk for thrombosis. *Alterations in the coagulation system can result from inflammatory factors, variations in the viscosity of blood and blood components, increased cytokines and prothrombotic proteins in circulation, or deficiencies of natural or endogenous anticoagulant factors.* Two types of hypercoagulability states occur: primary and secondary. Primary disorders are genetically inherited, and secondary disorders are acquired, including tissue damage such as surgery, fractures, burns, myocardial infarction, cancer, heparin-induced thrombocytopenia, and old age.

Thrombi may develop anywhere in the cardiovascular system. Based on their location, they are divided into arterial and venous thrombi. In descending order, the most common site of arterial thrombi is coronary, cerebral, and temporal arteries. Cardiac thrombi can be considered arterial thrombi.

13.10 Arterial Thrombosis

Normally, the rapid flow of arterial blood prevents the occurrence of thrombosis unless the vessel wall is damaged. Atheroma is by far the commonest predisposing lesion for arterial thrombosis. Atheromatous plaques produce turbulence and may ulcerate and cause endothelial injury, both of which can lead to thrombosis. These thrombi may narrow or occlude the lumen of arteries such as the coronary and cerebral arteries. Occlusion of these arteries will lead to myocardial infarction (MI) and cerebral infarction, respectively. *Cardiac thrombi can also be caused by infective endocarditis.* Bacteria or fungi can damage cardiac valves and develop small, infected thrombi on the valves (vegetation). In atrial fibrillation, a thrombus can form in the atrium.

The fate of the thrombus: A thrombus may accumulate more platelets and fibrin and cause blood vessel obstruction or dislodge and travel to other sites in the vasculature. The latter phenomenon is called embolisation. Total obstruction of the vessel by thrombus may cause the death of the tissue supplied by the vessel. This is called infarction. A thrombus may disappear by fibrinolytic activity (dissolution) or may get organised. The organisation of the thrombus occurs through the ingrowth of the fibrin-rich thrombus by endothelial cells, smooth muscle cells, and fibroblasts. The organisation of the thrombus may be accompanied by the formation of capillaries in the thrombus, thus re-establishing the lumen continuity. This process is called recanalisation.

Clinical effects of thrombi. An arterial thrombus may cause loss of pulse distal to the thrombus; over time, the tissue supplied by the artery may die. Myocardial infarction and stroke are examples of the formation of arterial thrombus. Venous thrombosis affects veins of the lower extremities in over 95% of cases. Superficial venous thrombosis is common in varicosities. When thrombosis occurs deep, it can cause deep venous thrombosis (DVT). *Superficial thrombi rarely embolise, whereas deep venous thrombosis can cause embolisation and serious consequences.* Pregnancy, malnutrition, cancer, and inflammation of veins (thrombophlebitis) are known to predispose to thrombosis.

13.11　Disseminated Intravascular Coagulation (DIC)

Disseminated intravascular coagulation (DIC) is a widespread hypercoagulable state that can lead to microvascular and macrovascular clotting and compromised blood flow, resulting in multiple organ dysfunction syndromes (MODS). DIC is not a specific illness; instead, it is a complication or an effect of the progression of other illnesses. This process begins consuming clotting factors and platelets, resulting in haemorrhage, which may be the presenting symptom of a patient with DIC. Disseminated intravascular coagulation is a rare but severe condition.

13.12　Embolism

An embolus is a detached intravascular solid, liquid, or gaseous mass carried by the blood to a site distant from its origin. The vast majority of emboli arise from thrombi. Other sources of emboli include air, nitrogen, fat, amniotic fluid, foreign bodies, and tumour cells. Unless otherwise specified, the term embolism should be considered to mean thromboembolism. *Approximately 99% of all emboli are a part of a thrombus that has been dislodged and is referred to as thromboembolism.* A thromboembolic event occurs when an embolus lodges in a vessel, rendering it unable to pass and causing partial or complete occlusion. If necrosis of the distal tissue results, it is referred to as infarction. An embolus will lodge in either the pulmonary or systemic circulation (depending on its site of origin), and the clinical outcome will depend on its resting place.

13.13　Pulmonary Embolism

The vast majority are caused by venous thromboembolism (VTE) arising from the deep veins of the lower limbs. Clinical signs/symptoms of pulmonary embolism vary depending on the size of the embolus. Suppose the embolus is very small (as in 60–80% of the cases), and the pulmonary emboli will be clinically silent. Embolic obstruction of medium-sized arteries manifests as pulmonary haemorrhage but usually does not cause infarction because of dual blood inflow to the area from the bronchial circulation. If the thrombus is large, it may block the outflow tract of the right ventricle, the bifurcation of the main pulmonary trunk (saddle embolus), or both branches, causing sudden death by circulatory arrest. *Sudden death, right-side heart failure (corpulmonale), or cardiovascular collapse occurs when 60% or more of the pulmonary circulation is obstructed with emboli.* The most common symptoms and signs of pulmonary embolism include pleuritic pain (sharp and stabbing pain, well localised and exacerbated by deep inspiration), breathlessness, hemoptysis, tachycardia, hypotension, and collapse. Recurrent thromboembolism can lead to pulmonary hypertension in the long run.

13.14　Systemic Thromboembolism

Systemic thromboembolism refers to emboli travelling within the arterial circulation and impacting the systemic arteries. *Most systemic emboli (80%) arise from intracardiac mural thrombi.* Two-thirds of intracardiac mural thrombi are associated with left ventricular wall infarcts, and a quarter with dilated left atria secondary to rheumatic valvular heart disease. Twenty percent of systemic emboli arise from an aortic aneurysm, thrombi on ulcerated atherosclerotic plaques, or fragmentation of valvular vegetation. Arterial emboli can travel to a wide variety of sites; the major sites are the lower extremities (75%) and the brain (10%), with the rest lodging in the intestines, kidneys, and spleen. The emboli may obstruct the arterial blood flow to the tissue distal to the site of the obstruction. This obstruction may lead to infarction. The infarctions, in turn, will lead to different clinical features, which vary according to the organ involved.

13.15 Infarction

Infarction is tissue death (necrosis) within the living body. It may be caused by blockage of the artery resulting in ischemia, rupture, mechanical compression, or vasoconstriction. The resulting lesion is referred to as an infarct. *Nearly 99% of all infarcts result from thrombotic or embolic events.* Other mechanisms include local vasospasm, expansion of atheroma due to haemorrhage into atheromatous plaque, external compression of the vessels (e.g. trauma), entrapment of vessels at hernial sacks, etc.

Morphology and classification of infarcts. The gross appearance of all infarcts is wedge-shaped, with the occluded vessel at the apex and the periphery of the organ forming the base of the wedge. The infarction will induce inflammation in the tissue surrounding the area of infarction. Following inflammation, some of the infarcts may show recovery. However, most are ultimately replaced with scars except in the brain.

Based on their gross appearance, infarcts are divided into white (pale) and red.

White infarcts occur in arterial occlusion in solid organs with a single arterial blood supply. Organs such as the heart, spleen, and kidney limit the amount of blood to percolate or seep into the area of ischemic necrosis from the nearby capillaries.

Red infarcts occur in venous occlusions (e.g. ovarian torsion), loose tissues (e.g. lung), and tissues with dual circulations (e.g. lung), in tissues that were previously congested because of sluggish outflow of blood, and when blood flow is re-established to a site of previous arterial occlusion and necrosis. Clinical examples include myocardial infarction, cerebral infarction, lung infarcts, kidney infarcts, and splenic infarcts.

Myocardial infarction usually results from occlusive thrombosis supervening an ulcerating atheroma of a major coronary artery. This is an example of a white infarct. Infarction is irreversible. Fibrosis replaces the damaged cells. Myocardial infarction can cause sudden death and cardiac failure.

Cerebral infarcts may appear pale or red. A fatal increase in intracranial pressure may occur due to swelling of a large cerebral infarction. Recent infarcts are raised above the surface, since hypoxic cells cannot maintain ionic gradients, absorb water, and swell. It is one cerebrovascular accident (CVA) type or stroke with various clinical manifestations. Necrotic brain cells cannot be replaced by regeneration.

Fibrosis cannot occur; the liquefied necrotic tissue is ultimately resorbed, leaving behind a cavity filled with clear fluid.

Pulmonary infarction is typically a dark red and conical (wedge-shaped) necrotic lesion. Pulmonary embolism is the most common aetiology for the development of infarction. Other diseases leading to pulmonary infarction include infection, malignancy, surgical iatrogenesis, amyloidosis, sickle cell disease, and vasculitis. Pulmonary infarction can cause chest pain and haemoptysis.

Renal infarction. Renal infarction is a rare condition, usually in individuals suffering from hypercoagulable states or with a history of atrial fibrillation or conditions predisposing to embolic events.

Splenic infarction. Splenic infarction occurs when blood flow to the spleen is compromised, causing tissue ischemia and eventual necrosis. Splenic infarction may be the result of arterial or venous occlusion. Bland or septic emboli and venous congestion by abnormal cells usually cause occlusion. Infarcts are conical and subcapsular. Initially, they are dark red, and later they turn pale.

13.16 Oedema

Oedema is a localised or generalised abnormal fluid accumulation in interstitial spaces and body cavities. *In oedematous conditions, capillary filtration exceeds the limits of lymphatic drainage.* The capillary hydrostatic and oncotic pressure gradients across the capillary regulate the fluid between the interstitial and intravascular spaces. The fluid accumulation occurs when local or systemic conditions disrupt this equilibrium, leading to increased capillary hydrostatic pressure, increased plasma volume, decreased plasma oncotic pressure (hypoalbuminemia), increased capillary permeability, or lymphatic obstruction.

When oedema is localised, it is designated descriptively. Examples include cerebral, ankle, periorbital, and pulmonary oedema. In the abdominal cavity, oedema is called ascites; in the pleural cavity, it is called hydrothorax. Generalised oedema is called anasarca. Patients with peripheral oedema usually present with painless swelling of the lower extremities. A residual indentation left by pressure on the site of the swelling indicates pitting oedema (figure). Bilateral lower limb pitting oedema is often a sign of cardiac failure, while generalised peripheral pitting oedema with swelling of the eyelids indicates hypoalbuminemia, as in Nephrotic syndrome. Non-pitting oedema is seen especially in patients with lymphatic and thyroid disorders.

Causes of oedema may include venous insufficiency, heart failure, kidney disease, low protein levels, liver disease, deep vein thrombosis, infections, lymphatic obstruction, certain medications, hereditary or acquired allergic reactions (angioedema), malnutrition, prolonged sitting, and pregnancy.

Forms of oedema. Oedema may be divided into inflammatory and non-inflammatory types.

Inflammatory oedema is due to inflammation-induced increased vascular permeability and leakage of plasma proteins. The resultant protein-rich fluid is called an exudate. This occurs in acute inflammation, chronic inflammation, and in angiogenesis. Inflammatory mediators, vascular dilatation, and increased blood flow cause increased vessel wall permeability.

Non-inflammatory oedema. This occurs in conditions characterised by increased hydrostatic pressure (e.g. hypertension and heart failure), reduced plasma osmotic pressure (e.g. Nephrotic syndrome), lymphatic obstruction (e.g. lymphedema due to obstruction by the tumour), and sodium retention (e.g. hyperaldosteronism). The fluid is called transudate.

Oedema of the lower extremities is typical of heart failure.

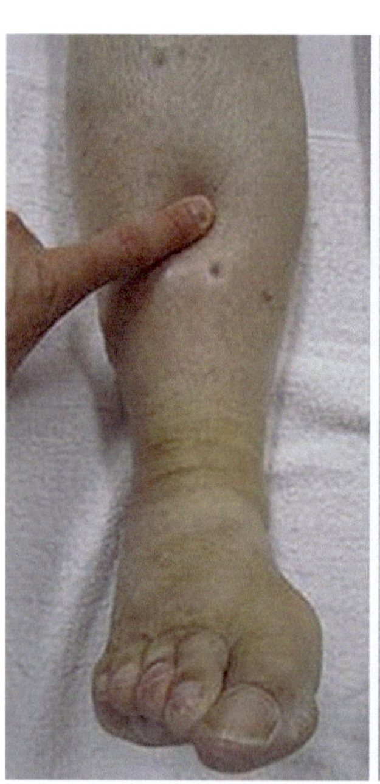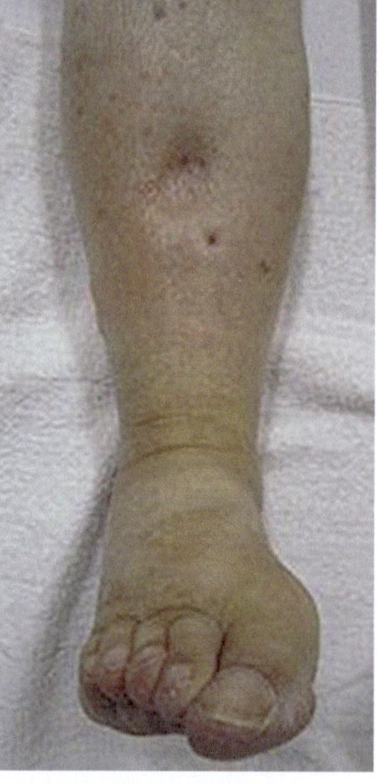

Pitting oedema during and after the application of pressure to the skin. This can occur due to standing or sitting too long, an allergic reaction, side effect of medicine, such as drugs for diabetes, high blood pressure, estrogen pills, or over-the-counter pain, and pregnancy. It can be a sign of congestive heart failure, deep vein thrombosis, liver failure, kidney failure, lymphoedema. A rise in hydrostatic pressure occurs in cardiac failure. A fall in osmotic pressure occurs in nephrotic syndrome and liver failure. Causes of oedema which are generalised to the whole body can cause oedema in multiple organs and peripherally. For example, severe heart failure can cause pulmonary oedema, pleural effusions, ascites and peripheral oedema. Pitting on pressure. Wikipedia.James Heilman. MD. https://en.wikipedia.org/wiki/Edema.

13.17 Shock

Shock is a state of organ hypoperfusion with resultant cellular hypoxia/anoxia and dysfunction. The fundamental defect in shock is reduced perfusion of vital tissues. Once perfusion declines and oxygen delivery to cells is inadequate for aerobic metabolism, cells shift to anaerobic metabolism with increased carbon dioxide production and elevated blood lactate levels. Cellular function declines, and if shock persists, irreversible cell damage and death occur.

There are several types of shock: septic shock caused by bacteria; anaphylactic shock caused by hypersensitivity or allergic reaction; cardiogenic shock from heart damage; hypovolemic shock from blood or fluid loss, and neurogenic shock from spinal cord trauma.

Septic shock is life-threatening when blood pressure drops dangerously low after an infection. Gram-negative bacterial infections are the major causes of septic shock syndromes, followed by Gram-positive bacterial infections. Fever (temperature higher than 38 C) or hypothermia (temperature less than 36 C), tachycardia (heart rate more than 90 beats per minute), tachypnoea (respiratory rate more than 20 breaths per minute), leucocytosis (WBC greater than 12,000/mm^3), or leukopenia (white blood cells (WBC) less than 4000/mm^3) are common features in septic shock syndrome. Sepsis results from an exaggerated systemic inflammatory response induced by infecting organisms. Inflammatory mediators are the key players in the pathogenesis of sepsis.

Cardiogenic shock is a clinical entity characterised by a low cardiac output state of circulatory failure that results in end-organ hypoperfusion and tissue hypoxia. The most common cause of cardiogenic shock is acute myocardial infarction. However, other disorders leading to impairment of the myocardium, valves, conduction system, or pericardium also can result in cardiogenic shock. Ischemia to the myocardium causes derangement to both systolic and diastolic left ventricular function, resulting in a profound depression of myocardial contractility.

Hypovolemic shock is characterised by severe hypovolemia (a condition in which blood plasma volume is too low) with decreased peripheral perfusion. This results from loss of circulatory volume, often due to major post-traumatic or surgical haemorrhagic events. Fluid loss due to vomiting, diarrhoea, and extensive burns are other causes of hypovolemic shock. The first changes in vital signs seen in hypovolemic shock include increased diastolic blood pressure with narrowed pulse pressure. As volume status continues to decrease, systolic blood pressure drops. As a result, oxygen delivery to vital organs cannot meet oxygen demand.

Cells switch from aerobic metabolism to anaerobic metabolism, resulting in lactic acidosis. As sympathetic drive increases, blood flow is diverted from other organs to preserve blood flow to the heart and brain. This propagates tissue ischemia and worsens lactic acidosis. If not corrected, the worsening hemodynamic compromise can eventually cause death.

Neurogenic shock is a devastating consequence of spinal cord injury (SCI) that can manifest as hypotension, bradyarrhythmia, and temperature dysregulation. It is mostly associated with cervical and high thoracic spine injury. Neurogenic shock is a combination of both primary and secondary injuries that lead to loss of sympathetic tone and, thus, unopposed parasympathetic response driven by the vagus nerve. Consequently, patients suffer from instability in blood pressure, heart rate, and temperature regulation.

13.18 Summary

Haemodynamic disorders are of clinical importance. These include hyperemia, congestion, haemorrhage, haemophilia, thrombosis, embolism, infarction, oedema, and shock.

Bibliography

Damjanov I. Hemodynamic disorders. BasicMedicalKey. 2016. https://basicmedicalkey.com/hemodynamic-disorders/.

Kemp WL, et al. Chapter 8. Hemodynamics. In: Kemp WL, Burns DK, Brown TG, editors. Pathology: the big picture. McGraw Hill; 2008. Accessed 20 Nov 2022. https://accessmedicine.mhmedical.com/content.aspx?bookid=499§ionid=41568291.

Kumar V, Abbas AK, Aster JC. Chapter 4. Hemodynamic disorders, thromboembolism, and shock. In: Robbins basic pathology. 10th ed. Philadelphia: Elsevier; 2018. p. 97–118.

McManus BM, et al. Hemodynamic disorders. In: Strayer DS, editor. Rubin's pathology. Philadelphia: Wolters Kluwer; 2020. p. 299–326.

Salim K. (2021). Hemodynamic disorders for students. https://doi.org/10.13140/RG.2.2.36185.03686.

14.1 Introduction

Fluid balance is essential in maintaining appropriate blood volume. Electrolyte balance is one of the key issues in maintaining homeostasis in the body. It also plays a critical role in protecting cellular function, tissue perfusion, and acid-base balance. *Most electrolyte imbalances include hypo and hyper states of sodium, potassium, calcium, and magnesium.* The kidney is principally responsible for the retention and excretion of electrolytes and fluid in healthy individuals. But other mechanisms like hormonal interactions of antidiuretic hormone, aldosterone, and parathyroid hormone, and other factors such as physiological stress also play essential roles in regulating fluid and electrolyte balance. *The body's balance between acidity and alkalinity is referred to as acid-base balance.* The blood's acid-base balance is precisely controlled, because even a minor deviation from the normal range can severely affect many organs.

14.2 Fluid Balance

Fluid balance is a term used to describe the balance of input and output of fluids in the body to allow metabolic processes to function correctly. Fluid balance is essential in maintaining appropriate blood volume. *Around 52% of total body weight in women and 60% in men is fluid.* Two-thirds of total body fluid is intracellular, and the remaining third is extracellular fluid divided into plasma and interstitial fluid. The fluid in body cavities, such as cerebral spinal and synovial, peritoneal, and pleural fluids, is known as "transcellular fluid." Fluid circulates between compartments by diffusion. Diffusion is the random movement of particles from regions where they are highly concentrated to areas of low concentration. The movement continues until the concentration is equally distributed. *Hydrostatic and osmotic pressures determine the distribution and movement of water between the intracellular and interstitial spaces.* Osmosis is water flow across a semipermeable membrane from a dilute solution to a more concentrated solution until stability is reached. Osmotic pressure is generated by the molecules present in a solution. When generated by protein molecules in solution, it is called colloid oncotic pressure. Osmotic pressure created by dissolved electrolytes in solution is called crystalloid oncotic pressure. In healthy people, protein molecules are usually too large to pass out of the capillaries into the interstitial fluid. Hydrostatic pressure, on the other hand, is created by the pumping action of the heart and the effect of gravity on the blood within the blood vessels.

Normally, the body regulates fluid volume within a narrow range. Low blood volume (hypovolaemia) due to excessive fluid loss causes low blood pressure (hypotension). In contrast, increased blood volume (hypervolemia) due to excessive water intake can cause high blood pressure (hypertension). To maintain homeostasis, hypovolaemia is compensated by tachycardia, and hypervolemia is compensated by bradycardia. Water balance is regulated by antidiuretic hormone (ADH).

14.3 Electrolyte Balance

Electrolytes are substances that have a natural positive or negative electrical charge when dissolved in a liquid such as blood. *Examples of electrolytes are sodium, potassium, chloride, magnesium, calcium, phosphate, and bicarbonate.* These electrolytes are derived from food and fluids. These compounds dissociate into particles that carry an electrical charge. In solutions, these electrically charged particles are called electrolytes. For example, sodium chloride (NaCl) dissolves in solution to form an equal number of positively charged sodium (Na^+) ions and negatively charged chlorine (Cl^-) ions.

Electrolyte imbalance, also known as water-electrolyte imbalance, is an abnormality in the body's electrolyte concentration. Examples of electrolytes include sodium, potassium, calcium, chloride, magnesium, and phosphate. The

S. R. Prabhu, *Textbook of General Pathology for Dental Students*, https://doi.org/10.1007/978-3-031-31244-1_14

most severe electrolyte disturbances involve abnormalities in the levels of sodium, potassium, and calcium.

Sodium (Na+) is responsible for maintaining the extracellular fluid volume and regulating the membrane potential of cells. Sodium regulation occurs in the kidneys. The proximal tubule is where the majority of sodium reabsorption takes place. In the distal convoluted tubule, sodium undergoes reabsorption. Hyponatremia develops when the serum sodium level is abnormally low, usually less than 135 mmol/L. Hypernatremia occurs when serum sodium levels are greater than 145 mmol/L. Hyponatremia patients may present with headaches, confusion, nausea, and delirium. In hypernatremia, symptoms include tachypnoea, sleeping difficulty, and feeling restless. Normal Range: (serum) 135–145 mmol/L. Mild-moderate Hyponatremia: 125–135 mmol/L, Severe: less than 125 mmol/L and Hypernatremia: Mild-moderate: 145 to 160 mmol/L, Severe: over 160 mmol/L.

Potassium (K$^+$) is mainly an intracellular ion. The primary responsibility for regulating sodium and potassium homeostasis is the sodium-potassium adenosine triphosphatase pump, which pumps out sodium in exchange for potassium, which moves into the cells. The filtration of potassium takes place at the glomerulus of the kidneys. The potassium reabsorption occurs at Henle's proximal convoluted tubule and thick ascending loop. *Hypokalaemia (low potassium) occurs when serum potassium levels are under 3.6 mmol/L*. Clinical features of hypokalaemia include weakness, fatigue, and muscle twitching. *Hyperkalaemia (excess potassium) occurs when the serum potassium levels are above 5.5 mmol/L*, which can result in cardiac arrhythmias. Muscle cramps, muscle weakness, rhabdomyolysis, and myoglobinuria. Normal Range (serum) is 3.6–5.5 mmol/L, Hypokalaemia: Mild Hypokalaemia under 3.6 mmol/L, Moderate: 2.5 mmol/L, Severe: greater than 2.5 mmol/L. Hyperkalaemia: Mild hyperkalaemia: 5–5.5 mmol/L, Moderate: 5.5–6.5, Severe: 6.5–7 mmol/L.

Calcium (Ca^{2+}) is involved in skeletal mineralisation, contraction of muscles, the transmission of nerve impulses, blood clotting, and secretion of hormones. It is present mainly in the extracellular fluid. Calcium absorption in the intestine is primarily controlled by the hormonally active form of vitamin D (1,25-dihydroxy vitamin D3). Parathyroid hormone also regulates calcium secretion in the distal tubule of the kidneys. Calcitonin acts on bone cells to increase the calcium levels in the blood. Hypocalcemia is the diagnosis when the corrected serum total calcium levels are less than 8.8 mg/dL (as in vitamin D deficiency or hypoparathyroidism). Normal : greater than 10.7 mg/dL, Severe: over 11.5 mg/dL. Hypercalcemia: less than 8.8 mg/dL.

Bicarbonate. (HCO$_3^-$.) *Kidneys predominantly regulate bicarbonate concentration and are responsible for maintaining the acid-base balance*. Kidneys reabsorb the filtered bicarbonate and generate new bicarbonate by net acid excretion, which occurs by the excretion of both titrable acid and ammonia. Diarrhoea usually results in loss of bicarbonate, thus causing an imbalance in acid-base regulation. Normal Range: 23–30 mmol/L. It increases or decreases depending on the acid-base status.

Magnesium (Mg^{2+}) is an intracellular cation. *Magnesium is mainly involved in ATP metabolism, contraction and relaxation of muscles, proper neurological functioning, and neurotransmitter release*. Hypomagnesemia occurs when the serum magnesium levels are less than 1.46 mg/dL. It can present with alcohol use disorder and gastrointestinal and renal losses, and ventricular arrhythmias. Normal Range (serum): 1.46–2.68 mg/dL. Hypomagnesemia: under 1.46 mg/dL. Hypermagnesemia: over 2.68 mg/dL.

Chloride (Cl$^-$) is an anion found predominantly in the extracellular fluid. The kidneys largely regulate serum chloride levels. Most chloride, filtered by the glomerulus, is reabsorbed by both proximal and distal tubules (majorly by proximal tubule) by both active and passive transport. *Hyperchloremia can occur due to gastrointestinal bicarbonate loss. Hypochloremia presents gastrointestinal losses like vomiting or excess water gain like congestive heart failure*.

Phosphorus (P) is an extracellular fluid cation. Eighty-five percent of the total body phosphorus is in the bones and teeth in the form of hydroxyapatite; the soft tissues contain the remaining 15%. *Phosphate plays a crucial role in metabolic pathways*. It is a component of many metabolic intermediates and, most importantly, of adenosine triphosphate (ATPs) and nucleotides. Vitamin D3, PTH, and calcitonin regulate phosphate simultaneously with calcium. The kidneys are the primary avenue of phosphorus excretion. Phosphorus imbalance may result from dietary intake, gastrointestinal disorders, and excretion by the kidneys. Normal Range: 3.4–4.5 mg/dL. Hypophosphatemia: less than 2.5 mg/dL and Hyperphosphatemia: greater than 4.5 mg/dL.

14.4 Acid-Base Balance

The body's balance between acidity and alkalinity is referred to as acid-base balance. Metabolic processes continually produce acid and, to a lesser degree, base. The blood's acid-base balance is precisely controlled because even a minor deviation from the normal range can severely affect many organs. The body uses different mechanisms to control the blood's acid-base balance. The body's acid-base mechanisms involve the lungs, kidneys, and buffer systems. Their role is briefly described below:

Role of the lungs: Carbon dioxide released from the lungs is mildly acidic. It is a waste product of the metabolism and is constantly produced by cells. It then passes from the cells into the blood. The blood carries carbon dioxide to the lungs, exhaled as carbon dioxide accumulates, and the pH of the blood decreases (acidity increases). *The brain regulates the amount of carbon dioxide exhaled by controlling the speed and depth of breathing.* By adjusting the speed and depth of breathing, the brain and lungs can regulate the blood pH minute by minute. An important property of blood is its degree of acidity or alkalinity. The acidity or alkalinity of any solution, including blood, is indicated on the pH scale. The pH scale ranges from 0 (strongly acidic) to 14 (strongly basic or alkaline). A pH of 7.0 is neutral in the middle of this scale. Blood is normally slightly basic, with a normal pH range of about 7.35–7.45. Usually, the body maintains the pH of blood close to 7.40.

Role of the kidneys: The kidneys can affect blood pH by excreting excess acids or bases. The kidneys can alter the amount of acid or base that is excreted. Still, because the kidneys make these adjustments more slowly than the lungs do, this compensation generally takes several days.

Buffer systems: Yet another mechanism for controlling blood pH involves using chemical buffer systems, which guard against sudden increases in acidity and alkalinity. The pH buffer systems are combinations of the body's naturally occurring weak acids and bases. These weak acids and bases exist in pairs that are in balance under normal pH conditions. The pH buffer systems work chemically to minimise changes in the pH of a solution by adjusting the proportion of acid and base.

The blood's most important pH buffer system involves carbonic acid (a weak acid formed from the carbon dioxide dissolved in the blood) and bicarbonate ions (the corresponding weak base).

14.5 Abnormalities in Acid-Base Balance

There are two abnormalities of acid-base balance: Acidosis and alkalosis.

Acidosis. *Acidosis is caused by an overproduction of acid* that builds up in the blood or an excessive loss of bicarbonate from the blood (metabolic acidosis) or a build-up of carbon dioxide in the blood that results from poor lung function or depressed breathing (respiratory acidosis). If an increase in acid overwhelms the body's acid-base control systems, the blood will become acidic. As blood pH drops (becomes more acidic), the parts of the brain that regulate breathing are stimulated to produce faster and deeper breathing (respiratory compensation). Breathing more rapidly and deeper increases the amount of carbon dioxide exhaled, which raises the blood pH back to normal. Acidosis is categorised depending on its primary cause as metabolic and respiratory:

Metabolic acidosis: Metabolic acidosis develops when the amount of acid in the body is increased through ingestion of a substance that is, or can be metabolised to, an acid—

such as wood alcohol (methanol), antifreeze (ethylene glycol), or large doses of aspirin (acetylsalicylic acid). Many other drugs and poisons can cause acidosis. Metabolic acidosis can also occur as a result of abnormal metabolism. *The body produces excess acid in the advanced stages of shock (lactic acidosis) and poorly controlled type 1 diabetes mellitus (diabetic ketoacidosis).* Even the production of normal amounts of acid may lead to acidosis when the kidneys are not functioning normally, as in kidney failure. It, therefore, cannot excrete sufficient amounts of acid in the urine. Metabolic acidosis also develops when the body loses too much base. For example, bicarbonate can be lost through the digestive tract due to diarrhoea or an ileostomy.

Symptoms of mild metabolic acidosis include fatigue, nausea, and vomiting. Breathing becomes more profound and slightly faster (as the body tries to correct the acidosis by expelling more carbon dioxide). As the acidosis worsens, people begin to feel extremely weak and drowsy and may feel confused and increasingly nauseated. Eventually, in severe cases, heart problems may develop, and blood pressure can fall, leading to shock, coma, and death.

Respiratory acidosis: *Respiratory acidosis develops when the lungs do not expel carbon dioxide adequately*, as in chronic obstructive pulmonary disease, severe pneumonia, heart failure, and asthma. Respiratory acidosis can also develop when disorders of the brain or the nerves or muscles of the chest, as in Guillain–Barre syndrome or amyotrophic lateral sclerosis. In addition, people can develop respiratory acidosis when their breathing is slowed due to oversedation due to opioids, alcohol, or potent sedatives. As a result of the slowed breathing, the level of oxygen in the blood may be low. Sleep-disordered breathing (e.g. sleep apnoea) can repeatedly pause breathing long enough to cause temporary respiratory acidosis.

Symptoms of respiratory acidosis include drowsiness and headache. Drowsiness may progress to stupor and coma as the oxygen in the blood becomes inadequate. Stupor and coma can develop within moments if breathing stops, is severely impaired, or over hours if breathing is less dramatically impaired.

14.5.1 Alkalosis

Alkalosis is excessive blood alkalinity caused by an overabundance of bicarbonate in the blood, a loss of acid from the blood, or a low level of carbon dioxide in the blood that results from rapid or deep breathing. Two types of alkalosis occur: metabolic and respiratory.

***Metabolic alkalosis** is a primary increase in bicarbonate (HCO_3^-) with or without a compensatory increase in carbon dioxide partial pressure (Pco2).* In metabolic alkalosis, pH may be high or nearly normal. Common causes include prolonged vomiting, hypovolemia, diuretic use, and hypokalaemia. Renal impairment of HCO_3^- excretion must be present to sustain alkalosis. Symptoms and signs in severe cases include headache, lethargy, and tetany. Diagnosis is clinical and with arterial blood gas and serum electrolyte measurement. Metabolic alkalosis is due to acid loss, alkali administration, the intracellular shift of hydrogen ion (H + —as in hypokalaemia), or renal HCO_3^- retention.

Respiratory alkalosis is a primary decrease in carbon dioxide partial pressure (Pco2) with or without a compensatory decrease in bicarbonate (HCO₃⁻). In respiratory alkalosis, pH may be high or near normal. Respiratory alkalosis can be acute or chronic. The chronic form is asymptomatic, but the acute condition causes light-headedness, confusion, paraesthesia, cramps, and syncope. Signs include hyperpnea or tachypnoea and carpopedal spasms. Diagnosis is clinical and with arterial blood gas (ABG) and serum electrolyte measurements.

Compensation for acid-base disorders. *Each acid-base disturbance provokes automatic compensatory mechanisms that push the blood pH back to normal.* The respiratory system generally compensates for metabolic disturbances, while metabolic mechanisms compensate for respiratory disturbances. At first, the compensatory mechanisms may restore the pH close to normal. Thus, if the blood pH has changed significantly, the body's ability to compensate is failing.

14.6 Summary

Fluid balance is essential in maintaining appropriate blood volume. Electrolyte balance protects cellular function, tissue perfusion, and acid-base balance. The most severe electrolyte disturbances involve abnormalities in the levels of sodium, potassium, and calcium. The body uses different mechanisms to control the blood's acid-base balance. Acidosis and alkalosis occur when the acid-base balance is abnormal.

Bibliography

Berkelhammer C, Bear RA. A clinical approach to common electrolyte problems: 3. Hypophosphatemia. Can Med Assoc J. 1984;130(1):17–23.

Boden SD, Kaplan FS. Calcium homeostasis. Orthop Clin North Am. 1990;21(1):31–42.

Cooper MS, Gittoes NJ. Diagnosis and management of hypocalcaemia. BMJ. 2008;336(7656):1298–302.

Hamm LL, Nakhoul N, Hering-Smith KS. Acid-base homeostasis. Clin J Am Soc Nephrol. 2015;10(12):2232–42.

Hopkins E, Sanvictores T, Sharma S. Physiology. Acid-base balance. Treasure Island (FL): StatPearls Publishing; 2023. https://www.ncbi.nlm.nih.gov/books/NBK507807/.

Lewis JL III. Acidosis - hormonal and metabolic disorders. MSD Manuals; 2022a. https://www.msdmanuals.com/en-au/home/hormonal-and-metabolic-disorders/acid-base-balance/acidosis.

Lewis JL III. Alkalosis - hormonal and metabolic disorders. MSD Manuals; 2022b. https://www.msdmanuals.com/en-au/home/hormonal-and-metabolic-disorders/acid-base-balance/alkalosis.

Liamis G, Liberopoulos E, Barkas F, Elisaf M. Spurious electrolyte disorders: a diagnostic challenge for clinicians. Am J Nephrol. 2013;38(1):50–7.

Palmer LG, Schnermann J. Integrated control of Na transport along the nephron. Clin J Am Soc Nephrol. 2015;10(4):676–87.

Turner JJO. Hypercalcaemia - presentation and management. Clin Med (Lond). 2017;17(3):270–3.

Veldurthy V, Wei R, Oz L, Dhawan P, Jeon YH, Christakos S. Vitamin D, calcium homeostasis and ageing. Bone Res. 2016;4:16041.

Viera AJ, Wouk N. Potassium disorders: hypokalaemia and hypersalemia. Am Fam Physician. 2015;92(6):487–95.

15.1 Introduction

Ageing can be defined as the time-related deterioration of the physiological functions necessary for survival and fertility. Ageing refers mainly to humans, many other animals, and fungi. Ageing is characterised by a progressive decline in physical, mental, and reproductive capacity and an increase in morbidity and mortality. Ageing in humans increases the risk of human diseases such as cancer, Alzheimer's disease, diabetes, cardiovascular disease, stroke, and many other diseases. At the biological level, ageing results from the impact of the accumulation of a wide variety of molecular and cellular damage over time. This leads to a gradual decrease in physical and mental capacity, a growing risk of disease, and, ultimately, death. Although some of the variations in older people's health are genetic, most are due to people's physical and social environments.

15.2 Theories of Ageing

Modern biological theories of human ageing currently fall into two main categories: programmed and error (damage) theories.

15.2.1 The Programmed Theories

The programmed theories imply that ageing follows a biological timetable (regulated by changes in gene expression that affect the systems responsible for maintenance, repair, and defence responses). The programmed theory considers ageing to result from a sequential switching on and off of certain genes. The genotype determines the variation in lifespan among species or individuals. Genetic influence on ageing is evident in members of the same family who tend to live to similar ages and age at an equal rate. People whose parents and ancestors have lived longer manage to live lon-

ger, and vice versa. Twin studies also support a genetic component, as identical twins (monozygotic twins) are much more similar in life expectancy than non-identical or dizygotic twins. Longevity appears to be inherited through the female line, since mitochondria come for the egg, not the sperm. Reports indicate that longevity genes are specific genes associated with living longer. Two genes that are directly associated with longevity are SIRT1 (sirtuin 1) and SIRT2. It is also possible that a gene may be present but can either be turned on or turned off.

Endocrine and immunological theories. These have been included under the programmed category. Endocrine theory points to biological clocks acting through hormones to control the pace of ageing. The immunological theory states that the immune system is programmed to decline over time, leading to an increased vulnerability to infectious diseases and, thus, ageing and death.

15.2.2 The Error (Damage) Theory

The error theory states that damage accumulation may cause biological systems to fail. This theory emphasises environmental assaults on living organisms that induce cumulative damage at various levels as the cause of ageing. Evidence suggests that about 2–3% of the oxygen atoms taken up by the mitochondria are reduced insufficiently to reactive oxygen species (ROS). These ROS include the superoxide ion, the hydroxyl radical, and hydrogen peroxide. ROS can oxidise and damage cell membranes, proteins, and nucleic acids. One major theory also proposes metabolism as the cause of ageing. According to this theory, ageing is a by-product of normal metabolism, and no mutations are required.

Genetics is not the sole factor in determining longevity. Other factors have a role to play. It is theorised that ageing may be related to either the depletion of stem cells or the loss of the ability of stem cells to differentiate or mature into dif-

S. R. Prabhu, *Textbook of General Pathology for Dental Students*, https://doi.org/10.1007/978-3-031-31244-1_15

ferent kinds of cells. Pluripotent stem cells are immature cells that have the potential to become any cell in the body. It's important to note that this theory refers to adult stem cells, not embryonic stem cells.

15.3 Normal Ageing

The ageing process is universal but not uniform. Awareness of age-related physiological changes is essential in clinical practice. Some features are described below.

Body: Normal ageing is associated with a reduction in height that is in turn related to a decrease in the height of the vertebral body, thinning of the intervertebral discs, a certain amount of flexing of the hips and knees, and flattening of the arch of the foot.

Skin: Normal structural changes of skin ageing include a thinning of the stratum corneum, a reduction in the number of Langerhans cells, melanocytes, and mast cells, and a reduction in the depth and extent of the subcutaneous fat layer. Skin wrinkles are prevalent. Sense of touch often declines due to skin changes.

Dental and Oral: Normal dental changes of ageing include increased dentin thickness, the diminished volume of the dental pulp, and a shift in the proportion of nervous, vascular, and connective tissues. Normal oral ageing changes include thinning the oral mucosa with the receding of the gums and a reduction in the number of lingual papillae as well as a decreased ability to detect salt, bitter, sweet, and sour. Atrophy of the alveolar bone occurs with normal ageing. Ageing affects the salivary glands and alters saliva's quantity (flow rate) and quality (ion and protein composition, e.g.).

Visual Acuity: Normal vision changes with ageing include presbyopia (i.e. the loss of accommodative amplitude), reduced contrast sensitivity, impaired adaptation to darkness or light, and delayed recovery time to glare.

Vestibular Function. Dizziness is a common multifactorial geriatric syndrome contributing to falls.

Hearing: Hearing loss (presbycusis) and increased cerumen production with ageing contribute to difficulty hearing. Presbycusis is usually sensorineural. It refers to a functional decline in the ability to hear and process sound associated with ageing.

Musculoskeletal: Normal ageing is characterised by decreased bone and muscle mass and increased adiposity. By age 85, approximately 20% of people meet the criteria for sarcopenia (significant loss of muscle mass and strength). Skeletal changes include bone architecture alterations, decreased bone height, and thinning.

Cardiovascular: Increase in left ventricular stiffness and decrease in compliance; decreased left ventricular diastolic filling and relaxation; increased stroke volume, reduced maximal cardiac output and vasodilator response to exercise.

Pulmonary: Chest wall stiffness; decreased arterial oxygenation and impaired carbon dioxide elimination; reduction of vital capacity and forced expiratory volume, increased residual volume and functional residual capacity.

Gastrointestinal: Decreased elasticity of connective tissue and reduction in phase I metabolism.

Renal/urogenital: Diminished proliferative reserve; apoptosis; loss of glomerular and tubular mass; decline in GFR, loss of tubular volume, and narrowed homeostatic control of water and electrolyte balance.

Neurologic: Decrease in size of hippocampus and frontal and temporal lobes; decreased number of receptors of all types in the brain with increased sensitivity; decrease in complex vasoconstrictive skills and logical analysis skills; decrease in processing speed, decrease in reaction time and decrease the ability to shift cognitive sets rapidly; memory distraction and decline in executive function; abnormal reflexes.

Hematologic: Decreased marrow cellularity, increase in bone marrow fat, and reduction in cancellous bone.

Neuroendocrine: Decrease or increase in hormone levels; inability to conserve or dissipate heat.

15.4 Age-Related Diseases

Ageing (senescence) increases vulnerability to age-associated diseases. While ageing is not a disease, it is a risk factor for different conditions. The following diseases are common in the elderly:

Cardiovascular disease. This category includes chronic ischemic heart disease, congestive heart failure, and arrhythmia. Ischemic heart disease may be underdiagnosed in the oldest old.

Hypertension, a major contributor to atherosclerosis, is the most common chronic disease of older adults.

Atherosclerosis. Vascular remodelling, plaque accumulation, and arterial elasticity loss are characteristic features of atherosclerosis. Older age is listed as a major risk factor for atherosclerosis.

Stroke. Advanced age is one of the most significant risk factors for stroke.

Cancer. Cancer is the second leading cause of death in older adults. However, by age 85, the death rate from cancer begins to fall. Slow-growing tumours seem to be common in this population.

Osteoarthritis is a common chronic condition among older adults and a common cause of chronic pain and disability.

Diabetes. Type 2 diabetes rates have increased as populations age and become more overweight. Diabetes remains a strong risk factor for cardiovascular disease at age 85. Diabetes is also associated with peripheral arterial disease and peripheral neuropathy, contributing to diabetic foot ulcers and amputations.

Osteoporosis. Many 85-year-old adults have osteoporosis, a severe weakening of bone density. Osteoporosis is associated with an increased rate of bone fractures.

Parkinson's disease. Three-quarters of all Parkinson's disease cases begin after the age of 60. This is a risk factor among older adults.

Chronic Obstructive Pulmonary Disease (COPD) is most common in people over 65.

Benign prostatic hyperplasia (BPH). By age 40, 10% of men will have signs of BPH; by age 60, this percentage increases by five-fold. Men over 80 have over a 90% chance of developing BPH, and almost 80% of men will develop BPH in their lifetime.

Cataracts and age-related macular degeneration are common in the older population.

Memory loss and dementia. Mild short-term memory loss, word-finding difficulty, and slower processing speed are normal parts of ageing—rates of dementia increase with age. Alzheimer's disease (AD) is the cause of 60–70% of cases of dementia.

15.5 Summary

Ageing results from the impact of the accumulation of a wide variety of molecular and cellular damages over time. This leads to a gradual decrease in physical and mental capacity, a growing risk of disease, and, ultimately, death. Common conditions in older age include hearing loss, cataracts, refractive errors, back and neck pain and osteoarthritis, chronic obstructive pulmonary disease, diabetes, depression, and dementia.

Bibliography

Belikov AV. Age-related diseases as vicious cycles. Ageing Res Rev. 2019;49:11–26. https://doi.org/10.1016/j.arr.2018.11.002. ISSN 1568-1637. PMID 30458244. S2CID 53567141

Cefalu CA. Theories and mechanisms of aging. Clin Geriatr Med. 2011;27:491.

Jaul E, Barron J. Age-related diseases and clinical and public health implications for the 85 years old and over population. Front Public Health. 2017;11(5):335. https://doi.org/10.3389/fpubh.2017.00335. PMID: 29312916; PMCID: PMC5732407

Lambard D. Ageing. In: Strayer DS, editor. Rubin's pathology. 7th ed. Philadelphia: Wolters and Kluwer; 2015. p. 477–87.

Pain: Basic Concepts

16.1 Introduction

The experience of pain is a subjective one and more than a simple sensation. The International Association for the Study of Pain (IASP) defines pain as "an unpleasant sensory and emotional experience associated with or resembling that associated with actual or potential tissue damage." In medical diagnosis, pain is a symptom of an underlying condition. Pain may be broadly classified into physiological and pathological pain.

16.2 Pathophysiology of Pain

Pain can be etiologically classified as nociceptive, neuropathic, or mixed. Nociceptive pain results from an injury or disease affecting somatic structures such as skin, muscle, tendons, bone, and joints. Nociceptive pain is the normal response to noxious (intense) stimulation. Depending on the responsible stimulus, this type of pain can range from sharp, pricking, or shock-like to dull, aching, or burning. Neuropathic pain is caused by a lesion or disease affecting the somatosensory system. Mixed pain contains significant portions of both neuropathic and nociceptive pain. Pathological pain is nonprotective and maladaptive. Nociception is the result of suprathreshold stimulation of peripheral nociceptors. Inflammatory pain is a type of nociceptive pain resulting from activating and sensitising nociceptors by inflammatory mediators. Nociceptive input is then transmitted to the spinal cord via primary afferents. Modulation of the nociceptive input occurs in the dorsal horn of the spinal cord, influenced by descending inhibitory systems. Central sensitisation is a neuromodulatory change resulting in secondary hyperalgesia development. The modulated nociceptive input then travels up the ascending tracts, mainly via the spinothalamic tract to the thalamus and subsequently to the brain's higher centres. Pathological pain, such as neuropathic pain and central nervous system dysfunctional pain, results from neuroplasticity of the peripheral and central nervous systems. The abnormal ectopic firing of neurons in the absence of a stimulus, increased neuronal hypersensitivity, changes within ion channels, and even alteration in gene expression and changes in the cortical representation are involved in the pathogenesis of these pain states.

16.3 Classification of Pain

Pain can be etiologically classified as nociceptive, neuropathic, mixed, and psychogenic.

16.3.1 Nociceptive Pain

Nociceptive pain is *the most common type of pain caused by nociceptive stimuli.* It is the normal response to noxious (intense) stimulation and the physiological response to potentially harmful environmental stimuli. Potentially damaging mechanical, thermal, and chemical stimuli are detected by nerve endings called nociceptors, which are found on external surfaces such as skin (Fig. 17.1), and mucous membranes and on internal surfaces such as the periosteum, joints, and some internal organs. *Nociceptive pain is associated with activating peripheral receptive terminals of primary afferent neurons in response to noxious chemical (inflammatory), mechanical, or ischemic stimuli.* Some nociceptors are unspecialised free nerve endings with cell bodies outside the spinal column in the dorsal root ganglia. Nociceptors are categorised according to the axons which travel from the receptors to the spinal cord or brain. In nociceptive pain, symptoms are local to the target tissue. Depending on the responsible stimulus, this type of pain can range from sharp, pricking, or shock-like to dull, aching, or burning. Toothache is an example of nociceptive pain.

Nociceptors are the specialised sensory receptors responsible for detecting noxious (unpleasant) stimuli, transforming

S. R. Prabhu, *Textbook of General Pathology for Dental Students*, https://doi.org/10.1007/978-3-031-31244-1_16

the stimuli into electrical signals, which are then conducted to the central nervous system. They are the free nerve endings of primary afferent Aδ and C fibres. *Aδ fibres transmit rapid, sharp, localised pain. C fibres transmit slow, diffuse, dull aches.* Distributed throughout the body (skin, viscera, muscles, joints, meninges), they can be stimulated by mechanical, thermal, or chemical stimuli. Inflammatory mediators (e.g.

bradykinin, serotonin, prostaglandins, cytokines, and H^+) are released from damaged tissue and can stimulate nociceptors directly. They can also act to reduce the activation threshold of nociceptors so that the stimulation required to cause activation is less. This process is called primary sensitisation. These pains respond well to primary analgesics, such as nonsteroidal anti-inflammatory drugs and opioids.

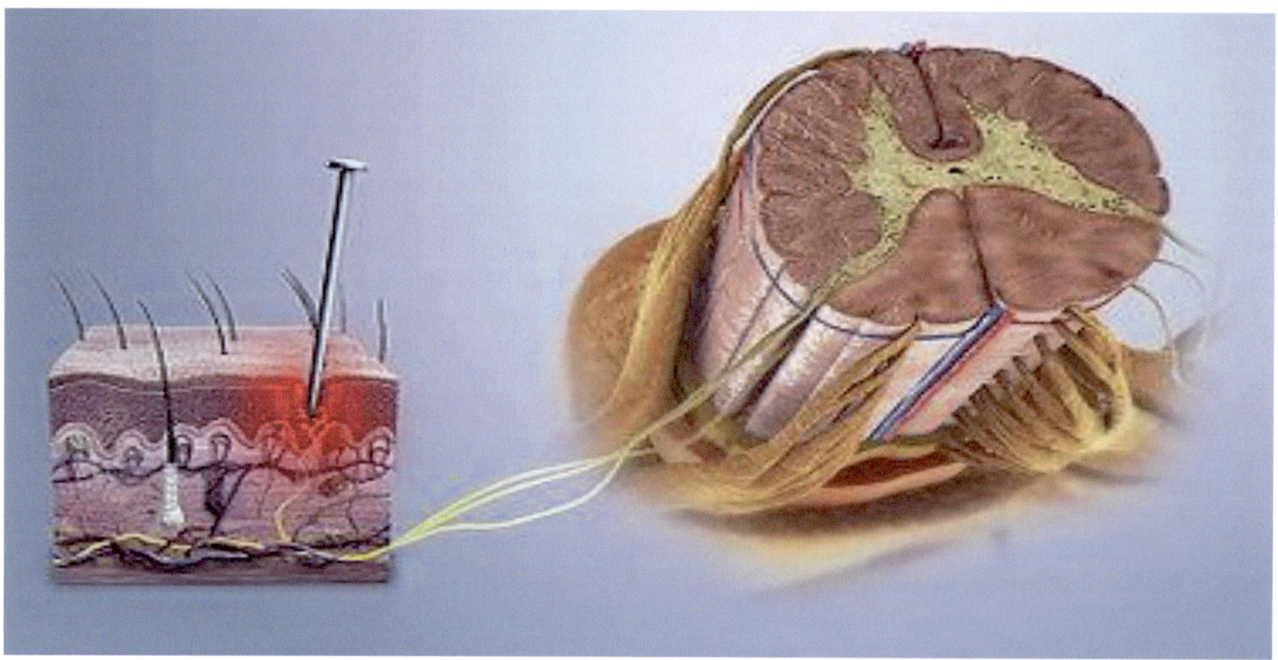

Mechanism of nociception via sensor afferents. Wikipedia. CC BY-SA 4.0

16.3.2 Neuropathic Pain

Neuropathic pain is caused by a lesion or disease of the somatosensory system, including peripheral fibres (Aβ, Aδ and C fibres) and central neurons. The somatosensory system allows for perceiving touch, pressure, pain, temperature, position, movement, and vibration. The somatosensory nerves arise in the skin, muscles, joints, and fascia. They include sensory receptors that respond to changes in temperature (thermoreceptors), mechanical stimulation (mechanoreceptors), chemical signals (chemoreceptors), and itchy sensations (pruriceptors). Nociceptors send signals to the spinal cord and eventually to the brain for further processing. Most sensory processes involve a thalamic nucleus receiving a sensory signal that is then directed to the cerebral cortex. Lesions or diseases of the somatosensory nervous system can lead to altered and disordered transmission of sensory signals into the spinal cord and the brain. Pathology of the peripheral disorders that causes neuropathic pain predominantly involves the small unmyelinated C fibres and the myelinated A fibres, namely, the Aβ and Aδ fibres.

16.3.3 Mixed Pain

The term "mixed pain" is increasingly applied for specific clinical scenarios, such as low back pain, cancer pain, and postsurgical pain, in which there "is a complex overlap of the different known pain types (nociceptive, neuropathic, nociplastic) in any combination, acting simultaneously and/or concurrently to cause pain in the same body area." The diagnosis of mixed pain is made based on clinical judgement following detailed history-taking and thorough physical examination.

16.3.4 Psychogenic Pain

Psychogenic pain does not conform to anatomical and neurophysiological knowledge. It is often attributed to psychopathology. *If the pain reported by a patient cannot be objectively confirmed as due to a physical cause, or if the complaint is recalcitrant to appropriate treatment, it is often assumed as psychogenic pain.* This is a diagnosis of exclusion. Psychological dysfunction has been proposed to cause phantom limb pain, orofacial pain, fibromyalgia, pelvic pain, abdominal pain, chest pain, and headache. Recent reports indicate that the role of "psychological" disturbances causing pain has been disputed and explained as dysfunctional peripheral and central neurophysiological mechanisms.

16.4 Conditions Associated with Peripheral and Central Neuropathic Pain

Common conditions associated with peripheral neuropathic pain include postherpetic neuralgia, trigeminal neuralgia, painful radiculopathy, diabetic neuropathy, leprosy, amputation (phantom pain), and peripheral nerve injury pain. *Central neuropathic pain is due to a lesion or disease of the spinal cord and brain.* Cerebrovascular diseases affecting the central somatosensory pathways include poststroke pain and neurodegenerative diseases such as Parkinson's disease. These are brain disorders. Spinal cord lesions or conditions that cause neuropathic pain include spinal cord injury, syringomyelia, and demyelinating diseases, such as multiple sclerosis, transverse myelitis, and neuromyelitis optica.

It is caused by damage to nerves in the central or peripheral nervous system. Damage can be due to several mechanisms, including trauma or surgery, diabetes mellitus, chemotherapy, radiotherapy, ischemia, infection, or malignancy. Common peripheral neuropathic pain states include diabetic neuropathy and radicular pain (such as sciatica). The pain of neuropathic origin, which arises from direct lesions or damage to the somatosensory system, is considered pathological. *The pain of neuropathic origin is often described as burning, aching, and electric shock-like in quality.* It is typically more severe and less responsive to conventional treatments than nociceptive and inflammatory pain.

Neuropathic pain can be peripheral or central. Peripheral neuropathic pain is initiated or caused by a pathophysiological mechanism associated with altered nerve functioning and responsiveness. Mechanisms include hyperexcitability, abnormal impulse generation, and mechanical, thermal, and chemical sensitivity. Central pain is initiated or caused by a primary lesion or dysfunction in the central nervous system (CNS).

Pain experiences. In clinical practice, various terminologies are used to describe the nature of pain, as listed below.

– **Acute pain** lasts for a short time, usually less than 3 months. This occurs following surgery, trauma, or other inflammatory conditions.
– **Sub-acute pain** is progressing towards chronic pain, but this progression may be prevented. This is known as the transition phase.
– **Recurrent pain** occurs cyclically, such as migraine or pelvic pain.
– **Chronic pain** lasts longer than 3 months.
– **Referred pain** is pain perceived as occurring in a region of the body topographically distinct from the region in which the actual source of pain is located.
– **Analgesia** is the absence of pain in response to a usually painful stimulus.
– **Hyperalgesia** refers to an increased response to a stimulus that is usually painful.

Examples of neuropathic pain and their probable causes:

– Trigeminal neuralgia (Cause: Compression of trigeminal ganglion or its branches)
– Postherpetic neuralgia (Cause: Shingles)
– Complex regional pain syndrome (Causes: Trauma/infection/surgery/inflammation)
– Diabetic neuropathy (Cause: Persistent hyperglycaemia)
– Central pain (Cause: Trauma to the spinal cord and Stroke)
– Phantom pain (Cause: Amputation Surgery)

16.5 Summary

Pain is an unpleasant sensory and emotional experience associated with or resembling that associated with actual or potential tissue damage. Nociceptive pain is the normal response to noxious (intense) stimulation. Neuropathic pain is caused by a lesion or disease affecting the somatosensory system. Mixed pain contains significant portions of both neuropathic and nociceptive pain.

Bibliography

Colloca L, et al. Neuropathic pain. Nat Rev Dis Primers. 2017;3:17002. https://doi.org/10.1038/nrdp.2017.2. PMID: 28205574; PMCID: PMC5371025

Cousins MJ & Gallagher RM (2011) Fast facts: chronic and cancer pain.

Fong A, Schug SA. Pathophysiology of pain: a practical primer. Plast Reconstr Surg. 2014;134(4 Suppl 2):8S–14S. https://doi.org/10.1097/PRS.0000000000000682. PMID: 25255013

International Association for the Study of Pain. 2023. www.iasp-pain.org.

Melzack R, Wall P. Pain mechanisms: a new theory. Science. 1965;150:171–9.

Nicholas M & Molloy A (2011) Manage your pain.

Siddall PJ, Cousins MJ. Persistent pain as a disease entity: implications for clinical management. Anesth Analg. 2004;99:510–20.

17.1 Introduction

Oral diseases, while largely preventable, pose a significant health burden. World Health Organisation estimates that oral diseases affect nearly 3.5 billion people worldwide. Untreated dental caries in permanent teeth is the most common health condition, according to the Global Burden of Disease 2019. Acquired oral diseases such as dental caries, periodontal diseases, and oral cancer are caused by various modifiable risk factors, including sugar consumption, tobacco use, alcohol use, poor hygiene, and their underlying social and commercial determinants. This chapter provides an overview of dental, oral, maxillofacial, and salivary gland diseases, which are part of the gastrointestinal system.

17.2 Common Developmental Disorders

Dental anomalies are common congenital malformations that can occur either as isolated disorders or as part of a syndrome. Some of these have a genetic basis. Congenitally missing teeth (hypodontia, oligodontia, and anodontia) and supernumerary teeth are seen in several syndromes.

Tooth agenesis. Hypodontia refers to the absence of one to six teeth, excluding third molars, whereas oligodontia refers to the lack of more than six teeth, excluding third molars. Third molars are excluded, as these are missing in up to 20% of patients, making this a prevalent finding. Anodontia is the complete absence of teeth in one or both dentitions. Together, these are referred to as tooth agenesis.

Abnormality in tooth number. A supernumerary tooth is an additional tooth that can be found in any region of the dental arch. The most common supernumerary tooth appears in the maxillary midline and is called mesiodens.

Abnormalities in tooth size, shape, and form are common in the general population. These are thought to result from disturbances in the morphodifferentiation (cap-bell) stage of tooth development. The most common abnormality

is a variation in the size of the upper lateral incisors and second premolars. In patients with hypodontia, the most common abnormality is a peg-shaped upper lateral incisor.

Structural changes in dental hard tissues can occur in both dentitions. These include amelogenesis imperfecta and dentinogenesis imperfecta. Amelogenesis imperfecta, an inherited disorder, results in the defective formation of tooth enamel. Dentinogenesis imperfecta is a genetic disorder causing the defective formation of dentin. Both diseases can affect deciduous and permanent teeth, leaving them weak, sensitive to temperature and pressure, and prone to quick wear.

Cleft Lip and Cleft Palate: The most common craniofacial deformity is the clefting of the lip and palate. Clefting, the incomplete fusion of the lip and palate, can appear alone or as part of a hereditary syndrome. A family history of clefting increases the chances of inheriting the disorder. A cleft lip or "harelip" usually appears on one side, most often on the left. A bilateral or two-sided cleft is less common. An incomplete cleft stops short of the nostril; a complete cleft goes into the nostril. Both cleft types often involve the palate. A typical patient with a cleft palate/cleft ridge has defects in the roof of the palate, with an opening into the nasal cavity.

17.3 Dental Caries and Pathology of the Dental Pulp

Dental caries is commonly known as tooth decay. It is one of the oldest and most common diseases in humans. It is a multifactorial dietary-microbial disease resulting from dental plaque (biofilm) associated cariogenic bacteria which metabolise fermentable dietary carbohydrates (glucose, fructose, maltose, and sucrose) to produce acid, which over time demineralises tooth structure. Two major groups of bacteria involved in the carious process are the mutans streptococci and the *Lactobacilli* species. The acids produced include lactic, acetic, formic, and propionic, all of which can readily

123

S. R. Prabhu, *Textbook of General Pathology for Dental Students*, https://doi.org/10.1007/978-3-031-31244-1_17

dissolve the mineral content of the enamel and dentine. The carious process is a continuum resulting from many cycles of demineralisation and remineralisation. This process continues as long as cariogenic bacteria, fermentable carbohydrates, and saliva are present. Demineralisation begins at the atomic level at the crystal surface inside the enamel or dentine. Remineralisation is the natural repair process for non-cavitated lesions and relies on calcium and phosphate ions assisted by fluorides.

Most dental pain occurs as a result of caries. Initially, caries presents as a painless white spot (decalcification of the enamel, which may be reversible), followed by cavitation and brownish discolouration. Once caries reaches the dentine, pain may result from thermal stimulation or sweet or sour food or drink. Untreated dental caries can present complications. These include apical periodontitis, periapical abscess, periapical granuloma, periapical cyst, cellulitis, periostitis, and osteomyelitis of the jawbone.

Pulpitis. Left untreated, dental caries usually destroys most of the tooth and invades the dental pulp leading to inflammation (pulpitis). Two types of pulpitis occur: acute and chronic.

- **Acute pulpitis** is characterised by a constant throbbing pain in the affected tooth (often made more severe by reclining). The pain is associated with the increased pulpal pressure caused by the influx of inflammatory cells, increased vascularity (hyperaemia), and the inability of the pulp chamber to expand. Bacterial invasion may follow the inflammatory response.
- **Chronic pulpitis** may result from a persistent low-grade irritation or may follow acute pulpitis. It is characterised by mild intermittent pain of varying intensity over a prolonged period which is difficult for the patient to localise. Pain is usually induced by thermal stimulation or sweet foods. There is a bacterial invasion with increased plasma cells and lymphocytes and an influx of macrophages. Chronic pulpitis can resolve itself, progress to acute pulpitis, or result in pulp necrosis following the accumulation of dead bacteria and necrotic debris. In an exposed pulp, the pulpal tissue may extrude through communication into the oral cavity (hyperplastic pulpitis) to form a pulp polyp; this is more common in primary teeth.

Condensing osteitis (Sclerosing osteitis). Condensing osteitis refers to focal areas of bone sclerosis associated with apices of teeth with pulpitis or pulpal necrosis.

Apical periodontitis and periapical granuloma. Apical periodontitis refers to inflammation of the periodontal ligament (PDL) surrounding the apex of the tooth caused by pulpal infection, bacterial products, or other irritants through the height of the root. Usually, this occurs due to acute inflammation (acute apical periodontitis). Periapical granu-

loma, also known as chronic apical periodontitis, refers to the formation of granulation tissue surrounding the apex of a non-vital tooth arising in response to pulpal necrosis.

Dental abscess. An odontogenic infection is characterised by the localisation of pus in the structures that surround the teeth. Secondary to dental caries, trauma, or failed root canal treatment. Bacteria and their toxic products enter the periapical tissues via the apical foramen and induce acute inflammation and pus formation.

Cellulitis. Acute inflammation of the soft tissue spaces of the facial and cervical region due to spreading of odontogenic infection. Causative organisms predominantly are anaerobic bacteria from odontogenic sources (mandibular molars in particular). If swelling is bilateral and involves parapharyngeal space, the condition is called Ludwig's angina which can be life-threatening.

17.4   Other Acquired Dental Disorders

Tooth wear. Tooth wear refers to non-carious tooth surface loss predominantly due to a combination of three processes: attrition, abrasion, and erosion. When these forms of tooth wear lead to "fractures" of the tooth surface due to stress exerted by extrinsic forces on the enamel, the condition is known as abfraction.

Attrition is the loss of tooth substance caused by physical tooth-to-tooth contact. Attrition mainly causes wear of the incisal and occlusal surfaces of the teeth—common in the elderly and those with parafunctional activity such as bruxism.

Abrasion is the loss of tooth substance caused by physical means other than teeth and is commonly seen as "shallow" concave or wedge-shaped notches on the cervical margins of teeth. Vigorous horizontal tooth brushing, pipe smoking, nail-biting, and improper use of floss and toothpicks are the major causes of abrasion.

Erosion is the chemical dissolution of tooth substance caused by acids unrelated to the acid produced by bacteria in dental plaque. Erosion may occur with excessive consumption of acidic foods and drinks or medical conditions involving repeated regurgitation and reflux of gastric acid, as in gastro-oesophageal reflux disease (GORD) and bulimia. Erosion is usually seen on the palatal surfaces of anterior maxillary teeth.

Abfraction is loss of tooth substance at the cervical margins purportedly caused by minute flexure of teeth under occlusal loading. Abfraction presents as triangular lesions along the cervical margins of the buccal surfaces of the teeth where the enamel is thinner and, therefore, in the presence of occluding forces, is prone to fracture.

Cracked tooth syndrome (CTS). This is defined as a fracture plane of unknown depth and direction that passes through tooth structure which, if not already involved, may progress to communicate with the pulp and or periodontal ligament. Patients suffering from cracked tooth syndrome classically present with a history of sharp pain when biting or consuming cold food/beverages. The symptom of pain on biting increases as the applied occlusal force is raised. Pain is due to the sudden movement of fluid in dentinal tubules, which occurs when the fractured portions of the tooth move independently. Activation of myelinated A-type fibres within the dental pulp accounts for the acute nature of the pain. Mandibular molars appear to be the most commonly involved in this condition, followed by maxillary premolars and maxillary molar teeth. Mandibular premolar teeth are the least affected. Some common causes of CTS include large carious lesions and restorations, bruxism, sudden excessive biting force (e.g. on a piece of bone), and restorative procedures using high-speed handpieces.

17.5 Periodontal Diseases

Periodontal diseases comprise a wide range of inflammatory conditions that affect the supporting structures of the teeth, such as the gingiva, alveolar bone, and periodontal ligament. Local factors cause most periodontal diseases; some may be manifestations of systemic conditions such as diabetes mellitus, leukaemia, or vitamin deficiency. Recent evidence indicates that periodontal inflammatory disease is also linked to atherosclerosis, a risk factor for coronary artery disease. Periodontal disease begins with gingivitis, the localised inflammation of the gingiva initiated by bacteria in the dental plaque, a microbial biofilm that forms on the teeth and gingiva. Usually, gingivitis refers to and is associated with plaque-induced inflammation of the gingiva.

Gingival diseases. Gingival diseases can be associated with plaque, endogenous hormonal fluctuations, drugs, systemic diseases, and malnutrition. Most gingival diseases are of inflammatory origin (gingivitis) and confined to the gingival tissues.

Gingivitis. Gingivitis is characterised by inflammation of the gingival tissues with no loss of attachment or bone. It occurs in response to the bacteria that live in biofilms (dental plaque) at the gingival margin and in the sulcus (plaque-induced gingivitis). Systemic or local risk factors or drugs can also mediate plaque-induced gingivitis. Dental plaque is a dense, non-mineralized complex mass of bacterial colonies living in a gel-like matrix that forms around the gingival margin and can be found both supra- and subgingivally. Non-biofilm-induced gingivitis can be due to traumatic, genetic, hormonal, metabolic, and specific infections. The clinical signs of gingivitis include erythema, bleeding on probing, and oedema. Gingivitis is reversible by the removal of dental plaque. While some cases of gingivitis may not progress to periodontitis, periodontitis is always preceded by gingivitis.

Periodontitis. Periodontitis is an inflammatory disease that progressively destroys the tooth-supporting apparatus (periodontal ligament and alveolar bone). Periodontitis usually develops when gingivitis is not treated. Periodontitis risk factors include dental plaque, smoking, diabetes, obesity, and vitamin C deficiency. In periodontitis, deep periodontal pockets form, harbouring anaerobic organisms. Colonising organisms include *Aggregatibacter actinomycetemcomitans, Porphyromonas gingivalis, Prevotella intermedia,* and many Gram-negative bacilli. The organisms trigger the chronic release of inflammatory mediators, including cytokines, prostaglandins, and enzymes from neutrophils and monocytes. The inflammation affects the periodontal ligament, gingiva, cementum, and alveolar bone. The gingiva progressively loses its attachment to the teeth, bone loss begins, and periodontal pockets deepen. With progressive bone loss, teeth may loosen, and gingiva recedes. Tooth migration is common in later stages, and tooth loss can occur.

17.6 Mucosal Diseases

Diseases of the oral mucosa are caused by various local and systemic causes and manifest as lesions, including vesicles, bullae, erosions, erythema, exophytic mass, or red and white patches. This chapter provides an overview of the pathology and clinical aspects of common oral mucosal disorders, such as lichen planus (LP), erythema multiforme (EM), mucous membrane pemphigoid (MMP), pemphigus Vulgaris (PV), candidiasis, herpes simplex viral infections, aphthous stomatitis, leukoplakia, and squamous cell carcinoma.

Lichen planus is a chronic systemic (mucocutaneous) disease. Oral presentations of lichen planus include reticular, papular, plaque-form, atrophic, ulcerative (erosive), and bullous forms. Mucosal lesions are usually multiple and almost always have a bilateral, symmetrical distribution. Buccal mucosa, tongue, and gingiva are the favoured sites of oral lichen planus (OLP). OLP is a T-cell-mediated inflammatory (immunologic) disorder. Both antigen-specific and non-specific mechanisms are hypothesised to be involved in the pathogenesis of oral lichen planus (OLP). Antigen-specific mechanisms in OLP include antigen presentation by basal keratinocytes and antigen-specific keratinocyte killing by CD8(+) cytotoxic T cells. Non-specific mechanisms include mast cell degranulation and matrix metalloproteinase activation in OLP lesions. These mechanisms may combine to cause T cell accumulation in the superficial lamina propria, basement membrane disruption, intra-epithelial T cell migration, and keratinocyte apoptosis in OLP.

Erythema multiforme (EM) is an immune-mediated, reactive mucocutaneous disorder that often presents with oral, especially labial mucosal erythema, blistering, and ulceration. The aetiology and pathogenesis of EM remain obscure. Herpes simplex virus (HSV) infection and medications have been implicated as possible triggers. The process is characterised by cytotoxic CD8+ T-cell-induced apoptosis and necrosis of the basal keratinocyte cells. Cytokines, mostly tumour necrosis factor-alpha (TNF-α), are found in the lesional tissue. In herpes simplex virus–associated EM, gamma-interferon (γ-IFN) predominates and mediates the epidermal damage.

Mucous membrane pemphigoid (MMP) is an antibody-mediated autoimmune disease characterised by the separation of the oral mucosal epithelium at the junctional basement membrane zone, giving rise to a sub-basilar split clinically appearing as a blister. MMP predominantly affects mucosa and rarely the skin. Ocular manifestations have been reported to occur in patients with oral lesions. Immunologically, MMP is characterised by the deposits of predominantly IgG antibodies with complement factor C3 and, to a lesser extent, with IgA or IgM antibodies directed at various antigens within the basement membrane zone.

Pemphigus Vulgaris (PV) is a group of autoimmune diseases characterised by intra-epithelial blistering, resulting in superficial vesicles or bullae that easily rupture, resulting in ulceration of mucosal and cutaneous sites. Pemphigus Vulgaris (PV) is the most common and clinically aggressive variant. PV commonly affects the oral mucosa and the skin. Other mucosal sites may also be involved, including the mucosa of the conjunctivae, nose, oesophagus, pharynx, larynx, and genitalia. Pemphigus Vulgaris is an autoantibody-mediated condition. In this disorder, the antibody-complement complexes are directed at the epithelial cells' inter-epithelial attachment (desmosomes), causing intraepithelial blisters. The main adhesion molecule antigen target in PV is desmoglein 3 (Dsg3).

Oral Candidiasis (Oral Candidosis). Oral candidiasis is one of the common fungal infections of the oral mucosa caused by the yeast *Candida albicans*. These organisms are components of normal oral microflora, and around 30% to 50% of the population carry this organism without causing any symptoms. Oral candidiasis is a common opportunistic infection. Predisposing factors include impaired salivary gland function, drugs, dentures, high carbohydrate diet, extremes of life, smoking, diabetes mellitus, Cushing's syndrome, malignancies, and immunosuppressive conditions. There are several clinical forms of coral candidiasis: (acute) pseudomembranous candidiasis, acute atrophic candidiasis, chronic candidiasis: chronic atrophic candidiasis (denture stomatitis), chronic hyperplastic candidiasis (candidal leukoplakia), median rhomboid glossitis, and angular cheilitis. Predisposing factors set the scene for fungal infection. Adhesion of candida to epithelial cell walls is an important step in initiating infection. This is promoted by certain fungal cell wall components such as mannose, C3d receptors, mannoprotein, and saccharins. Other factors implicated are germ tube formation, presence of mycelia, persistence within epithelial cells, endotoxins, induction of tumour necrosis factor, and proteinases.

Oral Herpes Simplex Viral Infections. Of the eight types of herpes simplex viruses (HSV), HSV-1 and HSV-2 can cause oral or genital infections. Most often, HSV-1 causes gingivostomatitis and herpes labialis. HSV-2 usually causes genital lesions. Herpetic gingivostomatitis is common in children and is generally spread through direct contact or via droplets of oral secretions or lesions. Oral HSV infection is characterised by high-grade fever and painful gingival and oral lesions. The pathogenesis of herpes gingivostomatitis involves the replication of the herpes simplex virus, cell lysis, and eventual destruction of mucosal tissue. Exposure to HSV-1 on abraded surfaces allows the virus to enter and rapidly replicate in epidermal and dermal cells. Sufficient viral inoculation and replication will enable the virus to enter the sensory and autonomic ganglia, which travels to the ganglionic nerve bodies. HSV-1 commonly infects the trigeminal ganglia, where the virus remains latent until reactivation. Reactivation causing lips or perioral infection (herpes labialis) is precipitated by overexposure to sunlight, febrile illnesses, physical or emotional stress, and immunosuppression.

Aphthous Stomatitis (Aphthous ulceration). Aphthous stomatitis is characterised by painful aphthous ulcers (commonly termed "canker sores") on the non-keratinized oral mucous membranes. If recurrence occurs frequently, it is called recurrent aphthous stomatitis. The precise aetiology remains unknown. Aphthous ulcerations are initially primarily the result of T cell-mediated immune dysfunction but may also involve neutrophil and mast cell-mediated destruction of the mucosal epithelium. Lesions can alter several intercellular mediators, such as elevations in interferon gamma, tumour necrosis factor-alpha, and interleukins (IL)-2, IL-4, and IL-5, as various adhesion molecules involved in cell communication and epithelial integrity. This inflammatory process results in a pseudomembrane containing fibrinous exudate, bacteria, inflammatory cells, and necrotic mucosal cells.

Oral Leukoplakia. Oral leukoplakia (OL) is a clinical term. OL is defined by the 2005 World Health Organisation (WHO) as a white plaque of questionable risk having excluded (other) known diseases or disorders that carry no increased risk for cancer. Frequently associated risk factors include tobacco use, alcohol consumption, chronic irritation, candidiasis, vitamin deficiency, endocrine disturbances, and possibly the human papillomavirus (HPV) virus. Often it is idiopathic. Any mucosal surface in the mouth may be affected by OL; common sites include lateral borders of the tongue, the floor of the mouth, and buccal mucosa. Oral leukoplakia carries an increased risk of malignant transformation.

Oral squamous cell carcinoma (OSCC) (Oral Cancer). Oral squamous cell carcinoma (OSCC), commonly known as oral cancer, is the sixth most frequent type of cancer. It is the malignancy arising in the oral squamous epithelial lining, which presents as red or white patches, non-healing ulcer or ulcero-proliferative growth involving the tongue, buccal mucosa, gingiva, palate, the floor of the mouth, or lip. OSCC has a multifactorial aetiology, with the most important risk factors being tobacco use and alcohol abuse, which have a synergistic effect. Solar radiation is a major risk factor for lip squamous cell carcinoma. Potentially malignant disorders include leukoplakia, erythroleukoplakia, erythroplakia, oral submucous fibrosis, actinic keratosis of the lip, palatal lesions associated with reverse smoking, chronic candidiasis, lichen planus, discoid lupus erythematosus, syphilitic glossitis, and dyskeratosis congenita that also carry a higher risk for the development of OSCC.

The cell of origin of OSCC is the oral keratinocyte. DNA mutations in these cells cause OSCC. This is often spontaneous but increased by exposure to a chemical, physical, or microbial mutagen that can induce carcinogenesis. The various changes in the DNA can progress from a normal keratinocyte to a potentially malignant keratinocyte characterised by an ability to proliferate in a less-controlled fashion than normal. The cells become autonomous and cancer results, characterised by invasion across the epithelial basement membrane and, ultimately, to lymph nodes, jawbone, and distant metastasis to the brain, liver, and other sites.

17.7 Diseases of the Jaw Bones

Diseases of the jaw can be divided into two main groups: those related to dentition and those restricted only to the bone. Tooth-related jawbone diseases can be divided into jaw cysts (odontogenic and non-odontogenic), jaw tumours (odontogenic and non-odontogenic), and fibro-osseous lesions.

17.7.1 Jaw Cysts

Cyst, by definition, is a pathological cavity lined by epithelium and contains liquid or semisolid material. The majority of cysts in the jaw bones are called odontogenic cysts as they are derived from odontogenic epithelium. A small group of jawbone cysts can be non-odontogenic because of the non-odontogenic epithelial origin.

Odontogenic cysts can be grouped as inflammatory and developmental.

Inflammatory cysts. In this group, inflammation stimulates epithelial odontogenic remnants to proliferate and transform into epithelium-lined cystic cavities. Two types of cysts are included in this group: radicular and residual.

- **Radicular cysts** are located at the root tips of non-vital teeth with necrotic pulp tissue.
- **Residual cyst** is a radicular cyst left behind in the jaw after the removal of the associated tooth.

Developmental odontogenic cysts. This group includes dentigerous cyst, eruption cyst, glandular odontogenic cyst, lateral periodontal cyst, gingival cyst, and odontogenic keratocyst (also known as an Odontogenic Keratocystic Tumor).

- **Dentigerous cyst.** This cyst surrounds the crown of an unerupted tooth, mostly the mandibular third molar tooth or the maxillary canine.
- **Eruption cyst.** This is associated with an erupting deciduous or permanent tooth and appears as dome-shaped bluish soft swelling shortly before the appearance of these teeth in the oral cavity.
- **Lateral periodontal cyst** is located between the roots of vital teeth. If these occur in the soft tissues of the gingiva, then it is called a gingival cyst.
- **Odontogenic keratocyst (OKC)** is a relatively common developmental odontogenic cyst representing approximately 10% to 14% of all jaw cysts. It is defined by its characteristic microscopic features, which include basilar nuclear palisading and keratin production (primarily in parakeratin). The odontogenic keratocyst is also known as the odontogenic keratocystic tumour (OKT).

Non-odontogenic cysts. These jaw cysts are derived from other epithelial sources in the jaws or neighbouring soft tissues. Two examples include nasopalatine cysts and nasolabial cysts.

- **Nasopalatine cyst.** Epithelial remnants of the nasopalatine duct are the source of the nasopalatine duct cyst. This cyst lies in the anterior palate just behind the central incisor teeth.
- **Nasolabial cyst.** Nasolacrimal duct is the origin of the nasolabial cyst. This cyst is located in the soft tissue just lateral to the nose at the buccal aspect of the maxillary alveolar process.

17.7.2 Jaw Tumours

Based on the tissue of origin, jaw tumours can be grouped as odontogenic and non-odontogenic.

Odontogenic tumours. This group of tumours arises from odontogenic tissues, which may be either epithelial, mesenchymal, or both.

Epithelial odontogenic tumours. These consist of ameloblastoma, calcifying epithelial odontogenic tumour (Pindborg tumour), adenomatoid odontogenic tumour, and squamous odontogenic tumour.

- **Ameloblastoma.** The most common epithelial odontogenic tumour is ameloblastoma. It is a benign, locally aggressive tumour derived from remnants of an enamel organ or dental lamina. Radiographically, ameloblastoma may be multilocular (common) or unilocular and more commonly occur in the mandible than the maxilla. Recent evidence regarding its pathogenesis points to the dysregulation of mitogen-activated protein kinase (MAPK) pathway signalling as a critical step in the pathogenesis of this tumour.
- **Calcifying epithelial odontogenic tumour (CEOT).** Also known as Pindborg tumour, this is a rare benign epithelial odontogenic neoplasm of slow growth that is locally aggressive and tends to invade bone and adjacent soft tissues. Radiographically, CEOT is characterised by uni- or multilocular lesion that often shows a mixed radiolucent-radiopaque pattern.
- **Adenomatoid odontogenic tumor (AOT).** This benign odontogenic epithelial tumour often assumes the clinical presentation of a dentigerous cyst, enclosing the crown part of an impacted tooth (mostly maxillary canine) to which it is connected at the level of the cementoenamel junction. Histologically, this tumour consists of epithelial nodules. Larger nodules also contain duct-like spaces (hence the name adenomatoid) lined by columnar cells and an extracellular eosinophilic matrix.
- **Calcifying cystic odontogenic tumour (Gorlin cyst).** Also known as a calcifying odontogenic cyst (COC), this is a rare odontogenic epithelial developmental lesion. Histologically, it shows the proliferation of odontogenic epithelium and scattered nests of ghost cells and calcifications that may form the cyst lining or present as a solid mass.
- **Squamous odontogenic tumour.** This odontogenic epithelial tumour comprises islands of well-differentiated non-keratinizing squamous epithelium surrounded by mature fibrous connective tissue.

Mesenchymal odontogenic tumours. This group of tumours consists of odontogenic myxoma, odontogenic fibroma, and cementoblastoma.

- **Odontogenic myxoma.** This is a benign odontogenic neoplasm histologically characterised by spindle- to stellate-shaped odontogenic mesenchymal cells set in a myxoid stroma. Radiographically, the tumour appears as a radiolucent lesion that can be uni- or multilocular, creating a soap bubble or honeycomb appearance.
- **Odontogenic fibroma.** The tumour histologically consists of fibroblasts lying in a background of myxoid material intermingled with collagen fibres that may vary from delicate to coarse and thus resemble the dental follicle.
- **Cementoblastoma.** Cementoblastoma is derived from the ectomesenchyme of the odontogenic origin and consists of a mass of cellular cementum connected with the root surface that may show signs of external resorption. Fibrous tissue with hyperplastic cementoblasts is present at the periphery of the cementoblastoma.

Mixed epithelial and mesenchymal odontogenic tumours. This group of odontogenic tumours consists of ameloblastic fibroma, ameloblastic fibro-odontoma, and odontoma.

- **Ameloblastic fibroma.** This tumour is histologically characterised by the proliferation of both odontogenic epithelium and mesenchymal tissue without the formation of enamel or dentin and thus resembles the immature tooth germ. The majority of tumours are seen in the premolar-molar region of the mandible in persons under the age of 20 years.
- **Ameloblastic fibro-odontoma.** Histologically this tumour is characterised by a combination of dentin and enamel together with soft tissues resembling the epithelial enamel organ and the mesenchymal dental papilla. Radiographically this tumour shows a mixed radiodense-radiolucent lesion.
- **Odontoma.** These are one of the most common mandibular lesions encountered and the most common odontogenic tumours of the mandible. They are hamartomas with lesions consisting of various tooth components (dentin, cementum, pulpal tissue, and enamel). Odontomas are divided histologically into two types: complex and compound odontomas. Complex odontoma consists of haphazard irregular calcified lesions with no distinct tooth components, and compound odontomas consist of multiple identifiable tiny teeth (denticles).

17.7.2.1 Giant Cell Tumours

- **Giant cell lesions** (GCLs) are rare lesions that prominently feature multinucleated giant cells in their histology. They include central giant cell granuloma (CGCG), giant cell tumour of bone (GCT), Brown tumour, peripheral giant cell granuloma (PGCG), and Cherubism (CHB).
- **Central giant cell granuloma (CGCG)** typically occurs in the second and third decades (mean age of approxi-

mately 25 years). Females are more frequently affected than males. CGCG has a predilection for the mandible, especially the body and anterior portions of the jaw. The lesion microscopically shows numerous osteoclast-like multinucleated giant cells interspersed between spindle- to oval-shaped fibroblasts with a highly vascular stroma and areas of haemorrhage and haemosiderin deposition. Mitoses can be identified. However, no atypical mitoses are seen.

- **Giant cell tumour of bone.** Giant cell tumours of the jaw are sporadic. It is an aggressive but benign neoplasm. The lesion generally manifests as multilocular radiolucency of bone with well-delineated margins. The lesion may resorb the alveolar ridge and displace the roots of the teeth. Microscopically giant cell tumour shows spindle-shaped stromal cells, mononuclear round to oval cells resembling histiocytes, and abundant, evenly distributed osteoclastic giant cells.

- **Brown tumour** is a manifestation of hyperparathyroidism. This is an osteolytic lesion affecting the jaws alongside other skeletal bones. Increased parathyroid hormone (PTH) leads to the activation of osteoclasts, releasing calcium and phosphorous from the bone and subsequent resorption of bone. This lesion typically presents as well-defined unilocular or multilocular radiolucency, with tooth displacement and resorption. Jaw lesions are typically erythematous with a brown tinge due to the presence of haemosiderin, hence the name of the lesion. Microscopic features include the replacement of bone with a fibrous stroma containing mononuclear cells alongside osteoclast-like giant cells. Abundant hemosiderin is typically noted, and reactive bone formation may also be seen.

- **Peripheral giant cell granuloma (PGCG).** The peripheral giant cell granuloma (PGCG) arises from the periodontal ligament and commonly occurs on the gingivae or in edentulous regions of the mandible and maxilla. Clinically PGCG appears as a solitary, sessile, red-to-purple swelling with a smooth or ulcerated surface. Microscopically, PGGC is characterised by an unencapsulated collection of spindle- to oval-shaped monocytes with scattered osteoclast-like multinucleated giant cells in a highly vascular stroma containing areas of hemosiderin deposits, haemorrhage, and immature bone.

- **Cherubism** is a rare genetic disorder affecting the jaws that typically presents in young patients (up to 6 years of age) and is limited to the jaws. Patients present with a bilateral, symmetrical expansion of the mandible, maxilla, or both jaws. If the maxilla is affected, the lesions may extend into the maxillary sinus and to the floor of the orbit, leading to a classical upward gaze. In most cases, Cherubism is due to a mutation in SH3BP2, a protein that encodes for a protein involved in osteoclastic differentia-

tion. Microscopic findings include the replacement of bone by fibrous connective tissue containing numerous multinucleate osteoclast-like giant cells within a well-vascularised stroma.

- **Aneurysmal bone cyst (ABC).** ABC primarily occurs in younger patients under 30 years of age, and the clinical features typically include swelling, mobile teeth, and pain. Radiologically, ABC presents as a well-defined, typically multilocular radiolucent lesion with the expansion of bone and displacement of adjacent teeth. Microscopically, multiple cystic spaces, blood filled fibrous septa are seen, containing multiple plump fibroblasts alongside numerous osteoclast-like multinucleated giant cells.

17.7.2.2 Non-Odontogenic Tumours

Compared to odontogenic tumours of the jawbone, non-odontogenic primary bone tumours are rare in the jaws. The list of non-odontogenic neoplasms is enormous. Only a few common primary bone tumours are described below. Tumours of fibrous, vascular, neural, and other tissues can involve jawbones. The following description is limited to only primary bone tumours.

- **Osteoma** is a benign bone tumour composed of compact or cancellous bone and is reportedly the most common osseous neoplasm of the jawbones. The tumour shows a predilection for the mandible, especially the ramus and the inferior border below the molars, rather than the maxilla. The major clinical manifestation caused by the growing osteoma is facial asymmetry.

- **Osteoblastoma** is a rare benign bone tumour. Osteoblastoma is more frequent in the mandible than in the maxilla. This tumour usually involves the posterior, tooth-bearing regions of the jawbones.

- **Osteosarcoma** is a primary sarcoma involving the jawbones. Osteosarcoma arising in the mandible predominates in the body of the bone and is followed in decreasing order of frequency by the symphysis, angle, and ascending ramus. The alveolar ridge and the maxillary antrum are the dominant affected sites in the maxilla. Pain and swelling are the most common symptoms. Radiographically, advanced cases of osteosarcomas may demonstrate a poorly defined osteolytic, osteoblastic, or mixed pattern of involvement.

- **Chondroblastoma** is a benign tumour which rarely involves the jawbones. The mandible is more commonly affected than the maxilla. Local pain, swelling, and tenderness are the most characteristic presenting symptoms. Radiographic changes include a well-defined radiolucent lesion, which may be surrounded by a thin sclerotic margin.

17.7.3 Fibro-Osseous Lesions

Fibro-osseous jaw lesions are microscopically characterised by a benign fibroblastic stroma in which new bone deposition occurs. This group of lesions includes ossifying fibroma, cementifying fibroma, fibrous dysplasia, and peripheral cemento-osseous dysplasia.

- **Fibrous dysplasia** is a self-limiting, slow-growing process that starts in childhood and is usually diagnosed by the age of 20 years. It may be limited to one bone (monostotic type), several bones (polyostotic type), or several bones with endocrine abnormalities and pigmented skin macules (McCune-Albright syndrome). Microscopically, fibrous dysplasia consists of a relatively vascular and loose benign fibrous connective tissue stroma surrounding immature fibrillar or woven bony trabeculae.
- **Ossifying fibroma** is a benign, slow-growing, well-circumscribed lesion with a predilection for the mandibular body and ramus of the jaw. Microscopically, ossifying fibroma is well demarcated from the surrounding resident bone. The tumour bone is seen as trabeculae and oval (spherical) islands distributed in a relatively uniform pattern throughout the lesion.
- **Cementifying fibroma** is considered a benign, osseous tumour arising from the periodontal ligament. Microscopically, it is composed of varying amounts of cementum, bone, and fibrous tissue.
- **Periapical cemento-osseous dysplasia** is a reactive/dysplastic process at the apices of vital mandibular (especially incisors) teeth, predominantly in middle-aged women. This lesion is self-limiting. Microscopically, this lesion shows a benign fibroblastic matrix containing a heterogeneous distribution of new and old bone in the form of islands and trabeculae.

17.8 Diseases of the Salivary Glands

Diseases of the salivary glands can be grouped into three major categories: sialolithiasis and mucoceles, salivary gland infections and inflammatory conditions, and salivary gland tumours.

- **Sialolithiasis and mucoceles:** Sialolithiasis (salivary calculus or salivary stones) is a common disorder. The pathogenesis of sialolithiasis is thought to be due to the stagnation of saliva that is high in calcium. Risk factors include dehydration, smoking, and various medications (most commonly anticholinergics and diuretics). Most calculi are found within the submandibular gland, likely due to its highly viscous saliva. The remaining calculi are located in the parotid gland (6%–20%) and sublingual/minor salivary glands.
- **Mucoceles.** Mucoceles can be differentiated into mucus extravasation phenomenon or mucus retention cysts and ranulas. Extravasation mucocele results from extravasation of saliva into the surrounding soft tissues and retention of mucoceles due to retention of saliva within the duct due to obstruction. These are common in the minor salivary glands. The ranula is an example of a large mucus extravasation cyst of the sublingual gland in the floor of the mouth.

Inflammatory-infectious conditions. These include acute and chronic bacterial sialadenitis, mumps, Human immunodeficiency virus–associated salivary gland disorder, postirradiation sialadenitis, and cheilitis glandularis.

- **Bacterial sialadenitis.** Bacterial sialadenitis is caused because of the retrograde spread of infection secondary to decreased salivary flow or ductal obstruction. *Staphylococcus aureus* is the most common etiologic agent for acute bacterial parotitis. Acute suppurative bacterial sialadenitis most often affects the parotid gland and, to a lesser extent, the submandibular glands. Fever and unilateral glandular enlargement of the parotid gland with purulent discharge through the Stenson's duct are common features of bacterial sialadenitis.
- **Viral sialadenitis.** Viruses that commonly cause sialadenitis are paramyxoviruses (mumps virus), typically affecting the parotid glands bilaterally. Children are most often affected, with peak incidence occurring at approximately 4 to 6 years of age.
- **Inflammatory disorders.** Chronic inflammation and fibrosis most commonly affect the parotid gland, often resulting from repeated acute infections with progressive damage to the ductal epithelium leading to stricture formation and acinar atrophy. Necrotising sialometaplasia is an inflammatory disorder of the salivary glands due to ischemic necrosis of minor salivary gland tissue. It is associated with smoking, local trauma, pressure from a denture, and local anaesthetic injection. This lesion is usually located in the posterior region of the hard palate.
- **Granulomatous disorders.** Less commonly, granulomatous disorders presenting with salivary gland swelling may occur. These include tuberculosis, cat scratch disease, sarcoidosis, actinomycosis, and Wegener's granulomatosis.
- **Autoimmune disorder.** Sjögren's syndrome is an autoimmune disorder that results in immunologically mediated destruction and inflammatory enlargement of the lacrimal and salivary glands. Sjögren's syndrome (SS) occurs predominantly in postmenopausal women and

presents with dryness of the eyes and mouth, leading to chronic mouth and ocular discomfort. Progressive symmetrical enlargement of the salivary glands may develop slowly in patients. Two types of SS occur Type1 (primary) and type2 (secondary). Sjogren's type 1 disease (Mikulicz's disease or "sicca syndrome without a connective tissue disorder") refers to autoimmune inflammation of the salivary glands without a systemic collagen vascular disorder. Sjogren's type 2 disease refers to autoimmune inflammation of the salivary glands with a systemic autoimmune process such as rheumatoid arthritis, systemic lupus erythematosus, and scleroderma.

- **Neoplastic salivary gland disease.** Salivary gland neoplasms are relatively uncommon and constitute only about 2% of all head and neck neoplasms, mostly (80%) occurring in the parotid gland. In comparison, the remaining 20% occur in the submandibular and minor salivary glands. About 80% of parotid tumours are benign; however, the incidence of malignancy in submandibular tumours is approximately 50%.

17.8.1 Medication-Induced Hyposalivation and Xerostomia

- **Xerostomia** (dry mouth) is the most frequent oral adverse effect of medications. Hyposalivation or xerostomia-causing medications include antihistamines, decongestants, antidepressants, anxiolytic drugs and sedatives, antihypertensive drugs, anticholinergic agents, and antipsychotic drugs.
- **Salivary gland tumours.** Most salivary gland tumours present as painless enlarging masses and are located in the parotid glands, most benign. Only 20% are malignant. The etiological agents of salivary gland cancers remain unclear. Some possible risk factors are therapeutic radiation for other head and neck cancers, occupational exposures in rubber manufacturing and woodworking, history of HIV infection, previous cancers related to the Epstein-Barr virus, immunosuppression, and radiation. Salivary gland tumours in the parotid or submandibular glands usually present as an enlarging mass with or without neurological symptoms such as facial nerve paralysis or pain if the tumour is malignant. Minor salivary gland tumours present as a submucosal intraoral mass which subsequently ulcerates. Ipsilateral facial nerve palsy, sudden tumour growth, pain, tumour fixation to the overlying skin or underlying muscle, and cervical lymphadenopathy are essential features of salivary gland neoplasms.

- **Benign and malignant tumours.** In both the major and minor salivary glands, the commonest type of benign tumour is pleomorphic adenoma (mixed salivary gland tumour). Among the malignant tumours, the commonest type is mucoepidermoid carcinoma. This predominantly affects the parotid glands. Adenoid cystic carcinoma is the commonest malignant tumour in the submandibular and minor salivary glands. A detailed description of these and other less common tumours is beyond the scope of this chapter.

17.9 Summary

Oral diseases, particularly dental caries, and periodontal diseases pose a great threat to public health. Some risk factors for dental and oral diseases include high sugar intake, tobacco use, and abuse of alcohol. Most oral diseases are preventable.

Bibliography

Featherstone JDB. Dental caries: a dynamic disease process. Aust Dent J. 2008;53(3):286–91. https://doi.org/10.1111/j.1834-7819.2008.00064.x.

Odell EW. Cawson's essentials of oral pathology and oral medicine. 9th ed. Edinburgh, UK: Elsevier; 2017.

Prabhu SR. Handbook of oral pathology and oral medicine. West Sussex, UK: Wiley Blackwell; 2022.

Pathology of Organ Systems of the Body

18

18.1 Introduction

Oral health is an integral part of general health. Most oral diseases and conditions share modifiable risk factors with the leading non-communicable diseases. There is a proven relationship between oral and general health. Several epidemiological studies have linked poor oral health with cardiovascular diseases, poor glycaemic control in people with diabetes, low-birth-weight preterm babies, and other diseases, including rheumatoid arthritis and osteoporosis. Oral disease is also a significant problem in medically or immunologically compromised patients suffering from various chronic conditions. Therefore, a dental clinician should have adequate knowledge of diseases of organ systems that present oral manifestations. This chapter deals with some common organ systems, psychiatric diseases, and disorders that have dental relevance.

18.2 Gastrointestinal Diseases

Dyspepsia. Dyspepsia is a collective term suggestive of indigestion, commonly known as "upset stomach." Some causes of dyspepsia include oesophagitis, drugs, alcohol, pregnancy, depression, anxiety neuroses, peptic ulcer, gastric carcinoma, pancreatic disease, Crohn's disease, and liver failure. Symptoms include burning or pain in the upper part of the abdomen related to eating, flatulence, heartburn, water brash, abdominal bloating, nausea, and vomiting.

Dysphagia. Difficulty in swallowing food or drinks is called dysphagia. Causes of dysphagia include gastroesophageal reflux disease (GORD), anxiety (globus hysterics), oesophageal spasm, pharyngitis, Barret's oesophagus, severe iron deficiency (Plummer Vinson syndrome), bulbar palsies, myasthenia gravis, and achalasia (a condition in which the muscles of the lower part of the oesophagus fail to relax, preventing food from passing into the stomach). Common symptoms include difficulty swallowing food and drinks, "lump in the throat," gurgling in the neck when drinking, and regurgitating food.

18.2.1 Gastroesophageal Reflux Disease (GORD)

Gastroesophageal reflux disease (GORD) is when acidic gastric fluid flows backwards into the oesophagus. This occurs when the lower oesophageal sphincter (LES) is compromised. LES is a ring of muscle that forms a valve at the lower end of the oesophagus, where it joins the stomach. The reflux of fluid into the oesophagus may cause inflammation, erosions, or ulcerations mediated by pepsin and hydrochloric acid. Patients complain of a retrosternal burning sensation ("heartburn") often triggered by food, coffee or alcohol, pregnancy, smoking, and drugs. Symptoms are aggravated by bending, lying flat, lifting weights, and straining. The pain of GORD often mimics that of angina.

Oral manifestations of GORD include erosion of the palatal aspects of the maxillary anterior teeth and premolars. Erosive lesions appear smooth, shiny, yellow, and sensitive to cold. Other symptoms include xerostomia, burning mouth syndrome, and halitosis.

Gastritis. This common condition is characterised by acute or chronic inflammation of the gastric mucosa, sometimes accompanied by erosions. Causes include overindulgence in alcohol and drugs. *Helicobacter pylori* infection is often the cause of chronic gastritis. Epigastric pain after eating, vomiting and indigestion, lack of appetite, and weight loss are common symptoms.

Hiatus hernia. Protrusion of the stomach through an aperture in the diaphragm (hiatus) causes a hiatus hernia. In many cases, constipation and GORD may be associated with a hiatus hernia. Many patients with hiatus hernia are symptomatic. Occasionally, chest pain is the only complaint.

S. R. Prabhu, *Textbook of General Pathology for Dental Students*, https://doi.org/10.1007/978-3-031-31244-1_18

Gastroenteritis. Gastroenteritis refers to inflammation of the mucosal surfaces of the stomach, small intestine, and large intestine. The leading cause of gastroenteritis is infection (bacteria, viruses, and parasites); drugs and chemicals may cause this in many cases. Causative bacteria include *Vibrio cholera, Escherichia coli, Shigella species, Salmonella spp, Clostridium deficile, and Campylobacter spp.* Viral agents include rotaviruses and adenoviruses. Parasitic agents include *Giardia lamblia* and *Cryptosporidium parvum.* Common symptoms include sudden nausea, vomiting, rumbling noises, diarrhoea, and abdominal cramps. Watery diarrhoea is a feature of viral gastroenteritis, and bloody diarrhoea with fever occurs in bacterial gastroenteritis. Severe gastroenteritis may lead to tachycardia, hypotension, and shock.

Peptic ulcer disease. Peptic ulcer disease (Peptic ulcers: Gastric and duodenal ulcers). Peptic ulcer disease is characterised by well-defined ulcers in the gastrointestinal mucosa. Causes include chronic acid-pepsin secretions, harmful effects of *Helicobacter pylori*, NSAIDs, and Crohn's disease. Peptic ulcers are divided into two groups: gastric and duodenal ulcers. Symptoms include epigastric pain and tenderness associated with eating in gastric ulcers. Pain between meals and during the night is a feature of a duodenal ulcer. Pain tends to wax and wane and aggravates during stress and with drugs and alcohol. Ingestion of food, milk, or antacids provides temporary relief. Protracted vomiting a few hours after meals indicates gastric outlet (pyloric) obstruction. Black tarry stools (melena) due to gastrointestinal haemorrhage. Weight loss is common.

Coeliac disease. Also known as gluten-sensitive enteropathy, Coeliac disease is characterised by the atrophy of the jejunal mucosa due to sensitivity to dietary gluten. Gluten has two components: glutenin and α-gliadin. The latter is antigenic. Genetic predisposition exists (HLA B8 and BR3). Symptoms include diarrhoea, steatorrhea, weight loss, abdominal pain, anaemia, muscle wasting, oral mucosal ulcers, skin pigmentation, peripheral oedema, and dermatitis herpetiformis (itchy, blistering skin disease). Oral manifestations of celiac disease include glossitis, angular cheilitis, bleeding tendencies, oral mucosal ulcers, dental enamel hypoplasia, delayed eruption, and oral mucosal signs of anaemia.

Crohn's disease. Crohn's disease is an inflammatory disease of any part of the GI tract due to unknown aetiology. The precise causes of Crohn's disease are unknown; it is believed to be caused by a combination of environmental, immune, and bacterial factors in genetically susceptible individuals. Symptoms include malaise, anorexia, weight loss, nausea, fever, abdominal pain, diarrhoea, arthralgia, rectal bleeding, pallor, finger clubbing, erythema nodosum, and perianal abscesses. Oral manifestations of Crohn's disease include diffuse labial, gingival or mucosal swelling, cobble-stoning of buccal mucosa and gingiva, aphthous ulcers, mucosal tags, angular cheilitis, and oral granulomas.

Ulcerative colitis is a chronic inflammation of a part or whole of the colon. The cause is unknown. Probable factors implicated are genetic, immunological, dietary, and psychological. Symptoms include diarrhoea with blood and mucous, malaise, lethargy and anorexia, weight loss, abdominal pain, erythema nodosum, arthritis, uveitis, pallor, and weakness. Oral manifestations of ulcerative colitis include aphthous ulceration or superficial haemorrhagic ulcers, angular stomatitis, and pyostomatitis vegetans.

Irritable Bowel Syndrome (IBS). Irritable bowel syndrome is characterised by constipation, diarrhoea, abdominal pain in the left iliac fossa, and frequent passage of stools. In most cases, the cause is psychological and stress related. Symptoms include pain in the left iliac fossa or epigastrium, aggravated by eating and relieved by defecation. Other symptoms include abdominal bloating, alternating diarrhoea and constipation and passage of mucus in stools, abdominal tenderness, and mucous on per rectal (PR) examination. There are no specific oral manifestations of IBS. Psychogenic facial pain and temporomandibular joint symptoms are sometimes present.

18.3   Liver Diseases

Infections, alcohol, autoimmunity, and malignancy cause most liver diseases. These include Viral hepatitis, Alcoholic liver disease, Fatty liver disease, Liver cirrhosis, and Hepatocellular carcinoma.

18.3.1 Viral Hepatitis

Hepatitis refers to inflammation of the liver. Causes of hepatitis include viral infections (viral hepatitis), alcohol (alcoholic hepatitis), and autoimmunity (autoimmune hepatitis). Common viruses involved in the causation of hepatitis include hepatitis A, B, C, D, and E.

Hepatitis A virus infection. Hepatitis A virus is an RNA virus. Transmission of infection occurs through the faecal-oral route. The risk group includes food handlers and day-care workers (with poor hygiene). The incubation period ranges from 15 to 50 days. Chronic hepatitis A viral infection does not occur and has no carrier state. People who get hepatitis A may feel sick for a few weeks to several months but usually recover completely and do not have lasting liver damage. Common symptoms may include jaundice, loss of appetite, and diarrhoea. Prophylaxis is through Immunoglobulin (Ig) and vaccines. Immunity following infection is probably a lifetime. Hepatitis A infection has no association with hepatocellular carcinoma.

Hepatitis B virus infection. Hepatitis B viruses are DNA viruses. Transmission of infection occurs through percutaneous, sexual, or perinatal routes. The risk group includes IV drug users, healthcare workers, haemodialysis patients, men having sex with men (MSM), and heterosexuals with multiple partners. The incubation period ranges from 30 to 180 days. Hepatitis B infection can cause both acute and chronic symptoms. Most people do not experience any symptoms when newly infected. However, some people have acute illnesses with symptoms that last several weeks, including jaundice, dark urine, extreme fatigue, nausea, vomiting, and abdominal pain. Hepatitis B infection has a carrier state. Chronic carrier state is 90% in infants (neonates) and 6–10% in adults. Prophylaxis is through Hepatitis B Immunoglobulin (HBIg) and vaccine. Immunity following infection lasts for over 20 years and probably a lifetime. Hepatitis B infection has an association with hepatocellular carcinoma.

Hepatitis C virus infection. Hepatitis C viruses are RNA viruses transmitted through percutaneous and occasionally via sexual and perinatal routes. The risk group includes IV drug users, healthcare workers, haemodialysis patients, men having sex with men (MSM), and heterosexuals with multiple partners. Incubation for hepatitis C infection ranges from 15 to 160 days. The virus can cause acute and chronic hepatitis, ranging in severity from mild to serious, lifelong illnesses, including liver cirrhosis and liver cancer. The chronic carrier state of Hepatitis C infection is 50–80%. Immunity following infection is very weak and ineffective.

Hepatitis D virus infection. Hepatitis D viruses (HDV) are defective RNA viruses. Hepatitis D infection cannot occur without the hepatitis B virus. HDV infection occurs when people become infected with both hepatitis B and D simultaneously (co-infection) or get hepatitis D after first being infected with hepatitis B (super-infection). The routes of HDV transmission, like HBV, occur through broken skin (via injection, tattooing, etc.) or contact with infected blood or blood products. Incubation ranges from 21 to 140 days. In acute hepatitis, simultaneous infection with HBV and HDV can lead to mild-to-severe hepatitis, with signs and symptoms indistinguishable from those of other types of acute viral hepatitis infections. There is a carrier state for HDV. Although the association with hepatocellular carcinoma is unknown, patients with HDV-induced cirrhosis are at an increased risk of hepatocellular carcinoma (HCC). Chronic infection does not occur in HDV infection, and a chronic carrier state occurs. No HDV prophylaxis, but the HBV vaccine offers some immunity for susceptible individuals.

Hepatitis E virus infection. Hepatitis E viruses (HVE) are defective RNA viruses. The virus is shed in the stools of infected persons and enters the human body through the intestine. It is transmitted mainly through contaminated drinking water. The infection is usually self-limiting and resolves within 2–6 weeks. Occasionally, a serious disease known as fulminant hepatitis (acute liver failure) develops, which can be fatal. The risk group includes travellers to endemic regions such as India, Asia, Africa, and Central America. Incubation ranges from 15 to 64 days. Cases of hepatitis E are not clinically distinguishable from other types of acute viral hepatitis. Chronic infection does not occur, and there is no chronic carrier state. The severity of infection is usually mild—20% fatality in pregnant women in the third trimester of pregnancy. There is no prophylaxis. Immunity following infection is probably a lifetime. There is no association with hepatocellular carcinoma.

Alcoholic liver disease (ALD) is liver damage from alcohol abuse. ALDs include fatty liver, alcoholic hepatitis, and cirrhosis. Oral manifestations of ALD may include advanced periodontal disease, jaundice of the oral mucosa, oral bleeding tendencies, parotid gland enlargement, and sweet, musty breath odour.

Fatty liver disease (FLD) refers to excess fat build-up in the liver. It is the mildest form of reversible liver injury. There are two types of fatty liver disease: non-alcoholic fatty liver disease (NAFLD) and alcoholic fatty liver disease (AFLD). NAFLD is made up of simple fatty liver. The primary risks for NAFLD include type 2 diabetes and obesity. In FLD, often, there are no or few symptoms. Occasionally, there may be tiredness or pain in the upper right side of the abdomen.

Alcoholic hepatitis is due to excessive intake of alcohol. Signs and symptoms of alcoholic hepatitis include jaundice, ascites (fluid accumulation in the abdominal cavity), fatigue, and hepatic encephalopathy (brain dysfunction due to liver failure).

Liver Cirrhosis. Liver cirrhosis is characterised by replacing liver tissue with fibrosis, scar tissue, and nodules, leading to loss of liver function. Some causes of liver fibrosis include hepatitis B and C infections, alcohol abuse, hemochromatosis, primary biliary cirrhosis, drugs (e.g. methotrexate), and sarcoidosis. Symptoms of liver cirrhosis include lethargy, jaundice, itching, ankle oedema, and ascites. Signs include enlarged liver and spleen, palmar erythema, finger clubbing, oesophageal varices, and dark urine. Oral manifestations include jaundice of the oral mucosa (soft palate and sublingual region), bleeding tendencies, and poor oral hygiene.

Hepatocellular carcinoma. This is a carcinoma of hepatocytes—common worldwide. Causes include liver cirrhosis from any cause and carriage of hepatitis B and C viruses. Symptoms include abdominal pain, weight loss, fever, jaundice, and enlarged liver. Oral mucosa may show signs of jaundice.

18.4 Cardiovascular Diseases

Angina pectoris (angina) is a common symptom of heart disease characterised by pain caused by heart muscle ischemia. In most cases, this is usually caused by obstruction or spasms of the coronary arteries. Major risk factors for angina include cigarette smoking, diabetes, high blood pressure, a sedentary lifestyle, and a family history of premature heart disease. Symptoms of angina include severe central chest pain, often with shortness of breath. Pain often radiates to the left arm, neck, and jaw. Pain is typically induced by physical exercise, emotion, heavy meals, or cold weather and relieved by rest and nitrates. This is called stable angina. If angina is of recent onset, severe, rapidly worsening on minimal or no exertion, and lasts longer than a few minutes, it is considered unstable angina. This is usually a forerunner of myocardial infarction. During the attack of angina or myocardial infarction, in addition to chest pain, the patient may complain of acute pain in the jaw. Jaw pain may resolve as soon as the chest pain is controlled.

Myocardial infarction. Myocardial infarction (MI) refers to necrosis (death) of a part of the heart muscle due to total occlusion of the coronary artery. The major cause of infarction is the embolism following the rupture of atheromatous coronary artery plaque, which may be precipitated by vigorous exercise, major surgery, or infections. Symptoms include severe central pain radiating to the left arm, neck, and jaw associated with nausea, vomiting, breathlessness, and sweating. Pain does not respond to nitrates. The patient may show signs of shock. In some cases, symptoms do not occur, and MI is discovered incidentally on an ECG performed at a later date. This is called silent infarction.

Heart failure (Cardiac failure). Heart failure is a clinical syndrome characterised by a change in the heart's pumping function accompanied by shortness of breath and weakness. Causes of heart failure include ischemic heart disease, hypertension, valvular heart disease, arrhythmias, pulmonary embolism, anaemia, cardiomyopathies, infective endocarditis, and thyrotoxicosis.

Cardiac arrhythmias. Cardiac arrhythmias are characterised by the loss of rhythm resulting in heartbeat irregularities. These may include palpitations, irregularly irregular pulse, ectopic heartbeats, bradycardia, and tachycardia. In some cases, cardiac arrest may occur. Cardiac causes of cardiac arrhythmias include ischemic heart disease, myocardial infarction, rheumatic heart disease, and congestive heart failure. Noncardiac causes include pneumonia, obstructive pulmonary disease, thyrotoxicosis, drug-related side effects, infections, and electrolyte imbalances.

Congenital Heart Disease. Congenital heart disease (CHD) is a general term for any defect of the heart, heart valves, or central blood vessels that is present at birth. There are two types of congenital heart diseases: acyanotic and cyanotic CHDs. Acyanotic defects include atrial septal defect (ASD), ventricular septal defect (VSD), patent ductus arteriosus (PDA), and coarctation of the aorta. The cyanotic form includes Fallot tetralogy, tricuspid atresia, and pulmonary atresia. Oral manifestations may include delayed tooth eruption, frequent positional anomalies of teeth, and hypoplastic enamel.

Rheumatic Fever/Infective Endocarditis. Rheumatic fever (RF) is a non-contagious acute fever marked by inflammation and joint pain caused by a streptococcal infection. Beta-haemolytic streptococcal infection of the throat produces cross-reacting antibodies that attack heart valves, joints, and the skin.

Infective endocarditis (IEC), also known as bacterial endocarditis, is an infection of the endocardial surface of the heart, heart valves, the mural endocardium, or a septal defect. The infective agent is *Staphylococcus aureus.* Common symptoms of RF include fever, polyarthritis, pericarditic pain, heart murmurs, and signs of heart failure. Common symptoms include pyrexia, night sweats, fatigue, joint pains, and, in some cases, haematuria and pleuritic chest pain.

Hypertension. Hypertension refers to abnormally high blood pressure characterised by sustained elevation of resting systolic blood pressure (>140 mmHg), diastolic blood pressure (>90 mmHg), or both. Some common causes of hypertension include obesity, dietary salt, stress, and hereditary factors (Primary hypertension). Secondary hypertension is associated with glomerulonephritis, Cushing's syndrome, hyperthyroidism, myxoedema, alcohol abuse, contraceptive pills, drugs (prednisolone), and pregnancy. The majority of patients with hypertension are asymptomatic. Some may complain of headaches, dizziness, fatigue, nose bleeds, and nervousness. There are no specific oral manifestations of hypertension. In hypertensive patients on medication, adverse effects of antihypertensive drugs include xerostomia, gingival hyperplasia (with nifedipine), salivary gland swelling (with clonidine), and increased postoperative bleeding (e.g. for those patients on aspirin or thrombolytic therapy). Calcium channel blockers can cause mucosal lichenoid reactions and gingival swellings.

18.5 Respiratory Diseases

Chronic Obstructive Pulmonary Disease. Chronic obstructive pulmonary disease (COPD) is a lung disease characterised by chronic obstruction of lung airflow that interferes with normal breathing and is not fully reversible. The terms "chronic bronchitis" and "emphysema" are no longer used but are now included within the COPD diagnosis. Pathological changes occur in large airways (chronic bronchitis), small airways (bronchiolitis), and lung parenchyma (Emphysema). Productive cough, breathlessness, cyanosis, and peripheral oedema are common in COPD. There are no significant oral manifestations in COPD; however, some patients may show signs of cyanosis of the lips.

Lung Abscess and Bronchiectasis. A lung abscess is a pus-filled cavity in the lung due to a necrotising infection. The cavity is usually surrounded by inflamed tissue. The most common pathogens are anaerobic bacteria. Symptoms include fever, productive cough, sweats, and loss of weight. Sputum is purulent with or without traces of blood and foul smelling. Periodontal health in these patients is usually poor.

Bronchiectasis refers to the permanent abnormal widening of the bronchi, causing a risk of infection. Causes include cystic fibrosis and immune defects. Symptoms include chronic cough, haemoptysis, and large amounts of purulent sputum. Periodontal disease and halitosis are common in these patients.

Asthma. Asthma is characterised by bronchial inflammation leading to bronchial constriction, oedema, and mucus plugging. Causes include sensitivity to antigens such as house dust mites, animal dander, and pollen. Intrinsic causes include atopy with raised IgE levels. Asthma is associated with cold weather, stress, exercise, beta-blockers, aspirin, smoking, environmental pollution, and viral infections. Signs and symptoms include audible expiratory wheeze, breathlessness, cough, chest hyperinflation, and tachypnoea.

Pneumonia. Pneumonia is characterised by infection of the lung parenchyma by *Streptococcus pneumoniae, Streptococcus aureus, Streptococcus pyogenes, Legionella pneumophila, Pneumocystis carinii,* and influenza viruses A and B. Signs and symptoms include productive cough with rusty sputum, rigours, breathlessness, chest pain, haemoptysis, pyrexia, and tachypnoea.

Pulmonary Tuberculosis. Pulmonary tuberculosis refers to the primary infection of the lungs by *Mycobacterium tuberculosis.* Typical symptoms of active tuberculosis are a chronic cough with blood-containing mucus, fever, night sweats, and weight loss. Extrapulmonary tuberculosis (of lymph nodes, bone, and brain, e.g.) may occur, but primary tuberculosis infection of the oral soft tissues is extremely rare; however, secondary involvement of oral tissues from pulmonary infection can occur. These may include chronic, painless tuberculous ulcers on the dorsum or lateral borders of the tongue. Ulcers disappear once the systemic infection is treated with antituberculosis medications.

Cystic Fibrosis. Cystic fibrosis (CF) is a hereditary disorder affecting the exocrine glands. The majority of patients present symptoms in infancy. Cough, wheezing, barrel-shaped chest, digital clubbing, and cyanosis are common signs and symptoms. Bulky, foul-smelling stools due to pancreatic insufficiency are common in cystic fibrosis children. In cystic fibrosis, disorders of the salivary glands can give rise to xerostomia. Increased calculus formation, enamel defects, gingivitis, and swelling of the lips are also reported in these patients.

Lung cancer. Lung cancer (carcinoma) is a common pulmonary disease worldwide. Cigarette smoking is the major cause. Susceptibility to lung cancer is high among patients with COPD and pulmonary fibrosis. In the early stages, lung cancer may be asymptomatic. As cancer advances, symptoms and signs include cough, dyspnoea, chest pain, haemoptysis (blood in the sputum), hoarseness of voice, pleural effusion, facial and extremity oedema, and weight loss.

18.6 Diseases of the Blood and Blood-Forming Organs

18.6.1 Anaemias

Anaemia refers to a decrease in the oxygen-carrying capacity of the blood caused by either decreased production of red blood cells, increased destruction of red blood cells, increased demand for iron, or formation of abnormal red blood cells. Anaemias can be classified as Haemolytic anaemia (autoimmune and non-autoimmune), Iron-deficiency anaemia (microcytic anaemia), Aplastic anaemia (normocytic anaemia), Pernicious anaemia (macrocytic anaemia), sickle cell anaemia, and thalassemia.

Haemolytic anaemia. Haemolytic anaemia is caused by excessive intravascular or extravascular (in the spleen) destruction of red blood cells due to several causes. The normal survival of RBCs is about 120 days. In haemolytic anaemia, it is much shorter. Causes include autoimmune causes, infections, splenomegaly, drugs, RBC membrane disorders (spherocytosis), enzymopathies (deficiency of glucose-6-phosphate dehydrogenase), and haemoglobinopathies (sickle cell disease and thalassemia). Drugs that trigger haemolysis in G-6-PD deficiency include acetylsalicylic acid, ascorbic acid, dapsone, and vitamin K. Malaria is the most common cause in the developing world. Symptoms and signs (of G-6-PD-associated haemolytic anaemia, e.g.) Jaundice, palpitations, dyspnoea, and dizziness are common. Signs include splenomegaly, cyanosis, and Reynaud's phenomenon.

Aplastic anaemia (normocytic anaemia). A decrease in haematopoietic bone marrow leading to pancytopenia (involving all blood cells) results in aplastic anaemia. Causes include Idiopathic (60%), hereditary (Fanconi's anaemia), viral hepatitis, irradiation, insecticides, and drugs (Sulphonamides, NSAIDS, antithyroid drugs etc.). Symptoms include anaemia (due to deficiency of RBCs), bleeding tendencies, purpura, haematuria, epistaxis, ecchymosis, gingival bleeding (due to thrombocytopenia), and susceptibility to infections (due to leucopenia). Headache and dyspnoea are common.

Pernicious anaemia (macrocytic anaemia). Pernicious anaemia is characterised by the failure of secretion of intrinsic factors in the stomach (due to an autoimmune process), which is responsible for the absorption of vitamin B12 (cobalamin). Causes include autoimmune disorders resulting in permanent atrophy of gastric mucosa and total gastrectomy. A higher incidence has been reported in individuals with blood group A. Symptoms and signs include general symptoms and signs of anaemia, neurological symptoms such as paraesthesia of fingers and toes, and dementia. Other features include glossitis, periodic diarrhoea, weight loss, and mild jaundice due to haemolysis.

18.6.2 Haemoglobinopathies (Sickle Cell Anaemia and Thalassemia)

Sickle cell anaemia (Sickle cell disease). Sickle cell anaemia is an inherited disorder. In this disorder, red blood cells become sickle-shaped, and the blood experiences lower oxygen tension (as during GA administration) or decreased pH or dehydration. These changes result in erythrocytosis, increased RBC adhesion and blood viscosity, and increased vascular occlusion. The disease is inherited in an autosomal-recessive fashion. The condition is common in equatorial Africa and among those Africans who have migrated from this region. Symptoms and signs include anaemia and lethargy, growth retardation, delayed puberty, increased susceptibility to infection, leg ulceration, and infarcts in the spleen, lungs, kidneys, bowel, bones, and fingers. Often these features are precipitated by dehydration or infection.

Thalassemia. Thalassemia is an inherited disorder in which the synthesis of one of the globin chains of the haemoglobin is either reduced or absent, resulting in haemolysis and anaemia. Normally, haemoglobin comprises four protein chains, two α and two β globin chains. Patients with thalassemia have defects in the α or β globin chain, causing abnormal red blood cell production. The thalassemias are classified according to which chain of the haemoglobin molecule is affected. In α thalassemia (also known as thalassemia major), production of the α globin chain is affected, while in β thalassemia (also known as thalassemia minor), production of the β globin chain is affected. Symptoms and signs include severe anaemia, failure to thrive, and early death. Those who survive show mongoloid appearance of the head and face due to bone marrow hyperplasia. Leg ulcerations and hepatosplenomegaly are common.

Thrombocytopenia. This is a bleeding disorder due to a circulating platelets (thrombocytes) count below 50,000 per microlitre (normal 150,000 to 450,000 per microlitre). Idiopathic thrombocytopenic purpura is a severe form of thrombocytopenia probably due to an IgG antibody attack that may follow a viral infection. Causes include various diseases and conditions leading to decreased marrow production, decreased platelet survival, increased platelet consumption, platelet sequestration, and platelet dilution. Symptoms and signs include purpuric spots and ecchymosis on the skin and mucous membranes, epistaxis, gastrointestinal bleeding and haematuria, headache, and dizziness.

Leukaemia. This disorder is a haematological malignancy characterised by the uncontrolled proliferation of (malignant) white blood cells derived from one of the haematopoietic precursor cells, resulting in the replacement of the normal bone marrow. Two significant types of leukaemia occur: acute and chronic. Acute leukaemia is common in children. A rapid increase in the number of immature blood cells characterises it. Chronic type is common in the elderly and is characterised by the excessive and slow build-up of relatively mature, but still abnormal, white blood cells. Acute and chronic leukaemias are further subdivided according to the type of white blood cells affected. This division includes lymphoblastic (or lymphocytic) leukaemias and myeloid (or myelogenous) leukaemias. Both types can present in acute or chronic forms. The causes of leukaemia largely remain unknown. Large doses of radiation, exposure to chemicals, infection with Epstein-Barr virus (EBV) and human lymphotropic virus (HTLV-1), and exposure to electromagnetic fields have been implicated as risk factors.

Acute Lymphoblastic Leukaemia (ALL). ALL is common in children and the elderly. It is a B-lymphocyte neoplasm. Malignant cells proliferate and infiltrate the bone marrow, resulting in granulocytopenia, thrombocytopenia, and anaemia. Malignant cells also enter the viscera, skin, and brain. Cause: Environmental causes may include infections (EBV and HTLV). Genetic factors may also play an essential role in the causation. Philadelphia chromosome (a shortened chromosome) is present in 25% of adults and 5% of children with ALL. ALL is more common in Down syndrome patients. Symptoms and signs: Flu-like symptoms, generalised lymphadenopathy, anaemia, bruising and bleeding tendencies (petechiae and ecchymoses), splenomegaly, and hepatomegaly. CNS involvement may result in cranial nerve palsies.

Chronic lymphocytic leukaemia (CLL). A chronic form of leukaemia involving mature clonal CD5 B- lymphocytes. This is the most common type of leukaemia in adults. Cause is unknown. Familial inheritance is a risk factor. Symptoms and signs include being asymptomatic at presentation. When symptomatic, fatigue, anorexia, and weight loss are common complaints. As the disease advances, anaemia, abdominal pain, thrombocytopenia, splenomegaly, lymphadenopathy, and hepatomegaly are noted.

Acute myeloid (myelogenous) leukaemia (AML). This is a neoplasm of myeloid (immature) white blood cells resulting in uncontrolled proliferation in the bone marrow. These cells appear in the peripheral circulation. Causes and risk factors include radiation exposure, chemotherapy, and exposure to chemicals (tobacco smoke, benzene, e.g.). Starting with flu-like symptoms, fatigue, easy bruising and bone pain, malaise, pallor, and dyspnoea on exertion are common. Other features include petechiae and ecchymoses in the skin and mucous membranes, delayed healing, infections, tonsils, lymph nodes, spleen, and gingiva enlargement. CNS involvement due to infiltration of neoplastic white blood cells occurs in 35% of cases.

Chronic myeloid (myelogenous) leukaemia (CML). This is a neoplasm of mature (differentiated) myeloid cell lines, less aggressive than AML. The cause is unknown. Radiation exposure is a risk factor. Shortened chromosome 22 (Philadelphia chromosome) is seen in 90% of cases. Many patients are asymptomatic at presentation. When symptomatic, myalgia, arthralgia, epistaxis, weight loss, gout, sweating, recurrent infections, and massive splenomegaly are common features.

18.6.3 Disorders of Coagulation

Haemophilias. Haemophilias are a group of genetic disorders resulting in a deficiency of one of the coagulation pathway factors. This group consists of three conditions: Haemophilia A, Haemophilia B (Christmas disease), and Von Willebrand's disease.

Haemophilia A. This is an inherited X–linked recessive disorder characterised by Factor VIII deficiency. This coagulation disorder affects males and is carried by females. The defective gene is located on the X chromosome (F8 gene). An affected male will not transmit the disorder to his sons, but all of his daughters will be carriers of the trait because they inherit his X chromosome. A female carrier will transmit the condition to half of her and carrier state to half of her daughters. Symptoms and signs include excessive bruising and hemarthroses from very early in childhood. Swelling, pain, and eventual deformity of the joints are common. Internal bleeding may occur. Spontaneous bleeding from oral soft tissues may occur in a severe form of the disorder. Excessive bleeding from trauma or surgery is common in these patients.

Haemophilia B (Christmas disease). Factor IX is defective or deficient in haemophilia B. This disorder is less common than Haemophilia A. Clinical features are identical to those of Haemophilia A. Detection of Factor IX is diagnostic.

Von Willebrand's disease. This is an autosomal-dominant inherited disorder characterised by defective platelet function and a deficiency or abnormality of factor VIII. Symptoms and signs include mucocutaneous bleeding and hemarthrosis.

18.7   Disorders of the Immune System

Diseases of the immune system can be grouped as hypersensitivity reactions, autoimmune diseases, and immunodeficiency diseases.

18.7.1 Hypersensitivity Reactions

Hypersensitivity reactions are characterised by the immune system's hyperfunction resulting in varying severity of allergic manifestations. Systemic manifestation resulting in anaphylaxis is a life-threatening condition, whereas those of skin and mucous membranes known as contact dermatitis (contact mucositis) are less dangerous.

Anaphylaxis. A severe life-threatening allergic (type 1 hypersensitivity) response to agents such as food, medications, and insect stings. Foodstuff includes shellfish, eggs, peanuts, soy, wheat, and milk. Medications include penicillins, aspirin, NSAIDs, tetracycline, local anaesthetics, and vaccines. Other causes include Venom from bees and wasps, X-ray contrast medium, latex, food additives, and food colours. Symptoms occur within minutes: Between 5 and 20 min if the allergen is injected and about 2 h if ingested. Skin/mucous membrane, respiratory, cardiac, and gastrointestinal symptoms result from allergic manifestations. These include skin hives, itchiness, swelling of lips, conjunctiva, throat or tongue and runny nose, shortness of breath, wheeze, or stridor cough, hoarseness of voice or painful swallowing, diarrhoea, vomiting, abdominal pain, low blood pressure, loss of bladder control, headache, confusion and fear, dysrhythmias and cardiac arrest.

Allergic contact dermatitis (ACD). Allergic contact dermatitis is an inflammatory condition of the skin which requires sensitisation to an antigen and is termed Type IV delayed hypersensitivity reaction involving a cell-mediated allergic response. (This is to be differentiated from contact dermatitis, which results from direct skin contact with an external agent without affecting immunologic mechanisms). Immunologic events in allergic contact dermatitis require interaction among antigens, antigen-presenting cells (Langerhans' cells) in the skin, and lymphocytes. The majority of contact allergens are of plant origin: poison ivy, poison oak, shells of cashew nuts, the resin of the Japanese lacquer tree, skin of mangoes, primrose, and chrysanthemums. Other allergens include nickel, gold, chromium, neomycin, cosmetic products, insecticides, soaps, household cleaners, hair dye, photographic developers, shampoos, and conditioners. Symptoms and signs include Itching, redness and vesiculation of the skin at the site of exposure within 12 h to 2 days after the contact with an allergen (in contact dermatitis, lesions appear soon after the exposure to an irritant).

Depending on the type of allergen involved, the lesions can ooze, drain, and crust or become scaled, raw, or thickened. Those who develop allergic contact dermatitis to a known allergen will continue to present skin manifestations on subsequent contacts throughout life.

Autoimmune disorders: Autoimmune disorders are characterised by the failure of the immune system to recognise 'self' from 'non-self' and cause clinical manifestations by forming autoantibodies against one's tissue antigens. Some autoimmune diseases are organ-specific, whilst others involve multiple body systems.

Sjögren's syndrome. Sjogren's syndrome (SS) is a chronic multisystem autoimmune disorder in which acinar tissue of exocrine glands (salivary and lacrimal glands in particular) is replaced and destroyed by lymphocytic infiltrate. Two types of SS occur: Primary and secondary. Primary causes dry eyes and dry mouth (Primary SS or SS-1). In the secondary SS (SS-2), a triad of dry mouth, dry eyes, and a connective tissue disorder such as rheumatoid arthritis (RA) or primary biliary cirrhosis (PBC), systemic lupus erythematosus (SLE) or primary systemic sclerosis (PSS) are present. The involvement of other exocrine glands may cause nasal dryness, tracheitis, pancreatitis, and vaginal dryness. The autoimmune process causes SS. Genetic predisposition may exist. In primary Sjogren's syndrome, symptoms include dryness of all mucosal sites, predominantly eyes (Keratoconjunctivitis sicca) and mouth (xerostomia). Oral manifestations include disturbances in taste sensation, fissured tongue, candidal infections, and extensive dental decay due to xerostomia. The risk of developing lymphoma of the parotid glands exists at a later stage of the primary disease. In secondary Sjogren's syndrome, in addition to dryness of the mucosal surfaces, joints (Rheumatoid arthritis), kidneys (interstitial nephritis), blood vessels (vasculitis), lungs (bronchitis), liver, pancreas, thyroid glands, peripheral nervous system (carpal tunnel syndrome and peripheral neuropathy) may be involved.

Systemic lupus erythematosus (SLE). SLE is an autoimmune disorder characterised by non-organ-specific antibodies predominantly affecting females. The cause is unknown. Sometimes, a variety of drugs may precipitate the condition. SLE is a multisystem disorder involving the skin, musculoskeletal system, renal system, nervous system, cardiovascular system, and respiratory system. Symptoms include joint pain (arthritis), myalgia, photosensitive skin rash on the face (malar "butterfly rash"), Raynaud's phenomena, vasculitis, purpura, oral white patches or ulcers, glomerulonephritis, peripheral neuropathy, cranial nerve palsies, seizures, hemiparesis, pancreatitis, abdominal pain, haemolytic anaemia, jaundice, abnormal liver function tests, splenomegaly, and lymphadenopathy. General symptoms include fever, malaise, and lethargy.

Giant cell arteritis (GCA). Also known as temporal arteritis, GCA is an autoimmune disorder involving large arteries of the head and neck (temporal artery in particular) in the elderly and is associated with polymyalgia rheumatica. The cause is not known. Cellular and humoral immunological systems are implicated. This is a disease of elderly Caucasian females in the majority of cases. Scalp tenderness, headaches, pulseless temporal arteries, ulcers on the scalp, and visual disturbances, including blindness in advanced cases due to the involvement of the retinal arteries. Temporal arteries are thickened and tender in this disorder. If basilar artery occlusion occurs, GCA is fatal.

Granulomatosis with polyangiitis. (Wagener's granulomatosis). This is an autoimmune disorder causing granulomatous vasculitis of small arteries. The cause is unknown. Familial predisposition in persons with previous viral or bacterial infections exists. Symptoms and signs include malaise, fever, arthralgia, and rhinitis as the first symptom. As the disorder advances, cough, haemoptysis, chest pain, dyspnoea, pleural effusion, skin purpura, haematuria, bloody nasal discharge, depressed nasal bridge, and ulcers on the palate and pharynx (painless or painful) occur. Strawberry gingivitis, underlying bone destruction with loosening of teeth, and non-specific ulcerations throughout oral mucosa are the orofacial features.

Reiter's syndrome (Reiter's arthritis). A triad of conjunctivitis, urethritis, and arthritis characterises this autoimmune disorder. The cause is unknown. It may develop in response to an infection in another part of the body (cross-reactivity). Symptoms and signs include inflammatory arthritis of large joints, inflammation of the eyes (conjunctivitis or uveitis), urethritis in men or cervicitis in women, mucocutaneous lesions, and psoriasis-like skin lesions. Enthesitis (inflammation of the sites where tendons or ligaments insert into the bone) can involve the Achilles tendon, resulting in heel pain. Not all affected persons have all the manifestations.

Bechet's disease. This multisystem autoimmune disorder is characterised by arthritis, iritis, and recurrent oral and genital ulceration. The cause is unknown. Association with an infective trigger may exist (cross-reactivity). Symptoms and signs include mouth ulcers, dysuria, epididymitis, erythema nodosum, anterior uveitis, keratitis, conjunctivitis, seizures, arthritis, arrhythmias, and encephalitis.

Immunodeficiency diseases: Immunodeficiency disorders fall under two categories: primary and secondary. Primary immunodeficiency disorders are of genetic origin, whereas those of secondary immunologic disorders are acquired. Individuals with immunodeficiencies have an increased susceptibility to infections.

Primary (genetic) immunodeficiency diseases. Primary immunodeficiency diseases are generally fatal, often resulting in death at an early age. They are either T-cell or B-cell defects. Examples of primary defects include congenital thymic dysplasia, severe combined immunodeficiency, and immunodeficiency with thrombocytopenia and eczema. Oral involvement in primary immunodeficiency disorders may include periodontal disease, oral ulcerations, and recurrent herpes infections.

Secondary (acquired) immunodeficiency diseases. HIV Disease. In HIV, immunodeficiency is due to a progressive reduction in CD4 lymphocytes from circulation caused by human immunodeficiency virus (HIV) infection. Bacterial, fungal, and viral infections, protozoal infestations, and malignancies resulting from the failure of antibody responses in HIV disease. In most cases, this is a sexually transmitted infection. Vertical transmission of infection from an infected mother to the infant can also occur. Depending on the stage of the HIV disease, malaise, fatigue, fever, weight loss, and diarrhoea are initial symptoms. Infection can lead to acquired immunodeficiency syndrome (AIDS). Signs include lymphadenopathy, wasting, immune thrombocytopenia, splenomegaly, anal herpes infections, and splenomegaly. Oral candidosis, oral hairy leukoplakia, oral herpes zoster infections, Kaposi sarcoma, and lymphomas are also seen in AIDS patients.

18.8 Diseases of the Renal System

Urinary tract infections (UTIs). This is a common bacterial infection of the urinary tract, which sometimes can also involve the kidney (pyelonephritis), bladder (cystitis), or prostate (prostatitis). 50% of women are infected and become symptomatic sometime during their lives. Bacteria involved include *E. Coli, Enterobacter spp, Klebsiella spp, Proteus spp, Pseudomonas aeruginosa, Enterococci, Staph spp, Strep group B, D, and G, and Strep viridans*. UTI is characterised by fever, incontinence, dysuria, chills, frequent urination, supra-pubic tenderness (cystitis), or tenderness over the renal angle (pyelonephritis), and haematuria.

Acute glomerulonephritis. Glomerulonephritis (GN) is a complex inflammatory disease of the glomeruli which can be caused by several factors and may manifest as acute GN, Nephrotic syndrome, and chronic GN. Acute GN is caused by preceding infection with *Streptococcus pyogenes* (presenting as sore throat in children,e.g). Occasionally, this may follow viral infections (including Hepatitis B virus infection) and renal involvement in multisystem disorders. **Symptoms and signs include** Headache, hypertension, vomiting, loin pain, facial oedema in the morning, haematuria, proteinuria, uremia, and reduced urine.

Nephrotic syndrome. A nephrotic syndrome is a form of glomerulonephritis characterised by the heavy leak of plasma proteins into the urine resulting in hypoalbuminemia. Causes include glomerulonephritis (GN), diabetes, systemic lupus erythematosus (SLE), infections, amyloidosis, drugs such as NSAIDs, penicillamine, and malignancies (such as lymphoma and leukaemia). Peripheral oedema and swelling of eyelids, ascites, pleural effusion, and frothy urine due to protein are common findings of nephrotic syndrome.

Renal Failure (RF). Renal failure is characterised by the loss of renal function leading to uremia. Two forms of Rf exist: acute and chronic. Chronic RF is characterised by gradual permanent loss of renal function. Causes include diabetes mellitus, glomerulonephritis, pyelonephritis, hypertension, renal stones, bladder outlet obstruction, and connective tissue disease. In acute RF, rapid deterioration of renal function occurs within hours or days. Dangerous levels of serum potassium may cause chronic RF, leading to apathy, confusion, drowsiness (due to accumulation of nitrogenous end products), ammoniacal breath odour, brown-coated tongue, metabolic acidosis leading to over-breathing, anorexia, nausea, vomiting, bleeding/bruising tendencies, anaemia, polyuria, peripheral oedema, increased pigmentation, ascites, pleural effusion, and pericarditis. In chronic RF, oral findings include mucosal pallor due to anaemia, the orange colouration of the mucosa due to the deposition of carotene-like pigments, xerostomia with or without candidiasis, metallic taste, ammoniacal salivary odour, uraemic stomatitis in severe cases with burning sensation and ulceration, petechiae, gingival bleeding, necrotising ulcerative gingivitis, radiological findings including ground glass appearance of alveolar bone, and tooth erosion due to persistent vomiting.

18.9 Diseases of the Endocrine System and Metabolism

Hyperparathyroidism (Primary and secondary). Due to glandular pathology, high parathyroid hormone (PTH) levels result in primary hyperparathyroidism. Causes include adenoma or hyperplasia of the parathyroid gland. Primary hyperthyroidism **is** often asymptomatic. When symptomatic, clinical features include polyurea, excessive thirst (due to hypercalcemia), anorexia, weakness, constipation, vomiting, renal colic, backache, hypertension, renal stones, peptic ulceration, giant cell tumour of the bone, and pancreatitis. (Classic symptoms: bones, stones, groans, and abdominal moans). Secondary hyperparathyroidism is characterised by prolonged hypocalcemia associated with renal failure and deficiency of dietary vitamin D.

Hypoparathyroidism. Hypoparathyroidism may be either primary due to autoimmune disease or secondary due to thyroid surgery. Symptoms and signs include peri-oral and peripheral paraesthesia and cramps. Abnormalities of hair, nails, and teeth occur in chronic cases. Tetany, in acute cases, is characterised by tingling in the extremities, spasms in the hands, facial twitching (Chvostek's sign: contracture of the facial muscles on tapping over the facial nerve), and fits.

Pseudohypoparathyroidism. Inherited disorder with resistance to PTH. Symptoms and signs include short stature, mental retardation, moon' face, cerebral calcifications, short fourth and fifth metacarpals, and hypothyroidism.

Hyperthyroidism. Also known as thyrotoxicosis, this common disorder is characterised by the overproduction of thyroid hormones. A common cause of hyperthyroidism includes an autoimmune disorder (Graves' disease). This occurs due to stimulating antibodies to the thyroid-stimulating hormone (TSH) receptors and less often due to a nodule within the multinodular goitre or a thyroid adenoma producing excessive thyroxine. Symptoms and signs include sweating, heat intolerance, sleep disturbances, irritability, amenorrhoea, palpitations, weight loss, increased appetite, and anxiety—tachycardia, atrial fibrillation, exophthalmos, fine tremor, goitre, and pretibial myxoedema.

Hypothyroidism. This is characterised by the underproduction of thyroid hormone. Causes include Iodine deficiency (the commonest worldwide cause) or autoimmune disorder (Hashimoto's disease). Thyroidectomy, or radiation to the gland. Rarely, also due to hypopituitarism. Symptoms and signs include weight gain, cold intolerance, depression, tiredness, constipation, slow relaxation of tendon reflexes, myxoedema (deposition of subcutaneous mucopolysaccharides), hair loss, hoarse voice, cold skin, and bradycardia.

Hypopituitarism. This is characterised by the deficiency of anterior or posterior pituitary hormones. Causes include anterior pituitary tumours, surgery on the pituitary for tumours, past head injury, tuberculosis, sarcoidosis, and radiation. Symptoms include myxoedema, infertility, amenorrhoea, depression, signs of hypoglycaemia, muscle weakness, and short stature.

Diabetes Insipidus (DI). This is characterised by the inability to produce concentrated urine due to complete or partial deficiency of antidiuretic hormone (ADH) (also called arginine vasopressin) or renal resistance to ADH action. These are known as cranial diabetes insipidus and nephrogenic Diabetes insipidus, respectively. Causes include Idiopathic, head injury, and sarcoidosis for cranial DI. Drugs, renal disease, and glycosuria can cause nephrogenic DI. Symptoms and signs include polyurea, nocturia, polydipsia, and dehydration.

Pituitary tumours. Adenomas of the pituitary gland can give rise to hypersecretion of growth hormone (GH) or prolactin and adrenocorticotropic hormone (ACTH). Resultant conditions may include acromegaly, hyperprolactinemia, and Cushing's disease.

Acromegaly: Clinical features include headache, coarsening of features, enlarged extremities, enlarged tongue, prognathism, sweating, hypertension, glucose intolerance, and heart failure.

Hyperprolactinemia may cause amenorrhoea, infertility, galactorrhoea, and impotence.

Cushing's disease: Clinical features include mood changes, central obesity, moon face, osteoporosis, hirsutism, hypertension, and oedema.

Cushing's syndrome (CS). This adrenal gland disorder is characterised by excess and prolonged exposure to circulating corticosteroids. Causes include ACTH-dependant and ectopic ACTH from tumours (bronchial carcinoma, e.g.) and non-ACTH-dependant tumours. Symptoms and signs include wasting of tissues, myopathy, thin skin, osteoporosis, easy bruising, obesity of trunk, head, and trunk (buffalo hump), moon face, hirsutism, increased susceptibility to infections, and poor wound healing.

Addison's disease (Primary adrenal insufficiency, adrenocortical failure, or hypoadrenalism). This disease of the adrenal glands is characterised by adrenocortical insufficiency. Causes include autoimmune destruction of the glands in about 80% of cases and TB, metastatic disease and hypoparathyroidism, diabetes mellitus, and Graves' disease in 20% of cases. Symptoms and signs include sudden withdrawal of steroids resulting in nausea, shock, and bowel disturbances. Other features of adrenal insufficiency include weakness, apathy, anorexia, weight loss, abdominal pain, infrequent periods, and constipation, hypotension, vitiligo, hyperpigmentation of mucous membranes, and those areas exposed to sunlight and pressure.

Adrenal crisis. If a patient with Addison's disease is challenged by extreme stress (of surgery or infection, e.g.), an adrenal crisis may occur. Features of this medical emergency include circulatory collapse, dehydration, hypoglycaemia, and hypotension. If not promptly treated, the condition is fatal.

Diabetes mellitus (DM) is a disorder of metabolism associated with the pancreas characterised by persistent hyperglycaemia due to deficiency of endogenous insulin or resistance to insulin action. Two types of DM exist: Type 1 and type 2 DM. Type 1 DM is insulin dependent, usually in children, often prone to ketosis. Type 2 DM Is non-insulin dependent. Usually, in obese older adults. Concordance in identical twins. Causes include an autoimmune process resulting in Beta-cell destruction of the pancreas for Type 1 DM. Obesity and genetic component are associated with Type 2 DM. Other factors associated with Type 2 DM include drugs such as corticosteroid therapy, thiazides, pancreatic disease, Cushing's disease, acromegaly, and thyrotoxicosis. Symptoms and signs include irritability, tiredness, thirst, dry mouth, weight loss, nocturia, blurring of vision, hyperphagia (excessive hunger and eating), dehydration, ketonuria, hyperventilation, ketone breath, obesity, lethargy, increased susceptibility to infections, and delayed wound healing that are common in type 2 DM. Polyphagia, polydipsia (excessive thirst), and polyuria (3Ps) are classic symptoms of type 1 DM. There is a bi-directional association between DM type 2 and periodontal disease.

18.10 Diseases of the Nervous System

Stroke. (Cerebrovascular Accident). Stroke, also known as cerebrovascular accident (CVA), is characterised by rapid loss of brain function due to disturbance in the blood supply, usually resulting from ischemic infarction or haemorrhage within the brain. Causes include thrombosis, embolism, haemorrhage, vasculitis, and hypoperfusion (general decrease in blood supply as in shock). Risk factors include old age, hypertension, previous attack of stroke, transient ischemic attack, diabetes, hyperlipidemia, tobacco smoking, excessive alcohol, oral contraceptive pills, and atrial fibrillation. Symptoms depend on the area of the brain involved. They may include hemiplegia and weakness of the face, numbness, vibratory or sensory sensation reduction, headache, vomiting, and initial flaccidity (hypotonicity replaced by spasticity (hypertonicity). In most cases, involvement is unilateral. Depending on the part of the brain affected, the defect in the brain is usually on the opposite side of the body.

If the brainstem is involved, symptoms include altered smell, taste, hearing, or vision, drooping of the eyelid, weakness of ocular muscles, decreased reflexes (such as gagging, swallowing, pupil reactivity to light), decreased sensation, and muscle weakness of the face, balance problems, and nystagmus, altered breathing and heart rate, inability to turn the head to one side, and inability to protrude the tongue and/or move from side to side.

If the cerebral cortex is involved, symptoms include difficulty with verbal expression (aphasia), auditory comprehension, reading and writing ability (Broca's area involvement), altered voluntary movements, memory deficit, and disorganised thinking.

If the cerebellum is involved, symptoms include altered walking gait, movement coordination, and vertigo.

Epilepsy. Epilepsy is characterised by a periodic disturbance in neurological function resulting in seizures due to abnormal excessive electrical discharge within the brain. In the majority of cases, the cause is not known. In infants, hypoxia, metabolic disorders, and infections; in adolescents, trauma, alcohol, drugs, infections, and tumours; in the elderly, cerebrovascular, metabolic, tumours, and infections may cause epilepsy. Symptoms and signs include changes in mood or behaviour during the prodromal period; this period may last for hours and is not a part of the seizure. The patient may also feel a strange feeling in the gut. This is called an aura.

Epileptic seizures: Partial and generalised. Partial epileptic seizures may include motor, sensory, psychic, and autonomic signs. Movement of the body parts, olfactory and visual changes, hallucinations, fear, tachycardia and dizziness, impaired consciousness lasting for a few seconds to 2 min, and repetitive movements of the face or limbs are common. Generalised seizures are divided into types: Tonic-clonic seizures (Grand Mal seizures), Status epilepticus, Petit-Mal seizures, Myoclonic seizures, Atonic seizures, Clonic seizures, and Tonic seizures.

Tonic-clonic seizures (grand mal type): Signs include an aura consisting of auditory, gustatory, and olfactory hallucinations, slurring of speech, frequent blinking, and irritability followed by the sudden loss of consciousness with an epileptic cry; this phase lasts for less than a minute, and the individual may show signs of cyanosis and tachycardia. This phase is the tonic phase. The clonic phase lasts for a few seconds to several minutes. Signs of the clonic phase include forceful jerking of the head, trunk, and extremities, loss of bladder control, and biting the tongue. In the postictal phase, the individual slowly returns to consciousness, followed by headache, sleepiness, and disorientation.

Status epilepticus: A tonic-clonic seizure of repeated episodes of epilepsy or an attack of a seizure lasting more than 5 min without recovery is called status epilepticus. The possibility of airway obstruction and aspiration may cause hypoxemia and acidosis, leading to death. This is a medical emergency.

Petit Mal seizures: Signs include facial twitching and minor movements of the hands without generalised muscular activity.

Myoclonic seizures: Signs include brief jerks of a finger, hand, or foot lasting a few minutes.

Atonic seizures (Drop seizures): Signs include sudden loss of tone of muscles resulting in hand dropping or individual falling to the ground.

Clonic seizures: Signs include rhythmic jerking movements of the body with impaired consciousness.

Tonic seizures: Signs include stiffening of the body or limbs with a risk of falling. It lasts up to 20 s and is followed by a postictal phase.

Parkinsonism and Parkinson's disease. Parkinsonism is a clinical condition characterised by slow movement (bradykinesia), speech, expressionless mask-like face, reduced movement (hypokinesia), rest tremor, rigidity, and postural instability. Parkinson's disease is one of the causes of Parkinsonism due to dopamine depletion within the basal ganglion of an unknown cause. Causes include the degeneration of dopaminergic neurons in the substantia nigra (Parkinson's disease). Less common causes include drugs, cerebral tumours, Wilson's disease, carbon monoxide poisoning, communicating hydrocephalus, and head trauma. Gait in Parkinson's disease is shuffling forwards with a flexed trunk (festinant gait). Limbs resist passive extension (lead-pipe rigidity/cog-wheel rigidity) during movement. The slow rest tremor gives a "pill-rolling" movement, which worsens during stress.

Multiple sclerosis (MS). This is a chronic inflammatory demyelinating disorder with the formation of plaques throughout the central nervous system. Peripheral nerves are not affected in MS. Cause is not known. A possible cause is an autoimmune process. MS is common in women. Symptoms include disturbances in visual function such as painful eyeball movements, nystagmus, double vision, distortion of the central image, and vision loss (predominantly optic nerve involvement). Sensory symptoms include numbness, coldness, pins and needles, swelling, and tightness in the arms and legs. Motor weakness includes paraplegia, difficulty walking, vertigo, and loss of balance. The relapsing-remitting course is common.

Myasthenia gravis (MG). This autoimmune disease causes the depletion of functioning muscle acetylcholine receptors in the neuromuscular junction, leading to muscle weakness. Association with thymic hyperplasia, hyperthyroidism, SLE, and rheumatoid arthritis has been reported in these patients. Symptoms and signs include muscle weakness of the neck, trunk, limbs, and ocular muscles resulting in ptosis. Dysphasia, diplopia, dysarthria, and "myasthenic snarl" on smiling are other significant features of this disorder.

Motor neuron diseases (MND). Motor neuron diseases (MNDs) are a group of degenerative neurological disorders that selectively affect motor neurons, the cells that control voluntary muscle activity, including speaking, walking, breathing, swallowing, and general body movement. Both upper motor neurons (UMN) and lower motor neurons (LMN) may be affected with no sensory abnormality. The cause of MNDs is unknown. Symptoms and signs include slurring speech, drooling of saliva, dysphagia, weakness, breathlessness, limb pain, dysphasia, dysarthria, wasting of the tongue with back jaw jerk, and neck weakness.

Bell's palsy. Bell's palsy is a form of facial paralysis resulting from a dysfunction of the cranial nerve VII (the facial nerve), resulting in an inability to control facial muscles on the affected side. Unilateral lacrimation (in the first month following Bell's palsy) is common when the patient eats (crocodile tears). Causes of Bell's palsy are idiopathic or viral infection (EBV or VZV) of the nerve, emotional and physical stress, exposure to cold, brainstem tumour, MS, stroke, trauma to the parotid gland, and parotid tumours, Symptoms and signs include unilateral sagging of the mouth, taste impairment, saliva dribbling, watering eyes, and inability to whistle and close lips or blow out cheeks. In these patients, the palpebral fissure is wide.

Neuralgias. Neuralgia is a sharp, shocking pain that follows the path of a nerve and is due to irritation or damage to the nerve. Under the general heading of neuralgias are trigeminal neuralgia (TN), atypical trigeminal neuralgia (ATN), occipital neuralgia, glossopharyngeal neuralgia superior laryngeal neuralgia, and post-herpetic neuralgia (caused by shingles or herpes). These are briefly described below.

Trigeminal neuralgia (TN). Symptoms and signs: Pain involves excitation of one or more trigeminal nerve branches (mandibular, maxillary, or ocular). Most pain is precipitated by touching, eating, or talking. Pain is of sudden onset, short duration, sharp/lightning-like or stabbing, and is unilateral. Repetitive episodes can occur. The area involved generally shows no signs of pathology between the attacks. The pain does not cross to the contralateral side.

Atypical trigeminal neuralgia (ATN). Symptoms include pain that can fluctuate in intensity from mild aching to a crushing or burning sensation. ATN pain can be described as heavy, aching, and burning. Sufferers have constant migraine-like headaches and experience pain in all three trigeminal nerve branches. Symptoms may include aching teeth, earaches, feeling of fullness in sinuses, cheek pain, pain in the forehead, and temples, jaw pain, pain around the eyes, and occasional electric shock-like stabs. Unlike typical neuralgia, this form can also cause pain in the back of the scalp and neck. Pain tends to worsen with talking, facial expressions, chewing, and certain sensations such as a cool breeze. Vascular compression of the trigeminal nerve, infections of the teeth or sinuses, physical trauma, or past viral infections are possible causes of ATN.

Occipital neuralgia: Occipital neuralgia is caused by damage to occipital nerves, usually due to trauma, physical stress on the nerve, repetitive neck contraction, flexion, or extension. Symptoms include aching, burning, and throbbing pain that typically starts at the base of the head and radiates to the scalp: Pain on one or both sides of the head, Pain behind the eye, Sensitivity to light, Tender scalp, and Pain when moving the neck.

Glossopharyngeal neuralgia. This involves unilateral irritation of the ninth cranial nerve (IX). Sensory vagal nerve afferents are also suspected to be involved in this pain syndrome. Symptoms and signs include cutting, stabbing, and shooting pain or sharp sensations in the throat. Throat pain can last minutes to hours. Ipsilateral ear sensations of "fullness" may occur before the throat's pain episode. Triggers include swallowing, talking, yawning, and coughing. Activation of the dorsal motor nucleus of the vagus nerve (X) during a glossopharyngeal neuralgia episode may result in bradycardia and syncope.

Superior laryngeal neuralgia. Symptoms include activation of the superior laryngeal nerve occurs via the general visceral afferent component of the vagus nerve. This rare pain syndrome is associated with lateral throat pain within the submandibular region. Pain may also present under the ear. Pain episodes can last minutes to days.

Postherpetic neuralgia (PHN). Nerve damage caused by herpes zoster is the cause of PHN. The damage causes nerves in the affected dermatomes of the skin to send abnormal electrical signals to the brain. These signals may convey excruciating pain and may persist or recur for months, years, or for life. Elderly and immunocompromised patients are susceptible. With a resolution of the HZ eruption, pain that continues for 3 months or more is defined as PHN. Pain varies from discomfort to severe and may be described as burning, stabbing, or gnawing. The area of the previous HZ may show evidence of cutaneous scarring. The sensation may be altered over the involved areas in the form of either hypersensitivity or decreased sensation.

18.11 Diseases of Bone and Joints

Diseases of bone and joints are common. These can have a developmental, inflammatory, immunological, infective, degenerative, or neoplastic origin. Only a few non-neoplastic disorders are dealt with below.

Rheumatoid arthritis (RA). Rheumatoid arthritis is a multisystem immunologically mediated disorder characterised by inflammatory changes involving mainly the synovial joints such as hands, wrists, ankles and knees, and circulating antibodies to IgG (Rheumatoid factor). The causes of RA are unknown. Often, patients are genetically predisposed individuals. Symptoms and signs include symmetrical joint pain, stiffness, redness, and swelling of joints of the hands, wrists and ankles, mainly in the morning, and "spindled" appearance of the fingers and "broadening" of the forefoot. As the disease progresses, shoulders, elbows, knees, cervical spine, and temporomandibular joints may be involved. Hips are usually not affected. General symptoms include fever, malaise, night sweats, and weight loss. Joint mobility and stability are impaired, and subluxation and ankylosis may occur. Deformities include ulnar deviation of fingers. Loss of finger function, "Z" deformity of the thumb, "swan necking" of fingers, clawing of toes with painful sensation (walking on pebbles), and subcutaneous nodules (Rheumatoid nodules) are common. Some patients may present signs and symptoms of Sjogren's syndrome or amyloidosis.

Osteoarthritis, also known as degenerative joint disease, is the most common form of inflammatory joint disease involving often-used joints such as hips, knees, feet, spine, hands, and temporomandibular joints. The exact cause is not known. Long-term wear and tear of joints are associated with the disorder. Other osteoarthritis-related factors include joint trauma, metabolic disorders, pre-existing structural defects, and obesity. Stiffness or pain in the joint(s) in the morning, lasting 15–20 min without any signs of redness or swelling, is a common feature. Other features include joint noises (crepitus) on the movement of the joint(s) appearance of Heberden's nodes (gelatinous cysts or bony outgrowths on the dorsal aspects of the distal interphalangeal joints). If nodes appear on the proximal interphalangeal joints, they are called Bouchard's nodes.

Osteoporosis is the loss of bone mass per unit volume causing increased porosity. Causes include advancing age, androgen/oestrogen deficiency (as in post-menopausal women), thyrotoxicosis, Cushing's syndrome, steroid use, inflammatory arthritis, chronic renal disease, and bone marrow replacement as in lymphomas and leukaemia. Symptoms and signs include bone pain, backache, kyphosis, crush vertebral fractures, and fractures with minimal trauma (particularly of the neck of the femur and distal radius).

Paget's disease of bone. Also known as osteitis deformans, Paget's disease of bone is a disorder characterised by excessive bone resorption followed by disorderly and excessive new bone formation leading to softening and painful enlargement of the bone(s) involved. The cause is unknown. Viral association (persisting measles or respiratory viral infection) with the disorder has been suggested in recent years. Common bones involved are the skull, vertebrae, pelvis, and long bones. Bone pain, especially at night, tenderness, deafness, nerve entrapment, pathological fractures, and impairment of vision are common. Rarely, development of osteosarcoma has been reported. Enlargement of the maxilla (leontiasis ossia) occurs in the maxillofacial region.

Fibrous dysplasia. Fibrous dysplasia is characterised by the replacement of an area of one bone (monostatic) or multiple bones (polyostotic) by the fibrous tissue and causing localised swelling(s).

18.12 Psychiatric Disorders

A psychiatric disorder is a psychological disorder potentially reflected in an individual's behaviour. It is generally determined by a combination of how an individual thinks, feels, acts, and perceives and the ability to relate to others. Symptoms (and signs) of psychiatric disorders include disorders of appearance and behaviour (self-neglect, depression, mania, tics, compulsion, etc.), disorders of speech (dysarthria, stammering, etc.), disorders of emotion (mood changes), and disorders of thought content (obsession, phobia, etc.), abnormal beliefs and interpretation of events (delusion, abnormal experiences, (hallucinations), and cognitive disorders (distractibility, amnesia, learning disability, etc.).Some common psychiatric disorders are dealt with below.

Anxiety neurosis is characterised by increased autonomic activity, which releases adrenaline. This leads to restlessness, dry mouth, palpitations, sweating, headaches, and diarrhoea. When certain objects provoke anxiety, the condition is called phobia. Fear of closed spaces (claustrophobia) and fear of spiders (arachnophobia) are common.

Depression is characterised by sleep disturbances resulting in early morning wakening, sadness of mood, loss of appetite, loss of weight, loss of interest in daily life activities, atypical facial pain, depersonalisation, and suicidal thoughts. Depression is generally reactive to adverse life events such as bereavement, retirement, separation, divorce, etc.

Hysteria is a subconscious effort used by the individual to resolve anxiety. Hyperventilation is a feature of hysteria. This may cause changes in acid-base balance, resulting in tetany and collapse.

Obsessive neurosis leads to repetitive actions or compulsions and obsessional thoughts. Some features include constant hand washing and returning home to check whether lights or gas burners have been switched off or doors locked.

Post-traumatic stress disorders (PTSDs) occur after dangerous and life-threatening experiences such as car crashes, battleground experiences, etc. Irritability, loss of concentration, and recurrent nightmares are common features of PTSD.

Delirium is characterised by clouding consciousness, leading to the disorientation of time and place. Fever can occur in alcohol withdrawal, chest infections that cause brain hypoxia, drug overdose, and stroke.

Dementia is characterised by an irreversible decline in mental capacity with short-term memory loss and slow-laboured thinking. This is common in senile dementia, as in Alzheimer's disease (due to neuronal atrophy) or after stroke.

Schizophrenia involves disorders of thought, emotion, and volition. Delusions and hallucinations are characteristic features of schizophrenia. Patients may become catatonic (motionless and speechless) as well.

Bipolar disorder is a mood disorder often referred to as manic depression and is characterised by alternating periods of mania and depression.

Dysthymia is a mood disorder characterised by a person reporting a low mood daily over 2 years.

Substance-induced mood disorders: Psychoactive drugs or other chemical agents can give rise to mood disorders. Alcoholism and chronic use of benzodiazepine (Valium) are included in this category.

Anorexia nervosa. This is an eating disorder characterised by deliberate weight loss induced by the individual (mostly adolescent girls) by self-induced vomiting, self-induced purging, use of appetite suppressants or diuretics, and excessive exercise. This leads to malnutrition and secondary endocrine and metabolic disturbances.

Bulimia nervosa. This eating disorder is characterised by repeated bouts of overeating to control body weight. Occasionally, the effects of repeated vomiting in these patients may give rise to tetany and electrolyte disturbances leading to cardiac problems.

18.13 Summary

Disorders of almost any body system can adversely impact oral health. Often, oral manifestations may be the first, only, or most severe feature of systemic disease. Numerous systemic conditions, including some autoimmune, haematologic, endocrine, and neoplastic diseases as well as chronic illnesses, cause manifestations in the oral cavity. Dental practitioners have a major role in participating in the diagnostic process as healthcare team members.

Bibliography

Odell EW. Cawson's essentials of oral pathology and oral medicine. 9th ed. Oxford: Elsevier; 2017.

Prabhu SR. Lecture notes on general medicine for dental practice. New York: Nova Science Publishers; 2014.

Prabhu SR. Handbook of oral diseases for medical practice. New Delhi: Oxford University Press; 2016.

Prabhu SR. Handbook of oral pathology and oral medicine. Oxford: Wiley Blackwell; 2022.

Glossary[1]

Abscess   A localised collection of pus in a cavity formed by the disintegration of tissues.

Achalasia   Failure to relax; mainly referring to smooth muscle fibres at any junction of the gastrointestinal tract (e.g. openings such as the pylorus, cardia, or other sphincter muscles); especially failure of the oesophageal sphincter to relax with swallowing.

Acinus (acini (pl.))   A small sac-like dilatation. Each acinus is supplied by a single terminal bronchiole, in the liver, the acinus is the smallest functional unit.

Acquired Immunodeficiency Syndrome (AIDS)   A virus that attacks the body's immune system.

Acute   A disease with sudden onset of signs and a short course.

Additives (food)   Additives are substances added to some food and drinks for functions such as colouring, sweetening, or preserving. Additives are allocated E numbers, which enables customers to quickly identify that the additive has been approved by the European Union (EU) after strict testing and that they are safe.

Allergen   A normally harmless substance, such as an ingredient in a foodstuff, that causes an allergic (immune) reaction in a susceptible person.

Amino acids   The building blocks that makeup proteins. The human body can produce some, whereas others can be obtained only through diet.

Adenocarcinoma   A malignant tumour originating in glandular tissue.

Adenoma   A benign tumour made up of glandular tissues.

Adenosis   A gland disease often marked by the abnormal formation or enlargement of glandular tissue.

Adherens junctions   Protein complexes that occur at cell-cell junctions in epithelial tissue.

Adhesion   In close proximity, joining of parts to one another may occur abnormally as in a fibrous band of scar tissue that binds together usually separate anatomical structures.

Adjuvant   A substance that enhances the immune response to the antigen with which it is mixed.

Adnexal   Appendages or accessory structures of an organ, for example, the uterus, including the uterine tubes, ligaments, and ovaries.

Aetiology (Aetiologic, Aetiological (adj.))   The science dealing with the causes of disease.

Afferent   Toward the centre, for example, afferent nerves carry impulses toward the central nervous system.

AFP (Alpha-Fetoprotein)   A substance commonly present only in foetal tissue. Its reappearance in some tumours enables it to be used as a marker.

Agenesis   Absence or failure of formation of any part or organ.

Agglutination   Clumping together of cells or particles.

Aggregation   A total or coming together of separate parts.

Air Pollution   Pollutants in the air that are detrimental to human health and the planet. It can include particulate matter, ozone, or noxious gases.

Akinesia (Akinetic (adj.))   Absence or loss of movement.

Allele   Any one of a series of genes may occupy the same locus on a chromosome.

Allergens   A substance that causes an allergic reaction.

Allergic Reaction   An abnormal physiological response by a sensitive person to a chemical or physical stimulus that causes no response in non-sensitive individuals.

Allodynia   Pain is due to a stimulus that does not normally provoke pain.

Amenorrhea   The absence of menstrual bleeding.

Amine   A chemical substance in the body whose structure is similar to ammonia; a family of hormones (adrenal medulla—epinephrine and norepinephrine) or neurotransmitters in the brain (dopamine, norepinephrine, epinephrine, serotonin).

Amino acid(s)   The basic building block of protein; there are 20 common amino acid types, and their sequence will determine the properties and function of each protein.

Amyloid   The extracellular protein substance deposited in amyloidosis. It is a waxy, amorphous, eosinophilic, hyaline-like material that exhibits red-green birefringence under polarised light when stained with Congo red.

---

[1] Sources: Underwood J C E and Cross SS. General and systematic Pathology. Fifth Edition. Churchill Livingstone. Edinburgh. 2012. *Modified from: Schulich School of Medicine and Dentistry, Western University, London, Ontario. Canada.*

Amyloidosis   A group of conditions of diverse aetiologies characterised by the accumulation of insoluble fibrillar proteins (amyloid) in various body organs and tissues—eventually compromises organ function. The associated disease states may be inflammatory, hereditary, or neoplastic, and the deposition may be local, generalised, or systemic.

Anaesthesia Dolorosa   Pain in an area or region that is anaesthetic.

Analgesia   Absence of pain in response to stimulation which would usually be painful.

Anaphylaxis   The immediate immunologic (allergic) reaction initiated by the combination of antigen (allergen) with mast cell cytophilic antibody (chiefly IgE). Anaphylactic (adj.)—as in anaphylactic shock—life-threatening respiratory distress, vascular collapse, and shock; manifesting extremely great sensitivity to a foreign protein or other material.

Anaplasia   Loss of differentiation of cells and their orientation to one another and their framework and blood vessels.

Anastomosis   A connection between two blood vessels or tubes.

Anencephaly   Markedly defective development of the brain, cerebral hemispheres absent or reduced to small masses, and the absence of the cranium bones.

Aneurysm   A ballooning out of the wall of a blood vessel or a heart chamber due to a weakening of the wall by disease or injury.

Angina   Spasmodic, choking, or suffocating pain. Angina pectoris, paroxysmal pain in the chest, often radiating to the arms; usually due to interference with the supply of oxygen to the heart muscle; often precipitated by excitement or effort.

Angiogenesis   The formation of new blood vessels.

Anomaly   An irregularity or deviation from normal; an abnormal structure.

Antibiotic   A compound that inhibits the growth and reproduction of bacteria. Antibiotics are not effective against viruses.

Antibody   A specialised protein produced by the immune system that helps destroy disease-causing organisms. An antibody is a component of humoral immunity. Antibodies can be effective defenders against both bacteria and viruses. An antibody must be made specifically for each pathogen.

Antigen   Any substance, almost always a protein, not normally present in the body which stimulates a specific immune response and the production of antibodies when introduced to the body.

Antigen-Presenting Cells (APC)   Cells that can process a protein antigen, break it into peptides, and present it in conjunction with class II MHC molecules on the cell surface where it may interact with appropriate T cell receptors.

Antiviral   A compound that inhibits the growth and reproduction of viruses.

Aphasia   Partial or complete loss of the ability to speak, write, or understand spoken or written language, resulting from damage to the brain by injury or disease.

Apnoea   Lack of breathing.

Apocrine   A form of secretion in which a portion of the cytoplasm leaves the cell together with the secretion product.

Apoptosis   Programmed cell death; is a specific "suicide" process in animal cells that includes fragmentation of nuclear DNA. Inducing apoptosis is a strategy to kill cancer cells.

Arrhythmia (s)   An irregular heartbeat.

Arthropod   An invertebrate animal with an external skeleton, a segmented body, and jointed appendages. This classification includes insects, spiders, and crustaceans. Some types, such as mosquitoes and ticks, can transmit diseases.

Ascites   Accumulation of serous fluid in the abdominal cavity.

Asymptomatic   Producing or showing no symptoms.

Ataxia   Failure of muscle coordination; unable to coordinate muscle movement resulting in jerkiness and incoordination.

ATP (adenosine 5-triphosphate)   An adenine-containing nucleoside triphosphate that serves as a store of free energy in the cell.

Atrophy   Wasting away; a decrease in the size and function of a cell, tissue, organ, or part.

Attenuate   To reduce the virulence of.

Atypical   Unusual, not characteristic.

Auscultation   Listening for sounds within the body; it may be performed with the unaided ear or with a stethoscope.

Autoantibody   An antibody that reacts with a naturally occurring antigenic molecule in the body; can cause autoimmune disease.

Autosomes and Chromosomes   Autosomes are non-sex chromosomes, while chromosomes are thread-like structures composed of DNA that carry the genetic information of an organism.

Aβ Fibres   Sensory nerve fibres with a thick myelin sheath, which insulates the axon of the cell and normally promotes the conduction of touch, pressure, proprioception, and vibration signals (35–90 metres per second).

Bacteraemia   The presence of bacteria in the blood.

Bacterium   A class of microorganisms is made of a single cell with a certain structure. While many bacteria are beneficial, some bacteria can cause disease. (Plural, bacteria).

Benign Growth/Tumour   A swelling or growth that is not cancerous and does not spread from one part of the body to another.

Bifurcation   The splitting of a tube or vessel into two branches or channels.

Biological Marker   A characteristic (such as the presence of a specific protein) by which a disease can be recognised.

Biopsy   Removal and examination, usually microscopic, of tissue from the living body, performed to establish a precise diagnosis.

Birefringent   It is the quality of transmitting light unequally in different directions.

Body Mass Index (BMI)   The body mass index (BMI) is a measurement that uses height and weight to assess whether someone's weight is healthy. BMI is calculated by dividing weight in kilograms (kg) by height in metres squared (m^2).

Bradycardia   Abnormally slow heart action.

BRCA1   A gene located on chromosome 17 normally helps to restrain cell growth. Inheriting an altered version of BRCA1 may predispose an individual to breast, ovary, or prostate cancer.

Bronchiectasis   Chronic dilatation of the bronchi. It may affect the tube uniformly or occur in irregular pockets.

BUN   Blood urea nitrogen: the urea concentration of serum or plasma, specified in nitrogen content; an important indicator of renal function (urea is the chief nitrogenous end-product of protein metabolism, formed in the liver from amino acids and ammonia compounds).

C fibres   Unmyelinated pain nerve fibres respond to warmth and a range of painful stimuli by producing a long-lasting burning sensation due to a slow conduction speed (0.5–2 metres per second).

Cachexia   Extreme loss of weight and body wasting associated with severe illness.

Cadherins   A type of cell adhesion molecule (CAM) that are important in the formation of adherens junctions to allow cells to adhere to each other.

Calculus   A stone developing in the body, for example, kidney or bile (not the branch of mathematics!).

Cancer   A group of diseases in which malignant cells grow out of control and spread to other body parts.

Carbohydrate   A molecule with the formula $(CH_2O)_n$. Carbohydrates include both simple sugars and polysaccharides.

Carbuncle   Deep-seated pus-producing infection of the skin and subcutaneous tissues.

Carcinogen   A substance that causes cancer.

Carcinoma *in situ*   A small, localised epithelial tumour that has not invaded surrounding normal tissue.

Carcinoma   Cancer of epithelial cells of either endodermal or ectodermal origin. The most common form of human cancer.

Cardiomegaly   Hypertrophy (enlargement) of the heart.

Caries   The destruction of bones or teeth.

Carrier   An individual capable of transmitting a pathogen without symptoms is referred to as a carrier.

Caseous   "Cheesy" or "cheese-like". As in caseous necrosis—cell death characteristic of certain inflammations (e.g. tuberculosis) where the affected tissue shows the crumbly consistency and dull, opaque quality of cheese. Based on casein—the principal protein of milk, the basis of curds and cheese.

Catarrh (Catarrhal (adj.))   Inflammation of a mucous membrane with increased flow of mucous

Caudal   Situated toward or about the tail; toward the inferior or posterior end of the body.

Causalgia   A syndrome of sustained burning pain, allodynia, and hyperpathia after a traumatic nerve lesion often combines vasomotor and sudomotor dysfunction and later trophic changes.

CD4+ T cell   A cell of the immune system, also known as a "helper" cell, helps other immune system cells produce antibodies. CD4+ T cells are the cell type that is infected and destroyed by HIV.

CEA. Carcinoembryonic Antigen   A tumour marker is present in patients' blood with certain types of cancer.

Cell Cycle   An ordered sequence of events in which a cell duplicates its chromosomes and divides into two.

Cell-Adhesion Molecule (CAM)   The molecule on the surface of the cell mediates cell-to-cell binding.

Cell-Mediated Cytotoxicity   Killing (lysis) of a target cell by specialised white blood cells called lymphocytes.

Cell-Mediated Immunity   Part of the immune system in which specific immune system cells, such as cytotoxic T cells, directly attack infected cells.

Cellulitis   Inflammation of the soft or connective tissue in which a thin, watery exudate spreads through the tissue spaces.

Cephalic   Pertaining to the head or the head end of the body.

Checkpoint   Any of several points in the cell cycle at which the progression of a cell to the next stage can be halted until conditions are suitable. These regulatory mechanisms are essential in preventing the formation of cancerous growths.

Chemoreceptors   Receptors that transduce chemical signals.

Chemotaxis (Chemotactic (adj.))   The movement of cells or organisms in response to chemical stimulation.

Cholangitis   Inflammation of a bile duct or the entire biliary tree.

Cholelithiasis   The presence of concretions ("gall stones") in the gallbladder or bile ducts.

Cholesterol   A lipid consists of four hydrocarbon rings. Cholesterol is a principal constituent of animal cell plasma membranes and the precursor of steroid hormones.

Chromatin The fibrous complex of eukaryotic DNA and histone proteins.

Chromosome Translocation Exchange of segments between nonhomologous chromosomes.

Chromosome A thread-like structure consisting of genetic material, known as DNA, with associated proteins and located in the nucleus of a cell.

Chronic A condition with slow onset, mild but continuous manifestations, and long-lasting, often progressive effects.

Cicatrisation The process of scar formation.

Ciliated Cilia are tiny hair-like structures that help transport secretions along a cell's surface.

CIN Cervical intraepithelial neoplasia; one of the terminologies used to describe precancerous or dysplastic changes in the cervical epithelial cells…IS—carcinoma in situ; a neoplasm where the tumour cells are still confined to the epithelium of origin without invasion of the basement membrane (likelihood of subsequent invasive growth is presumed high).

Clade A group of organisms that includes all descendants of one common ancestor.

Clone A group of identical genes, cells, or organisms derived from a single ancestor.

Cloning The process of making genetically identical copies.

Clubbing A proliferation of soft tissue about the ends (terminal phalanges) of fingers and toes.

CMV Cytomegalovirus.

Coagulate (Coagulative (adj.)) To cause to clot or become clotted; to convert a fluid or substance in solution into a solid or a gel. As in coagulative necrosis—a type of necrosis in which affected cells or tissue are converted into a dry, dull, homogeneous eosinophilic mass without nuclei as a result of the coagulation of protein.

Cognitive Impairment Cognitive impairment refers to problems with cognition and mental abilities such as memory or thinking. These difficulties are worse than would normally be expected for a healthy person of the same age. However, the symptoms are not severe enough to interfere significantly with daily life and are not defined as dementia.

Collagen The major structural protein of the extracellular matrix.

Collateral (Blood Supply) New vessels develop following chronic interruption of blood supply.

Columnar (Cells) Refers to the shape of cells that often line ducts or glands within the body.

Coma A state of profound unconsciousness from which one cannot be roused.

Comorbidity The simultaneous presence of two or more medical conditions.

Complex Regional Pain Syndromes Also known as causalgia and reflex sympathetic dystrophy, complex regional pain syndromes are conditions that are characterised by the presence of chronic, intense pain (often in one arm, leg, hand, or foot) that worsens over time and spreads in the affected area. These conditions are typically accompanied by skin colour or temperature changes where the pain is felt.

Conditioned Pain Modulation A reduction of a painful test stimulus under the influence of a conditioning stimulus.

Congenital It means "born with".

Congestion Abnormal accumulation of blood or fluid in part (e.g. of blood—passive congestion—obstruction of the escape of blood from a part (as in the liver); pulmonary congestion—engorgement of pulmonary vessels, with transudation of fluid into alveolar and interstitial spaces).

Contact Inhibition Contact inhibition enables noncancerous cells to cease proliferation and growth when they contact each other.

Contralateral The opposite side of the body.

Control Centre Also known as an integrator, the control centre consists of an error detector and controller.

Controller Receives errors from the error detector and sends output signals to increase or decrease the activity of effectors.

Contusion A bruise; an injury of a part without a break in the skin, characterised by swelling, discolouration, and pain.

Cor Pulmonale Eight-sided heart failure occurs due to long-standing lung disease.

Creatine Kinase An enzyme that catalyses the phosphorylation of creatine by ATP to form phosphocreatine. It occurs as three isozymes (specific to the brain, cardiac and skeletal muscle, respectively). Each isozyme has two components composed of muscle (M) and brain (B) subunits—CK1 (BB) is found primarily in the brain, CK2 (MB) in cardiac muscle, and CK3 (MM) primarily in skeletal muscle. Differential determination of isozymes is used in clinical diagnosis.

Creatine An amino acid; found in muscle. Phosphorylated creatine is an important storage form of high-energy phosphate—an energy source for muscle contraction.

Cribriform Perforated, sieve-like pattern.

Cruciate Shaped like a cross.

Cryptorchid A person with undescended testes.

Cryptorchism (Cryptorchidism) Failure of one or both testes to descend into the scrotum.

CT (Computerised Tomography) Sophisticated radiologic technique yielding a detailed image of internal body structures. Also, CAT—computerised axial tomography.

Cyanosis (Cyanotic (adj.)) A bluish discolouration of the skin, lips, nail beds, or mucous membranes due to excessive concentrations of reduced haemoglobin in the blood and hence deficient oxygenation.

Cyst   Any closed epithelium-lined cavity or sac, normal or abnormal, usually containing liquid or semi-solid material; a bladder.

Cystectomy   Removal of a cyst; removal or resection of the bladder.

Cytokine   Numerous secreted, small proteins are produced by white blood cells (e.g. interferons, interleukins) that bind to cell-surface receptors on specific cells to trigger their differentiation or proliferation. Some cytokines also called lymphokines regulate the intensity and duration of the immune response.

Cytology   The study of cells, their origin, structure, function, and pathology; the microscopic examination of cells to detect malignancy and microbiologic changes. Cells can be obtained by aspiration, washing, smear, or scraping.

Cytoplasm   The entire region between the plasma membrane and the nuclear envelope, consisting of organelles suspended in the gel-like cytosol, the cytoskeleton, and various chemicals.

Cytoskeleton   The network of protein fibres that collectively maintain the shape of the cell, secures some organelles in specific positions, allows cytoplasm and vesicles to move within the cell, and enables unicellular organisms to move.

Cytosol   The gel-like material of the cytoplasm in which cell structures are suspended.

Cytotoxic T cell   Also known as "killer" T cells, a type of immune system cell that can directly attack infected cells.

Cytotoxin (Cytotoxic (adj.))   A toxin or antibody having a specific toxic action upon the cells of particular organs.

Dander   Tiny scales from hair, feathers, or skin that may cause allergies and affect indoor air quality; household pets are sources of saliva and animal dander.

Degenerative Diseases   Diseases that occur as a consequence of damage and loss of specialised cells.

Degenerative   Progressive and often irreversible deterioration.

Dehiscence   A partial or total separation of previously approximated wound edges.

Dementia   Dementia describes symptoms associated with an ongoing decline of the brain and its abilities. This includes problems with memory loss, thinking speed, mental agility, language, understanding, and judgement.

Deoxyribonucleic Acid (DNA)   The primary material of life. DNA is a long, chain-like chemical found in the nucleus of all cells. The nucleotide segments of the chain define the genetic code that guides the development of every cell.

Deoxyribonucleic Acid (DNA)   The molecule that carries the genetic information for the development and functioning of an organism.

DES   Diethylstilbesterol, a synthetic nonsteroidal oestrogen; females exposed to it in utero are subject to increased risk of vaginal and cervical carcinoma.

Dialysis   A procedure by which a machine replaces kidney functions in patients with diseased kidneys.

Diapedesis   The passage of leukocytes (white blood cells) through capillary walls to the site of inflammation.

Diaphoresis   Perspiration, especially profuse perspiration.

Differentiation   The process usually involves gene expression changes by which a precursor cell becomes a specialised cell type.

Dilatation   The condition of being stretched beyond normal dimensions.

Dilation   The act of dilating or stretching.

Disorder   A disorder is a functional abnormality.

Diuresis   An excessive amount of urine; diuretic—produces an increase in urine.

Diverticulitis   An inflammation of a diverticulum, especially in the colon's wall, fills with faecal matter and becomes inflamed. It may cause bleeding or obstruction or may burst.

Diverticulosis   The presence of diverticula.

Diverticulum (Diverticula (pl.))   A pouch or sac occurring normally or created by the bulging of a membrane through a defect in the muscular coat of a tubular organ, such as the intestine.

DNA Repair   Cells contain enzymes to repair damage to their DNA by agents such as chemicals and radiation. If these enzymes or pathways are defective, mutation and cancer may result.

Duct   A passage with well-defined walls, especially a tubular structure, for selecting excretions or secretions.

Dynamic Mechanical Allodynia   A type of mechanical allodynia that occurs when pain is elicited by lightly stroking the skin.

Dysesthesia   It is an unpleasant abnormal sensation, whether spontaneous or evoked.

Dysmenorrhoea   Painful menstruation.

Dysphagia   Painful or difficulty swallowing.

Dysplasia   Abnormality of development; in pathology, alteration in size, shape, and organisation of adult cells.

Dyspnoea   Laboured or difficult breathing.

Dysrhythmia   Defective heart rhythm; also see arrhythmia.

Ecchymosis (Ecchymoses, (pl.))   A small haemorrhagic spot in the skin or mucous membrane, larger than a petechia, forming a non-elevated, rounded, or irregular blue or purplish patch.

Ectasia   Dilatation, expansion, or distention. For example, duct ectasia = dilatation of duct plugged with secretion, accompanied by a periductal and interstitial inflammatory infiltrate.

Ectopic Out of place; an object or organ situated in an unusual location away from its normal position.

Effector A component whose activity determines the t value of any variable in the system.

Efferent Moving away from the centre, for example, efferent nerve fibres carry motor impulses to muscles.

Effusion(s) The escape of a fluid into a part; the effused material (see exudate).

Electrolyte A compound, when dissolved in water, separates into charged particles. Electrolytes play an essential role in the workings of cells, maintaining fluid and acid-base balance.

Electromagnetic Fields Invisible areas of energy that are associated with the use of electrical power and various forms of natural and artificial lighting.

Embolus (Emboli (pl.) A detached intravascular solid, liquid, or gaseous mass carried by the blood to a site distant from its origin, thus obstructing blood flow. Most (99%) arise from thrombi (thromboembolic)—embolism–the sudden obstruction or blocking of a vessel by an embolus.

Emesis The act of vomiting.

Empyema Accumulation of pus in a body cavity.

Encephalitis Inflammation of the brain.

Endemic A disease is consistently present but limited to a particular region.

Endocarditis Inflammation of the endocardium.

Endocardium The innermost tunic of the heart (includes endothelial and subendothelial connective tissue).

Endogenous Originating from within the body.

Endomembrane System The group of organelles and membranes in eukaryotic cells that work together to modify, package, and transport lipids and proteins.

Endometriosis Benign glands and uterine stroma (connective tissue elements) outside the uterus.

Endoplasmic Reticulum (ER) A series of interconnected membranous structures within eukaryotic cells that collectively modify proteins and synthesise lipids.

Endoscope An instrument to visually examine the interior of a hollow organ such as the colon, intestine, or bladder; endoscopy is the procedure.

Enzyme A substance, usually a protein, that initiates and accelerates a chemical reaction.

Eosin Any of a class of rose-coloured stains or dyes; bromine derivatives of fluorescein; used in histology as a stain.

Epicanthus (Epicanthal (adj.)) A vertical fold on either side of the nose; a normal characteristic in persons of certain races but absent in others.

Epidemic An unexpected increase in disease cases in a specific geographical area.

Epidemiology The study of the relationships of various factors determining the frequency and distribution of diseases in the human community; also, the field of medicine deals with the determination of specific causes of localised outbreaks of infection, poisoning, or other diseases of recognised aetiology.

Epidermal Growth Factor (EGF) A protein found in the blood that stimulates cell growth.

Epidermal Growth Factor Receptor (EGFr) A protein located on the surface of some breast and other cancer cells to which epidermal growth factor attaches. The receptor enables the epidermal growth factor to stimulate cell growth.

Epigastrium The upper and middle region of the abdomen, located within the sternal angle. Epigastric is the adjective.

Epigenetic Factors that affect gene expression without changing the genome sequence.

Error Detector The error detector generates the error signal used to determine the output of the control centre.

Error Signal The error signal is one of the input signals to the controller.

Erythema Diffuse or patchy skin redness, blanching on pressure, due to congestion of cutaneous capillaries.

Erythrocyte(s) Red blood cell (s).

Eukaryotes Organisms whose cells have a nucleus enclosed within a nuclear envelope.

Exogenous Originating from outside of the body.

Expectancy-Induced Analgesia A reduction of pain experience due to anticipation, desire, and belief of hypoalgesia or analgesia.

Extracellular Matrix Secreted proteins and polysaccharides fill spaces between cells and bind cells and tissues together.

Exudate A fluid with a high concentration of protein and cellular debris which has escaped from blood vessels and been deposited in tissues or on tissue surfaces, usually due to inflammation.

Facies The face; or the expression or appearance of the face.

Febrile Having or showing symptoms of a fever.

Fibrillation A slight, local, involuntary muscular contraction due to spontaneous activation of single muscle cells or muscle fibres whose nerve supply has been damaged or cut off.

Fibrin An insoluble protein essential to blood clotting, derived from fibrinogen; a component of thrombi, vegetations, and acute inflammatory exudates.

Fibrinogen A coagulation factor.

Fibrinoid Resembling fibrin; an eosinophilic, homogeneous, proteinaceous material frequently formed on the walls of blood vessels and connective tissue in some patients (e.g. disseminated lupus erythematosus, scleroderma). Fibrinoid necrosis—results in acidophilic (eosinophilic) deposits with staining reactions that resemble fibrin in connective tissue, blood vessel walls, and other sites.

Fibrosis (Fibrotic (adj.))   Formation of fibrous tissue, usually in the repair or replacement of cellular elements.

Fine Particulate Matter   A complex air pollutant mixture that can include metals, organic chemicals, acid droplets, and soil or dust particles.

Fistula (Fistulas, Fistulae (pl.))   An abnormal passage or communication from one organ to another or from an internal organ to the body surface; may be caused by disease or injury or created surgically.

Fossil Fuels   A fuel (such as coal, oil, or natural gas) formed in the earth from plant or animal remains; fossil fuels are the nation's principal source of electricity; they cannot be replenished once they are extracted and burned.

Friable   Easily crumbled.

Fungi   A diverse group of single-celled or multicellular eukaryotic organisms that decompose and feed on organic matter. Examples include yeasts, mushrooms, and mould.

Gangrene   Necrosis due to obstruction, loss, or diminution of blood supply.

Gene Silencing   Reducing or switching off single genes' activity or expression.

Gene   The fundamental physical and functional unit of heredity. A gene is an ordered sequence of nucleotides located in a particular position in DNA and on a particular chromosome that encodes a specific functional product (i.e. a protein or RNA molecule).

Genetic Code   Set of rules specifying the correspondence between nucleotide triplets (codons) in DNA or RNA and amino acids in proteins.

Genetic Diseases   Inherited conditions in which a defective gene causes the disease.

Genome   Total genetic information is carried on chromosomes in the nucleus of a cell.

Genotype   The entire genetic constitution of an individual, or the alleles present at one or more specific loci. The actual genes carried by an individual.

Glomerulonephritis   Nephritis with inflammation of the capillary loops in the renal glomeruli.

Golgi Apparatus   A eukaryotic organelle made up of a series of stacked membranes that sorts, tags, and packages lipids and proteins for distribution.

Gram-Negative Bacteria   A category of bacteria that do not produce a positive result with a violet dye staining technique (bacteria that appear violet are referred to as Gram-positive). Gram-negative bacteria include Escherichia coli, Acinetobacter, Pseudomonas, and Klebsiella.

Gram-Positive Bacteria   A category of bacteria that produce a positive result with a violet dye staining technique due to the presence of a thick layer of peptidoglycan in their cell walls (bacteria that do not appear violet are referred to as Gram-negative). Gram-positive bacteria include streptococci, staphylococci, and the bacterium that causes anthrax.

Granulation Tissue   The tissue consists of fibroblasts, vascular endothelial cells, and macrophages within a matrix of collagen and fibrin.

Granuloma   A term applied to any small nodular aggregation of mononuclear inflammatory cells or a collection of modified macrophages resembling epithelial cells, giant cells, and other macrophages (usually surrounded by a rim of lymphocytes).

Greenhouse Gas   Any gas that absorbs infrared radiation in the atmosphere.

Growth Factors   Molecules capable of stimulating various cellular processes, including cell proliferation, migration, differentiation, and multicellular morphogenesis during development and tissue healing.

Gyrus (Gyri (pl.))   One of the convolutions on the brain's surface caused by infolding of the cortex.

H & E   Hematoxylin and eosin—A mixture of hematoxylin in distilled water and an aqueous eosin solution; a stain used routinely to examine tissues.

Haematuria   The presence of blood in the urine.

Haemoglobin   The oxygen-carrying pigment of the red blood cells (erythrocytes). It is a conjugated protein containing four heme groups and globin. A haemoglobin molecule has four globin polypeptide chains—alpha, beta, gamma, and delta. In the adult, Haemoglobin A predominates (alpha-2, beta-2).

Haemorrhage (Haemorrhagic (adj.))   To bleed; an escape of blood from the blood vessels.

Hamartoma   A benign tumour-like nodule composed of an overgrowth of mature cells and tissues normally present in the affected part but with disorganisation and often with one element predominating.

Haematemesis   The vomiting of blood.

Haematochezia   The presence of red blood in the stool.

Haematoma   A localised mass of blood, usually clotted, trapped in an organ, space, or tissue, resulting from a break in the wall of a blood vessel.

Haematoxylin   An acid-colouring matter from the heartwood; used as a histological stain—stains nuclei.

Hemianopia   Loss of vision or blindness in half the visual field of one or both eyes.

Hemiparesis   Weakness on one side of the body.

Hemiplegia   Paralysis of one side of the body.

Haemolysis   The liberation of haemoglobin, separating the haemoglobin from the red cells and its appearance in plasma.

Haemoptysis The spitting of blood or blood-stained sputum.

Haemosiderin A product of the decomposition of haemoglobin, found mainly intercellularly in areas of old haemorrhage.

Haemostasis The arrest of bleeding by the physiological properties of vasoconstriction and coagulation or by surgical means; interruption of blood flow through any vessel or to any anatomical area.

Hepatomegaly Enlargement of the liver.

Hereditary (familial) It is derived from one's parents.

Hernia The protrusion of an organ or tissue portion through an abnormal opening.

High-Density Lipoprotein (HDL) cholesterol is often referred to as "good" cholesterol, as it retrieves the "bad" cholesterol from the body and carries it to the liver, so that too much doesn't build up in the bloodstream.

Hilum or Hilus (Hila (pl.)) The part of an organ where blood vessels and nerves enter and leave.

Histologic Grade Estimating a tumour's likely "aggressiveness" is based on a microscopic examination of the tumour's tissue structure and cellular appearance.

HIV Human immunodeficiency virus; the biological agent is causing AIDS (acquired immune deficiency syndrome).

HL-A Human Leukocyte Antigens These tissue-compatibility antigens appear on white blood cells and cells in almost all other tissues and are analogous to red blood cell antigens (A, B, etc.). By typing for HL-A antigens, donors and recipients of white blood cells, platelets, and organs can be "matched" to ensure good performance and survival of transfused and transplanted cells.

Homeostasis The maintenance of a relatively stable internal environment by an organism in the face of a changing external environment and varying internal activity using negative feedback mechanisms to minimise an error signal.

Homologous Chromosome It pertains to one of a pair of chromosomes with the same gene sequence, loci, chromosomal length, and centromere location.

HPV Human papillomavirus; subtypes have been associated with the development of cervical cancer.

Human Immunodeficiency Virus (HIV) The most advanced stage of HIV infection.

Human Leukocyte Antigen (HLA) Glycoproteins that reside on the surface of almost every cell in the body and serve as recognition molecules in initiating an immune response.

Humoral Immunity Part of the immune system that provides immunity against disease-causing organisms in body fluids. The immunity is conferred by circulating antibodies produced by B lymphocytes and plasma cells. The main functional unit of humoral immunity is an antibody A

Hyperalgesia Increased pain from a stimulus that normally provokes pain.

Hyperaemia An excess of blood in a body part.

Hyperesthesia Increased sensitivity to stimulation, excluding the special senses.

Hyperplasia A controlled increase in the number of normal cells in normal arrangement in an organ or tissue, causing a corresponding increase in tissue mass.

Hypersensitivity A state of altered reactivity in which the body reacts with an exaggerated immune response to a foreign agent.

Hypertension High arterial blood pressure. Various criteria for its threshold have been suggested, ranging from 140 mm Hg systolic and 90 mm Hg diastolic to as high as 200 mm Hg systolic and 110 mm Hg diastolic.

Hypertrophy An increase in individual cell size, which increases tissue mass/organ size.

Hyphae Long, branching, filamentous structures of a fungus that are the main mode of vegetative growth.

Hypoalgesia Diminished pain in response to a normally painful stimulus.

Hypoesthesia Decreased sensitivity to stimulation, excluding the special senses.

Hypoplasia Incomplete development or underdevelopment of tissue, usually due to a decrease in the number of cells.

Hypotension Low blood pressure. Hypovolemia—decreased blood volume.

Hypoxia Reduced oxygen supply to tissues (below physiologic levels) despite normal blood perfusion.

Hysterectomy Surgical removal of the uterus.

Iatric About medicine or a physician.

Iatrogenic Resulting from the activity of physicians; usually used for any adverse condition in a patient resulting from treatment by a physician or surgeon and derived from data(o) (Gr)—medicine, physician.

Idiopathic Occurring without a known cause.

Ileum The distal portion of the small intestine, extending from the jejunum to the caecum.

Ileus An intestinal obstruction.

Immune Response The body's immune system responds by defending against attacks from disease-causing agents. The body can produce two immune responses—humoral and cell-mediated immunity.

Immune Response The body's immune system responds by defending against attacks from disease-causing agents. The body can produce two immune responses—humoral and cell-mediated immunity.

Immunity Prior exposure to the pathogen or vaccination can develop resistance to an infectious disease agent.

Immunogen A substance that produces an immune response.

Immunogenicity The ability to induce an immune response in the host.Immunoglobin (Ig) The term is used for antibodies that have specific antigen-binding capacity. These are glycoprotein molecules produced by plasma cells.

Immunoreactive Participating in an immune response, such as by reacting with a specific antibody, as determined by some immunological assay or technique.

Immunosuppression Weakening of the immune system causes a lowered ability to fight infection and disease.

In situ It means "in its original place"; may be used descriptively for cancer (e.g. c, carcinoma in situ) or to refer to experiments conducted in place, for example, in situ hybridisation).

Incubation It is the time between exposure to the virus and the onset of the disease. During this usually asymptomatic period, implantation, local multiplication, and spread (for disseminated infections) occur.

Indurated Hardened, firm.

Infant Botulism A very rare but life-threatening form of botulism in babies under 12 months caused by Clostridium botulinum bacteria spores in contaminated food.

Infarct A localised area of ischaemic necrosis produced by blockage of the part's arterial supply or venous drainage.

Infarction The formation of an infarct; acute myocardial infarction (AMI)—circulation to a heart region is obstructed, and tissue necrosis occurs.

Infective Diseases Result from the invasion of the body by pathogenic microbes.

Infectivity The ability of the infectious agent to pass from a sick to a susceptible healthy individual and cause disease.

Inflammatory Diseases Due to excess inflammatory cell activity in an organ.

Innate Lymphoid Cells (ILC) Innate counterparts of T cells that contribute to immune responses by secreting effector cytokines and regulating the functions of other innate and adaptive immune cells.

Insecticides Substances intended to repel, kill, or control insects.

Inspissation Drying-out; in histologic sections, inspissated secretions appear dense, amorphous, deeply staining material within the lumen of ducts or glands.

Insulin Insulin is a hormone made in your pancreas, which lies just behind your stomach. It helps our bodies use glucose for energy.

Integrins A protein found on the surface of cells helps them attach to, and communicate with, nearby cells.

Interferon A group of small proteins released from macrophages following stimulation or many cells after virus infection can induce changes in gene expression, leading to an antiviral state or other cellular changes important in the immune response.

Interferon-Gamma (IFN-γ) A pleiotropic molecule with associated antiproliferative, pro-apoptotic, and antitumour mechanisms.

Interleukin (IL) A naturally occurring molecule produced by the body that stimulates the growth of white blood cells and helps to signal and stimulate other cells.

Intussusception When a segment of one part of the intestine becomes telescoped into an immediately adjacent part.

Ipsilateral Same side of the body.

Iron Deficiency Anaemia A condition where a lack of iron in the body reduces the number of red blood cells.

Ischaemia (Ischaemic (adj.)) Deficiency of blood in part, usually due to functional constriction or actual obstruction or blockage of a blood vessel.

Jaundice Yellowness of the skin, sclera, mucous membranes, and excretions due to increased bilirubin in the blood and deposition of bile pigments.

Kaposi's Sarcoma A highly vascular tumour is occurring primarily in the skin. Formerly rare, it now occurs frequently as a complication of AIDS; a herpes virus is suspected of contributing to its occurrence in AIDS patients.

Karyolysis The dissolution of the nucleus—the nucleus swells and gradually loses its chromatin.

Karyorrhexis Rupture of the cell nucleus in which the chromatin disintegrates into formless granules extruded from the cell.

Karyotype (karyotyping) The chromosomal constitution of the cell nucleus; the photographic representation of the chromosomes for analysis.

Keloid Growth of extra scar tissue.

Keratoconjunctivitis Inflammation of the cornea and conjunctiva.

Kyphosis Abnormally increased convexity in the curvature of the thoracic spine as viewed from the side.

Lactation Lactation is the medical term for milk production for breastfeeding.

Lacuna (Lacunae (pl.)) A small space or depression, for example, lacunae are cavities in the bone tissue in which bone-forming cells are found.

Latency The viral genome's persistence that does not produce an infectious virus.

Leptomeninges The two delicate membranes of the meninges, the arachnoid, and pia mater.

Leucocytosis A transient increase in the number of white blood cells (leukocytes); due to various causes.

Leukocyte(s) White blood cell(s).

Leukocytosis A transient increase in the number of white blood cells (leukocytes); due to various causes.

Leukoplakia A white patch of oral mucous membrane that cannot be wiped off.

Lipids　Hydrophobic molecules function as energy storage molecules, signalling molecules, and the major components of cell membranes.

Lipopolysaccharides (LPS)　The major component of the outer membrane of Gram-negative bacteria.

Liquefaction　Conversion into a liquid form.

Liquefactive Necrosis　A type of necrosis characterised by dull, opaque, partly, or completely fluid remains of tissue, observed in abscesses and frequently in infarcts of the brain.

Low-Density Lipoprotein (LDL) Cholesterol　This type of cholesterol is often referred to as "bad" cholesterol, as too much can be harmful to health as it can build up in blood vessels and cause them to narrow, increasing the risk of blood clots which can lead to heart attacks or strokes.

Lumen　Opening, for example, of a blood vessel through which blood flows or in a gland or organ.

Lyme Disease　A multisystem disease affecting the skin, joints, and nervous system—caused by bacteria carried by certain kinds of ticks (most commonly found in areas of the north-eastern US).

Lymphadenopathy　A disease of the lymph nodes.

Lysosome　An organelle in an animal cell that functions as the cell's digestive component; it breaks down proteins, polysaccharides, lipids, nucleic acids, and even worn-out organelles.

Macrophage　A cell of the immune system that functions as one of the body's first defenders against disease-causing organisms. Macrophages can engulf and destroy pathogens. White blood cell is specialised for the uptake of particulate material by phagocytosis.

Major Histocompatibility Complex (MHC)　A group of genes that code for proteins found on the surfaces of cells that help the immune system recognise foreign substances.

Malignant Tumour　A cancerous tumour invades adjacent tissues and metastasises to other organ sites.

Mechanoreceptors　A sensory receptor that transduces mechanical stimulations.

Melanoma　Cancer of the pigment-forming cells (melanocytes).

Melena　Black blood in the stool; the source of blood is typically from the stomach or duodenum and is thus acted upon by digestive enzymes that break down the blood and create its black appearance.

Menarche　The first menstrual period, usually occurring during puberty.

Menorrhagia　Hypermenorrhoea or profuse menstruation.

Menorrhoea　The normal discharge of the menses.

Menses　The monthly flow of blood from the genital tract of a woman.

Mesoderm　The middle of the three primary germ layers of the embryo. It gives rise to all connective tissue; the musculoskeletal, cardiovascular, and lymphatic systems; most of the urogenital system; the blood; and the linings of some body cavities.

Metabolic Disorders　Arise due to abnormalities within metabolic pathways.

Metaplasia　The change in the type of adult cells in a tissue to a form abnormal for that tissue.

Metastasis　(Metastases (pl.); Metastatic (adj.)) Transfer of disease from one organ or part of the body to another not directly connected with it, due either to transfer of pathogenic organisms or to transfer of cells; all malignant tumours are capable of metastasising.

Metrorrhagia　Continuous or non-cyclical uterine bleeding.

Microbiome　Also known as the microbiota, it refers to the collection of microbes that inhabits the body.

Microlitre　One-millionth of a litre.

Micronutrients　A nutrient required by the body in tiny amounts for normal growth, development, and health maintenance, for example, vitamins and minerals.

Microorganism　Also called a microbe, an organism of microscopic size.

Mitochondria (Singular: Mitochondrion)　The cellular organelles responsible for carrying out cellular respiration, resulting in the production of ATP, the cell's primary energy-carrying molecule.

Mitosis　Nuclear division.

Monounsaturated Fat (Monounsaturated)　Monounsaturated fat is an unsaturated fat with one double bond in the fatty-acid chain. It can be found in olive oil, rapeseed oil, its spreads, avocados, nuts, and seeds.

Morbidity　A diseased state, disability, or poor health due to any cause that denotes the rate of disease in a population.

Mortality　Refers to the relative frequency of deaths in a specific population or location in a given time or place.

mRNA Messenger RNA　RNA molecule produced as a complimentary copy of DNA specifies a protein's amino acid sequence. It is translated into protein in a process catalysed by ribosomes.

Mutation　A permanent, hereditary change in the genetic code of DNA can be caused by exposure to chemicals or ultraviolet light or by mistakes that occur during DNA replication. Mutations can lead to cancer or birth defects.

Mycelium　The vegetative part of any fungus, consisting of a mass of branching, thread-like hyphae.

Myocyte(s)　(a) Muscle cell(s).

Myoepithelium　Flattened to stellate cells, believed to be contractile, which lie in many forms of externally secreting glands between the secreting cells and the basement membrane on which they lie.

Na⁺-K⁺ pump An ion pump that transports Na^+ out of the cell and K^+ into the cell.

Nares The nostrils, the external openings of the nasal cavity.

Natural Killer Cells (NKC) A group of innate immune cells that show spontaneous cytolytic activity against cells under stress, such as tumour cells and virus-infected cells.

Necrosis The morphological changes indicative of cell death caused by progressive enzymatic degradation.

Negative Feedback A control mechanism where the action of the effector (response) opposes a change in the regulated variable and returns it toward the set point value.

Neoplasm Any new or abnormal growth, specifically in which cell multiplication is uncontrolled. Neoplasms may be benign or malignant.

Neuralgia Pain in the distribution of a nerve or nerves.

Neuritis Inflammation of a nerve or nerves.

Neuropathic Pain Pain caused by a lesion or disease of the somatosensory nervous system.

Neutropenia Diminished number of neutrophils in the blood.

Neutrophil A granular leukocyte has a nucleus with 3 to 5 lobes connected by threads of chromatin and cytoplasm containing excellent granules: any cell, structure, or element readily stainable with neutral dyes.

Nitro-glycerine When compounded in tablets, is used to treat and prevent angina pectoris—used sublingually (under the tongue). A vasodilator.

NMR (Nuclear Magnetic Resonance) Scan More commonly now as MRI (magnetic resonance imaging)—is a sophisticated radiologic technique yielding a detailed image of internal body structures.

Nociception It is the neural process of encoding noxious stimuli.

Nociceptors A peripheral nervous system receptor is responsible for transducing and encoding painful stimuli.

Nocturia Excessive urination at night.

Nosocomial About or originating in a hospital.

Nuclear Envelope The double-membrane structure that constitutes the outermost portion of the nucleus.

Nucleolus The darkly staining body within the nucleus that is responsible for assembling ribosomal subunits.

Nucleotide Nucleic acid chains are composed of subunits called nucleotides.

Nucleus The most prominent organelle of eukaryotic cells; contains the genetic material.

Obesity Obesity is classified as a BMI of 30kg/m² or higher and is associated with various health problems, including type 2 diabetes, cardiovascular disease, and some cancers.

Obtund To dull or blunt (significantly to blunt sensation or dull pain) or to reduce alertness

Obtundation A clouding of consciousness.

Occlusion Closing or shutting off, for example, shutting off a blood vessel by a blockage of the opening.

Occult Not visible to the naked eye or hidden from view.

Oedema The accumulation of excess fluid in the intercellular or interstitial tissue spaces or body cavities.

Oliguria Diminished urine output about fluid intake.

Oncogene(s) Giving rise to tumours or causing tumour formation; genes that contribute to the formation of tumours.

Opportunistic Pathogens Potentially infectious agents that rarely cause disease in individuals with healthy immune systems.

Organelles Minute, intracellular structures that serve a specific function in the cell's life processes.

Orthotopic Occurring at the normal place.

Osteoarthritis A degenerative disease of joint cartilage.

Osteoporosis A common disease of the formation of bone leading to fragile bones and fractures.

Overweight Being overweight is classified as having a BMI of 25kg/m² to 29.9kg/m².

Oxidative Damage This is caused when there is a state of "oxidative stress" when there are excessive levels of highly reactive molecules called free radicals in the cell or a lack of molecules called antioxidants that can eliminate those free radicals.

p53 Gene A normally occurring tumour suppressor gene that is frequently inactivated in a variety of human neoplasms.

Pain Threshold The minimum intensity of a stimulus that is perceived as painful.

Palsy Paralysis, for example, cerebral palsy = persisting motor disorders in young children resulting from brain damage caused by birth trauma or intrauterine pathology.

Pandemic Disease A disease is a pandemic when its outbreak exponentially occurs in a wide geographic area.

Pandemic A disease occurring over a wide geographic area and affecting a very high proportion of the population. This term is often used to describe large outbreaks of influenza that occur worldwide and cause a high death rate.

Pap (Papanicolaou) Smear A specimen for microscopic examination of cells for detection of various conditions of the female genital tract (e.g. malignant and premalignant conditions), prepared by spreading the material across a slide.

Paraparesis Weakness affecting the lower extremities.

Paraplegia Paralysis of the lower limbs.

Parenchyma (Parenchymal (adj.)) An organ's essential (working) tissue as distinguished from the supporting connective tissue, vessels, nerves, etc.

Paresis Slight or partial paralysis.

Paraesthesia Any abnormal sensation, such as burning, tingling, or a "pins and needles" feeling, often in the absence of external stimuli.

Paroxysmal   Recurring "sudden attacks" of symptoms.

Pathogen   A disease-causing microorganism or agent.

Pathogen-Associated Molecular Patterns (PAMP)   PAMPs are conserved molecular structures produced by microorganisms and recognised as foreign by the receptors of the innate immune system.

Pathogenesis   The development of disease, specifically, the cellular events, reactions, and mechanisms occurring in disease development.

Pathogenic   Capable of causing disease.

Pathogenicity   Refers to the ability of an organism to cause disease. This ability represents a genetic component of the pathogen and the overt damage done to the host due to host–pathogen interactions. Commensals and opportunistic pathogens lack this inherent ability to cause disease.

Pathogens   Microorganisms that are capable of causing disease.

Pathognomonic   Characteristic or indicative of a disease; denoting symptoms or findings specific to a given disease and not found in any other condition.

Pathology   The branch of medicine that deals with the essential nature of the disease and the changes in body tissues and organs which cause or are caused by disease, the structural and functional manifestations of the disease.

Pattern Recognition Receptors (PRR)   Proteins capable of recognising molecules frequently found in pathogens.

Peptide   A protein with a small number of amino acids.

Perfusion   Transport of blood through blood vessels from the heart to internal organs, tissues, etc.

Pericarditis   Inflammation of the pericardium—the sac enclosing the heart and the roots of the great vessels.

Perikaryon (Perikarya (pl.))   The cell body; applied particularly to neurons.

Periorbita (Periorbital, (adj.))   The periosteum of the bones of the orbit or eye socket.

Periosteum   A specialised connective tissue is covering all bones and having bone-forming potential.

Peristalsis   A wave of contractions and relaxations of the digestive tract propelling its contents toward the anus.

Peritoneum   The membrane lining the walls of the abdominal and pelvic cavities and surrounding the contained organs; the two layers create a potential space—the peritoneal cavity.

Peritonitis   Inflammation of the peritoneum due to chemical or bacterial irritation.

Peroxisome   A small, round organelle that contains hydrogen peroxide, oxidises fatty acids and amino acids, and detoxifies many poisons.

Perturbation   Any change in the internal or external environment that causes a shift in a homeostatically regulated variable.

Petechia(e) ((Petechial (adj.))   A minute red spot(s) due to a small amount of blood escaping.

Phagocytosis   A process by which particulate material is engulfed by a cell.

Phenotype   This means an individual's observed biochemical, physiological, and morphological characteristics as determined by their genotype and the environment in which it is expressed.

Phosphorylation   The addition of a phosphate group to a molecule.

PID   A pelvic inflammatory disease.

Plant Sterols and Plant Stanols   Sterols and Stanols occur naturally in small amounts in some seeds, nuts, plant oils, and whole grains. Stanols and sterols are sometimes added to foods and beverages specially designed to lower cholesterol, such as certain spreads and yogurts.

Plasma Membrane   A membrane made of phospholipids and proteins that separates the internal contents of the cell from its surrounding environment.

Pleura (Pleural (adj.))   The serous membrane covering the lungs and lining the walls of the thoracic cavity; the two layers thus enclose a potential space—the pleural cavity.

Pleural Effusion   Increased amounts of fluid within the pleural cavity, usually due to inflammation.

Pleuritis   Inflammation of pleura.

PMN   Polymorphonuclear leukocyte; neutrophil.

Pollen   A fine powdery substance, typically yellow, consisting of microscopic grains discharged from the male part of a flower.

Polyarteritis   Inflammation involving several arteries simultaneously.

Polycyclic Aromatic Hydrocarbons (PAHs)   A class of chemicals that result from burning coal, oil, gas, wood, garbage, or tobacco. They bind to or form tiny particles in the air. High heat when cooking meat and other foods will also form PAHs.

Polymerase Chain Reaction (PCR)   A technique to amplify a single or few copies of a piece of DNA by several orders of magnitude, generating millions or more copies of a particular DNA sequence.

Polymorphonuclear   Having a nucleus so deeply lobed or divided as to appear multiple.

Polyp   A general term for any mass of tissue that projects outwards from a usually smooth surface.

Polyphenols   The name given to a broad group of compounds naturally present in plants that have been suggested to have some health benefits.

Polyunsaturated Fat (Polyunsaturated)   Polyunsaturated fat is an unsaturated fat with more than one double bond in the fatty-acid chain. Polyunsaturated fats include omega 6 (n-6) and omega-3 (n-3). They are termed "essential" fats as the body cannot make them, and we need to obtain them from our diet. Polyunsaturated fat can be found in the oils of nuts and seeds (and foods made from these) and in oily fish.

Positive Feedback   Positive feedback occurs when a change in a variable triggers a response which causes more change in the same direction.

Primary Cancer   The original site where cancer occurs.

Primary Disease   A disease that arises spontaneously and is not associated with or caused by a previous infection, injury, or event but may lead to a secondary illness.

Primipara   A woman who has born her first child.

Probiotic   Live microorganisms are intended to have health benefits. They consist of members of the microbiota that have beneficial effects and may be used to counter the damaging effects of harmful bacteria. For example, they may help prevent diarrhoea caused by some infections and antibiotics.

Prognosis   A forecast of the course and probable outcome of a disorder.

Programmed Cell Death   A standard physiological form of cell death characterised by apoptosis.

Prophylaxis   To prevent disease; preventive treatment.

Prostate-Specific Antigen (PSA)   A protein in the blood produced by prostate tissue that serves as a tumour marker.

Protease   An enzyme that splits proteins into their constituent peptides.

Proteinuria   An excess of serum proteins in the urine.

Proteolysis   Degradation of polypeptide chains.

Proto-Oncogene   A normal cellular gene that encodes a protein is usually involved in regulating cell growth or proliferation that can be mutated into a cancer-promoting oncogene, either by changing the protein-coding segment or altering the regulation of the protein.

Provoked Pain   Pain provoked by applying a stimulus.

Pruriceptors   Sensory receptors that transduce itchy sensations.

Pruritus   Intense itching.

Pseudohermaphroditism   A condition in which a person has the internal sexual organs (testes or ovaries) of one sex but, due to endocrine abnormalities, their external appearance is that of the opposite sex. Contrast with true hermaphroditism, where both types of internal sexual organs are present.

Psychogenic   Having an emotional or psychologic origin.

Puerperal   Relating to childbirth; the interval including the time of labour and recent post-delivery period.

Purpura (Purpuric (adj.))   A small haemorrhage in the skin, mucous membrane, or serosal surface; a group of disorders characterised by purpuric lesions, ecchymoses, and a tendency to bruise easily.

Pus   A protein-rich liquid inflammation product made up of cells (white blood cells or leukocytes), a thin fluid, and cellular debris.

Pyknosis   A thickening, especially degeneration, of a cell in which the nucleus shrinks in size and the chromatin condenses to a solid, structureless mass.

Pyogenic   Producing pus.

Pyothorax   An accumulation of pus in the thorax. See also empyema.

Pyrexia   A fever or febrile condition.

Pyrogen (Pyrogenic (adj.))   A fever-producing substance.

Quadriplegia   Being paralysed in all four limbs; unable to use arms and legs.

Radiation   The transmission of radiant energy in the forms of electromagnetic waves, streams of particles, sound, or heat.

Radioactivity   The quality of emitting or the emission of particulate or electromagnetic radiation resulting from the decay of the nuclei of unstable elements.

Rb Gene   A tumour-suppressor gene identified by genetic analysis of retinoblastoma, and also frequently inactivated in sarcomas and lung carcinomas that encodes a protein involved in the regulation of the process of making RNA from a DNA template in the nucleus of a cell.

Receptor   Any cell-associated protein that binds a specific extracellular signalling molecule that induces a cellular response.

Refractory Disease   A disease that resists treatment.

Regeneration   Regeneration is the natural process of replacing or restoring damaged or missing cells.

Repair   Restoration of diseased or damaged tissues naturally by healing processes.

Regulatory T cell (T reg)   T cells that have a role in regulating or suppressing other cells in the immune system.

Regurgitation   Flow in the opposite direction than normal, for example, throwing up of undigested food; backflow of blood through a defective heart valve.

Relapse   is when over some time, signs and symptoms of the same disease may reappear.

Remission   Remission is the process of conversion from active disease to quiescence.

Reperfusion   The flooding of tissue with blood after it has suffered ischaemia or a loss of blood supply.

Retrovirus   A type of virus containing an RNA genome that replicates in cells by first making a DNA copy of the RNA, a process termed reverse transcription. The virus uses RNA as its genetic material (rather than DNA). Examples include HIV and HTLV.

Rheumatoid Arthritis   A common chronic inflammatory disease primarily causing pain in the joints.

Rhinitis   Inflammation of the nasal mucous membrane.

Ribonuclease (RNase)   An enzyme that splits RNA into smaller units.

Ribonucleic Acid (RNA)   A nucleic acid in all living cells that has structural similarities to DNA.

Ribosome   A cellular structure that carries out protein synthesis.

RNA   Ribonucleic acid is a chemical structure that is related to DNA but has only one strand and somewhat different chemical composition. RNA performs various functions in the cell and can act as a messenger to carry the genetic code from the DNA to other parts of the cell. RNA can also serve as the genetic material of some viruses.

Rough Endoplasmic Reticulum (RER)   The region of the endoplasmic reticulum that is studded with ribosomes and engages in protein modification.

Sanguineous   Bloody; relating to blood.

Sarcoma   Cancer of connective tissue arising from cells of mesodermal origin.

Saturated Fat   Many food sources of saturated fat come from animal sources, including meat and dairy products, and is the kind of fat found in butter and lard, pies, cakes and biscuits, fatty cuts of meat, sausages, and bacon, and cheese and cream. Some vegetable oils, such as palm oil and coconut oil, are rich sources of saturated fat. Consuming too much-saturated fat can lead to high levels of cholesterol in the blood, which, in turn, can increase the risk of cardiovascular disease.

Sedentary   People described as sedentary spend much time sitting down and do very little physical activity.

Sclerosis   Abnormal hardening of the tissue.

Scurvy   A disease caused by insufficient intake of vitamin C.

Secondary Disease   A disease after or a consequence of another disease.

Second-Order Nociceptive Neurons   Nociceptive neurons in the central nervous system are activated by the $A\beta$, $A\delta$, and C afferent fibres and convey sensory information from the spinal cord to other spinal circuits and the brain.

Sedimentation Rate (ESR/ZSR)   A non-specific test that measures the settling of red blood cells per unit time in a column of fresh blood—a rough measure of increased amounts of fibrinogen and globulin which may occur in certain pathologic or physiologic states (e.g. heart attacks, cancer, pregnancy). ESR—erythrocyte sedimentation rate.

Seizure   An attack; the sudden onset or recurrence of a disease or certain symptoms, for example, an epileptic attack or convulsion.

Sepsis   Bacteria (pathogenic organisms) or toxins in the blood or tissues.

Sepsis   The body's extreme immune response to an infection causes damage to tissues and organs and can lead to death. Its incidence appears to be increasing, in part due to drug-resistant infections.

Sepsis   The body's extreme immune response to an infection that causes damage to tissues and organs and can lead to death. Its incidence appears to be increasing, in part due to drug-resistant infections.

Sequela(e)   The consequence(s) following a disease.

Serum   The clear, amber-coloured liquid separates when blood coagulates. It is protein-rich and contains antibodies.

Set Point   The set point refers to the "desired value". The set point is generally not a single value; it is a range of values.

Shock   A sudden disturbance of mental equilibrium; a profound haemodynamic and metabolic disorder characterised by failure of the circulatory system to maintain adequate perfusion of vital organs.

Sign   An objective indication or evidence of disease discovered on examination of a patient. Contrast with the symptom.

SIL   Squamous intraepithelial lesion; one of the terminologies used to describe precancerous or dysplastic changes in the cervical epithelial cells.

Smooth Endoplasmic Reticulum (SER)   The region of the endoplasmic reticulum that has few or no ribosomes on its cytoplasmic surface and synthesises carbohydrates, lipids, and steroid hormones; detoxifies chemicals like pesticides, preservatives, medications, and environmental pollutants, and stores calcium ions.

Somatic Mutations   Alterations in genes that occur within individual cells may accumulate throughout an individual's lifetime.

Spasm   A sudden, violent, involuntary muscle contraction; a sudden tightening of a passage or canal. Spastic—characterised by spasms or other uncontrolled contractions of the skeletal muscles; muscles are stiff, and the movements awkward. Spasticity—the condition characterised by spasms.

Splenomegaly   Enlargement of the spleen.

Spore   A form of a microorganism, such as a bacterium, that is dormant and stable in the environment but can become capable of reproducing after infecting an animal or person.

Squamous (Cells)   Cell type is often seen in areas exposed to significant irritation or trauma, for example, skin.

Static Pain   Another kind of mechanical hyperalgesia in those with neuropathic pain is when pain is provoked after gentle pressure is applied to the symptomatic area.

Steatosis   Fatty degeneration.

Stenosis (Stenoses, (pl.))   Narrowing or contraction of a duct or canal.

Steroid   A class of hormones with a particular chemical structure consisting of four interlocking carbon rings.

Stricture   An abnormal narrowing of a duct or passage.

Stridor   A harsh, high-pitched respiratory sound.

Stroma   The connective tissue framework of an organ or other structure, as distinguished from the tissues performing the unique function of the organ.

Subcutaneous Beneath the skin.

Sulcus (Sulci (pl.)) A groove, trench, or furrow; in neuroanatomy, for instance, a depression or groove on the brain surface separating the gyri.

Sulphur Dioxide A colourless, water-soluble, acidic gas produced from fossil fuel combustion.

Suppuration (Suppurative (adj.)) Formation or discharge of pus.

Symptom Subjective evidence of disease as perceived and reported by a patient.

Syncope Fainting; temporary loss of consciousness due to reduced oxygen delivery to the brain.

Synovia The transparent, viscid fluid secreted by the synovial membrane and found in joint cavities, bursae, and tendon sheaths.

Synovitis Inflammation of a synovial membrane, usually painful, particularly on motion, and characterised by fluctuating swelling (due to effusion in a synovial sac).

Systemic Lupus Erythematosus (SLE) A chronic autoimmune disease of unknown cause that can affect virtually any body organ.

Systole The heart's contraction during which blood is pumped into the heart; systolic is the blood pressure in the arteries when the heart pumps blood through the body.

Tachycardia Abnormally fast heartbeat.

T Cell Receptor (TCR) Located on the surface of T cells, TCR is responsible for recognising the antigen-major histocompatibility complex, leading to the initiation of an inflammatory response.

T Cell A type of white blood cell that plays an essential role in the immune system. The "T" stands for thymus, the organ where the cells mature (as opposed to another type of white blood cell, called B cells, which mature in the bone marrow). Subsets of T cells express different receptors on the cell's surface and perform specific functions. Also known as a T lymphocyte.

Telomerase An enzyme that will elongate the telomere of a chromosome but not other parts or genes.

Telomere The end portion of a chromosome. This part does not contain any genes that code for proteins.

Temporal Summation The phenomenon in which progressive increases in pain intensity are experienced during the repetition of identical nociceptive stimuli.

Teratogen A substance or condition that impairs the normal development of the embryo or foetus in utero, causing a congenital abnormality.

Thermoreceptors Sensory receptors that respond to changes in temperature.

TNM Staging The determination of distinct phases or periods in the course of a disease, the life history of an organism, or any biological process; the classification of neoplasms according to the extent of the tumour (e.g. TMN staging—staging of tumours according to three basic components: primary tumour (T), regional nodes (N), and metastasis (M)—from 0 (undetectable) to 4).

Thrombocytopaenia An abnormally small number or decrease of circulating platelets in the blood.

Thrombosis The inappropriate or pathological formation of a solid mass (from the blood constituents) within a blood vessel or organ.

Thrombus (Thrombi (pl.)) A solid mass formed from blood constituents within the blood vessels or the heart. Thrombi that form within the rapidly moving arterial circulation are mainly composed of fibrin and platelets with only a few trapped red and white cells.

Toxin Refers to molecules produced by microorganisms that may affect cells in the infected host.

Toxin A poison produced by a living organism.

Trait A genetically determined characteristic.

Trans Fats (Trans Fatty Acids) Trans fatty acids naturally occur in small amounts in some animal foods, including meat (like beef and lamb) and dairy products. They also happen through processing (industrial trans fats) when unsaturated oils are partially hydrogenated, making them more solid and better for processing. Hydrogenated fats must be declared on the ingredients label. Consuming a diet high in trans fats can lead to high cholesterol levels in the blood, which can cause health conditions such as heart disease, heart attacks, and strokes. In the UK, the food industry has largely removed industrial trans fats from their products, and the UK population currently consumes less than the target level.

Transcription One strand of a DNA molecule is used as a template for the synthesis (transcription) of a complementary RNA (mRNA). RNA polymerase and various accessory proteins called transcription factors to form a complex that initiates transcription.

Transcription The process by which the genetic information encoded in DNA is copied into a complimentary copy in RNA.

Transient Of short duration, momentary.

Transmissibility The probability of an infection, given contact between an infected host and a noninfected host.

Tropism Refers to the ability of a given pathogen to infect a specific location.

Troponin A protein of muscle that, together with tropomyosin, forms a regulatory protein complex controlling the interaction of actin and myosin and that, when combined with calcium ions, permits muscular contraction; when cardiac muscle cells are damaged, troponin is released into the bloodstream and provides a valuable indicator of cardiac cell death and evidence of myocardial infarction.

Tumour Marker A chemical substance found in increased amounts in the body fluids of some cancer patients. A tumour marker in the blood for specific cancer can indicate cancer in the body. Tumour markers can be used as part of the diagnostic process but generally cannot provide a definitive diagnosis. Tumour markers are also used to monitor treatment progress and the possible recurrence of cancer after treatment.

Tumour Necrosis Factor (TNF) A naturally occurring protein (a pro-inflammatory cytokine) that is produced by the phagocytic cells (macrophages).

Tumour Progression The development of increasing malignancy during the pathogenesis of a neoplasm.

Tumour Promoter A compound that stimulates the proliferation of cells that have already sustained carcinogen-induced mutations leads to neoplasm development.

Tumour Suppressor Gene A normal cellular gene whose loss of function leads to tumour development. These genes check cell-cycle progression and can hold cells in a static condition, thereby preventing cells from becoming cancerous. The p53 gene and Rb gene are examples.

Ulcer A local defect or excavation of an organ or tissue surface produced by the sloughing of necrotic inflammatory tissue.

Unsaturated Fat Unsaturated fats (monounsaturated and polyunsaturated fats) provide essential fatty acids and fat-soluble vitamins. UK guidelines encourage us to swap saturated fats for unsaturated fats.

Urea is the chief nitrogenous end-product of protein metabolism, formed in the liver from amino acids and ammonia compounds found in urine, blood, and lymph. Also, see BUN—blood urea nitrogen.

Uraemia An excess of the nitrogen-containing end-products of protein and amino acid metabolism in the blood; the entire constellation of signs and symptoms of chronic renal failure.

Vaccination Injection of a weakened or mild form of a disease-causing agent to produce immunity.

Vaccine A preparation of killed or weakened microorganisms is administered to produce or increase immunity to a particular disease.

Vacuole A membrane-bound sac, somewhat larger than a vesicle, that functions in cellular storage and transport.

Vape The action or practice of inhaling and exhaling the vapour produced by an electronic cigarette or similar device.

Vasculitis Inflammation of a vessel.

Vasodilator An agent that causes dilatation of the blood vessels.

Vector A segment of genetic material that is used as a vehicle to introduce specific genes into cells.

Ventricular Fibrillation Rapid, irregular twitching of heart muscle which prevents coordinated contraction of the heart.

Vertigo A sensation of spinning or whirling motion.

Vesicle A small, membrane-bound sac that functions in cellular storage and transport; its membrane can fuse with the plasma membrane and the membranes of the endoplasmic reticulum and Golgi apparatus.

Viromes The total collection of viruses associated with an organism or ecosystem is usually described through metagenomics sequencing of viral nucleic acids.

Virulence (Virulent (adj.) The degree of pathogenicity of a microorganism as indicated by the severity of the disease produced and the ability to invade the tissues of the host.

Virus A microscopic particle comprises genetic material (either DNA or RNA) and protein that can replicate only inside living cells.

Virus-Like Particle A particle assembled from multiple copies of the capsid protein that, like a virus, can produce an immune response. Unlike a virus, it is not infectious because it does not contain genetic material.

Volvulus A twisting of a loop of the intestine causing an obstruction may impair blood supply resulting in infarction.

Zoonosis A disease that is transmitted from animals to humans. The incidence of zoonoses (plural) increases when humans exist in close contact with animals and when humans encounter animals in new geographical regions.

Index